AF644743

South Asian Edition of

BIOPSY INTERPRETATION SERIES

BIOPSY INTERPRETATION OF THE LYMPH NODE

South Asian Edition of

BIOPSY INTERPRETATION SERIES

BIOPSY INTERPRETATION OF THE LYMPH NODE

Rebecca L. King, MD
Professor
Division of Hematopathology
Mayo Clinic
Rochester, Minnesota

Anamarija M. Perry, MD
Professor
Department of Pathology
University of Michigan
Ann Arbor, Michigan

Lauren B. Smith, MD
Professor
Department of Pathology
University of Michigan
Ann Arbor, Michigan

Wolters Kluwer

Philadelphia • Baltimore • New York • London
Buenos Aires • Hong Kong • Sydney • Tokyo

First edition

Copyright © 2024 Wolters Kluwer.

All rights reserved. This book is protected by copyright. No part of this book may be reproduced or transmitted in any form or by any means, including as photocopies or scanned- in or other electron-ic copies, or utilized by any information storage and retrieval system without written permission from the copyright owner, except for brief quotations embodied in critical articles and reviews. Ma-terials appearing in this book prepared by individuals as part of their official duties as U.S. govern-ment employees are not covered by the above- mentioned copyright. To request permission, please contact Wolters Kluwer at Two Commerce Square, 2001 Market Street, Philadelphia, PA 19103, via email at permissions@lww.com, or via our website at shop.lww.com (products and services).

This work is provided "as is," and the publisher disclaims any and all warranties, express or implied, including any warranties as to accuracy, comprehensiveness, or currency of the content of this work.

This work is no substitute for individual patient assessment based upon healthcare professionals' examination of each patient and consideration of, among other things, age, weight, gender, current or prior medical conditions, medication history, laboratory data and other factors unique to the patient. The publisher does not provide medical advice or guidance and this work is merely a reference tool. Healthcare professionals, and not the publisher, are solely responsible for the use of this work including all medical judgments and for any resulting diagnosis and treatments.

Given continuous, rapid advances in medical science and health information, independent professional verification of medical diagnoses, indications, appropriate pharmaceutical selections and dosages, and treatment options should be made and healthcare professionals should consult a variety of sources. When prescribing medication, healthcare professionals are advised to consult the product information sheet (the manufacturer's package insert) accompanying each drug to verify, among other things, conditions of use, warnings and side effects and identify any changes in dosage schedule or contraindications, particularly if the medication to be administered is new, infrequently used or has a narrow therapeutic range. To the maximum extent permitted under applicable law, no responsibility is assumed by the publisher for any injury and/or damage to persons or property, as a matter of products liability, negligence law or otherwise, or from any reference to or use by any person of this work.

First Indian Reprint, 2024
Second Indian Reprint, 2026

Indian Reprint ISBN: 978-81-19877-57-7
Original ISBN: -978-1-975184-62-9

Restricted Distribution: *This edition is licensed for sale and distribution in India, Pakistan, Sri Lanka,Bangladesh, Nepal, Bhutan, and the Maldives. This edition is not authorized for export outside these territories. Circulation of this edition outside these territories is illegal and strictly prohibited.*

Published by Wolters Kluwer (India) Pvt Ltd, New Delhi
Printed and bound at Replika Press Pvt. Ltd.

If you have difficulty buying LWW books,
please write to us at: marketing@wolterskluwerindia.co.in

DEDICATION

To Dr. Ivan Damjanov, pathologist and teacher extraordinaire, who I proudly call my mentor. The "One" who always believes in me. And to Andrea Damjanov, for all the care, compassion, and advice that she selflessly gave me (and to so many others who came before and after me). With love and deepest gratitude.

A.M.P.

To Dr. Bertram Schnitzer, my mentor, colleague, and friend who taught me about lymphomas and reactive lymph nodes with great enthusiasm and wisdom. I will be forever grateful for his mentorship.

L.B.S.

CONTRIBUTORS

Rebecca L. King, MD
Professor
Division of Hematopathology
Mayo Clinic
Rochester, Minnesota

Daniel P. Larson, MD
Assistant Professor
Division of Hematopathology
Mayo Clinic
Rochester, Minnesota

Daniel S. Martig, MD
Pathologist, Hematopathology
Hospital Pathology Associates
Minneapolis, Minnesota

Anna B. Owczarczyk, MD, PhD
Associate Staff Hematopathologist
Robert J. Tomsich Pathology and Laboratory Medicine Institute
Cleveland Clinic
Cleveland, Ohio

Anamarija M. Perry, MD
Professor
Department of Pathology
University of Michigan
Ann Arbor, Michigan

Kyle D. Perry, MD
Senior Pathologist
Pathology and Laboratory Medicine
Henry Ford Health System
Detroit, Michigan

Lauren B. Smith, MD
Professor
Department of Pathology
University of Michigan
Ann Arbor, Michigan

Anjanaa Vijayanarayanan, MD
Hematopathology Fellow
Department of Laboratory Medicine
University of California at San Francisco
San Francisco, California

PREFACE

The evaluation of lymph nodes and classification of lymphomas and non-neoplastic lymphoid proliferations begins with an understanding of the morphologic clues. In addition to histology, modern lymph node pathology requires a host of additional ancillary studies, which have become routine in diagnostic hematopathology. This multidisciplinary approach to lymph node pathology has also become the foundation of modern lymphoma classifications. This has enabled pathologists from different parts of the world to use standardized approaches to diagnosis. It has also improved our communication with practicing clinical hematologists and oncologists, and ultimately contributed to improved treatment of lymphoid neoplasia.

In this book, we present neoplastic lymph node pathology according to the 2022 International Consensus Classification (ICC). However, since both the ICC and the fifth edition of the World Health Organization (WHO) Classification are likely to be widely used during this transitional period in our field's history, we have included both classifications in the appendix.

Recent advances in hematopathology have been presented in several voluminous textbooks. In contrast to these comprehensive compendiums, we present here our own practical diagnostic approach tested over multiple years in our respective busy academic hematopathology practices. We hope that hematopathologists, as well as general surgical pathologists and pathology trainees, will find this book useful in their sign-out rooms.

In contemporary medical practice the prevailing trend is to use less invasive methods for obtaining diagnostic material. Accordingly, the specimens submitted to pathologists are often small core biopsies. However, as morphologists first, we recognize that no amount of ancillary testing can replace an adequate specimen for morphologic review in most instances. This book seeks to provide a foundation for morphologic assessment of both excisional and core needle lymph node biopsies and emphasize the challenges of small specimens. Cognizant of our diagnostic limitations under these conditions, we advocate a balanced approach and good communication with clinicians. We realize that sometimes more tissue may be required for a definitive diagnosis.

Targeted and judicious use of ancillary studies is emphasized throughout the text. Most notably we focus on the most useful immunohistochemical panels, which form the backbone of our daily lymph node evaluations. From numerous cytogenetic and molecular findings in different entities, we have chosen to highlight more relevant ones for diagnosis and prognostication, while recognizing that this is a rapidly evolving field.

Although we strove to include all of the pertinent information in describing the various neoplastic and nonneoplastic entities involving lymph nodes, the true focus of the book is morphology and pattern recognition, the importance of which cannot be overemphasized in lymph node pathology. We have sought to share our everyday experience and practice of lymph node pathology in this text and we hope that you will enjoy reading it.

Online resources are not available with this text.

ACKNOWLEDGMENTS

The authors would like to acknowledge the contributions of the following members of the Mayo Clinic Hematopathology team: Mechelle Miller, Greg Otteson, Reid Meyer, Matthew Howard, MD, Andrew Feldman, MD, and Ellen McPhail, MD.

CONTENTS

1

LYMPH NODE EVALUATION

ANAMARIJA M. PERRY and KYLE D. PERRY

PATTERN-BASED APPROACH TO LYMPH NODE EVALUATION

Lymph node pathology is a challenging and rapidly evolving field of pathology with many neoplastic and nonneoplastic entities to consider, as well as numerous nonhematopoietic conditions that can also involve the lymph node. Modern classification of lymphomas requires integration of the morphologic findings with ancillary studies (ie, immunohistochemistry, flow cytometry, cytogenetics, and molecular studies) in order to properly classify different entities.[1] Currently, two classifications of lymphomas exist–the 2022 International Consensus Classification (ICC)[2] and the 5th edition of the World Health Organization Classification.[3] In this book, 2022 ICC is used, and both classifications are provided in Appendix 1. One of the most important factors in a lymph node evaluation is an adequate tissue biopsy that provides sufficient tissue for morphologic evaluation and potential ancillary studies.

A lymph node evaluation starts with a hematoxylin and eosin (H&E)-stained slide. The importance of the H&E evaluation cannot be overemphasized. A properly fixed, cut, and stained section is critical for successful interpretation (as discussed in Chapter 2). The diagnosis (or differential diagnosis) is essentially formed on the H&E section and confirmed by ancillary studies. Performing immunohistochemical stains "blindly," with no idea of differential diagnosis frequently leads to confusion rather than correct diagnosis. The most common approach to a lymph node evaluation is a pattern-based approach, as different entities have distinct morphologic patterns that can be recognized on H&E section (Table 1.1). Much information can be gained from a low-power (2×) magnification, allowing a pathologist to answer the following questions:

- *Is the lymph node architecture preserved or effaced?* When the lymph node architecture is preserved, the different compartments (cortex, paracortex, medulla) are clearly defined, the lymph node sinuses are open, and the lymph node capsule is thin and intact.

TABLE 1.1 The Patterns of Lymph Node Involvement With Their Associated Differential Diagnosis

Patterns and Differential Diagnoses
Nodular/Follicular Pattern
Reactive
• Nonspecific follicular hyperplasia[a]
• Infections (eg, acute HIV lymphadenitis, syphilitic lymphadenitis, toxoplasma lymphadenitis)
• Autoimmune disorders (eg, rheumatoid lymphadenopathy)
• Kimura lymphadenopathy
• IgG4 disease-related lymphadenopathy (type II)
Neoplastic
• Follicular lymphoma
• Mantle cell lymphoma
• Marginal zone lymphoma colonizing follicles
• Small lymphocytic lymphoma
• Follicular T-cell lymphoma
• Pediatric-type follicular lymphoma
Macronodular Pattern
Reactive
• Progressive transformation of germinal centers
• IgG4 disease-related lymphadenopathy (type IV)
Neoplastic
• Nodular lymphocyte-predominant Hodgkin lymphoma
• Classic Hodgkin lymphoma, lymphocyte rich subtype
• Follicular lymphoma, floral variant
• Pediatric nodal marginal zone lymphoma
• Follicular T-cell lymphoma
• Pediatric-type follicular lymphoma
Angiofollicular Lymphoid Hyperplasia
Reactive
• Castleman disease, hyaline-vascular variant[b]
• HIV lymphadenitis, burn-out phase
• IgG4 disease-related lymphadenopathy (type I)
Neoplastic
• Angioimmunoblastic T-cell lymphoma (pattern II)

TABLE 1.1 The Patterns of Lymph Node Involvement With Their Associated Differential Diagnosis (Continued)

Interfollicular/Paracortical Expansion and/or Mixed Follicular and Paracortical Patterns

Reactive

- Infections (eg, infectious mononucleosis, CMV lymphadenitis)
- Dermatopathic lymphadenopathy
- Drug-induced lymphadenopathy
- IgG4 disease-related lymphadenopathy (type III)
- Autoimmune lymphoproliferative syndrome (ALPS)

Neoplastic

- Angioimmunoblastic T-cell lymphoma
- Peripheral T-cell lymphoma, not otherwise specified
- Mycosis fungoides involving lymph node
- Classic Hodgkin lymphoma
- Marginal zone lymphoma

Diffuse Pattern

Reactive

- Infections (eg, infectious mononucleosis)

Neoplastic

- B-cell non-Hodgkin lymphomas (eg, mantle cell lymphoma, diffuse large B-cell lymphoma, Burkitt lymphoma, high-grade B-cell lymphoma)
- T-cell non-Hodgkin lymphomas (eg, peripheral T-cell lymphoma, not otherwise specified, anaplastic large cell lymphoma)
- Classic Hodgkin lymphoma
- Nodular lymphocyte-predominant B-cell lymphoma, diffuse variant

Lymphomas With Prominent Fibrosis ("Sclerotic Pattern")

- Follicular lymphoma
- Classic Hodgkin lymphoma, nodular sclerosis subtype
- Primary mediastinal large B-cell lymphoma
- Anaplastic large cell lymphoma, ALK-positive (Hodgkin-like pattern)

(Continued)

TABLE 1.1 The Patterns of Lymph Node Involvement With Their Associated Differential Diagnosis (Continued)

Distended Sinuses ("Sinus Pattern")

Reactive

- Nonspecific sinus histiocytosis[a]
- Foreign body lymphadenopathy (eg, silicone lymphadenopathy, debris from prosthesis, lymphangiography)
- Tumor-reactive lymphadenopathy

Neoplastic

- Sinus histiocytosis with massive lymphadenopathy (Rosai-Dorfman disease)
- Anaplastic large cell lymphoma
- Langerhans cell histiocytosis
- Lymphoplasmacytic lymphoma

Granulomas +/− Necrosis

Nonnecrotizing (epithelioid) granulomas

- Sarcoidosis
- Common variable immunodeficiency
- Non-Hodgkin lymphomas (eg, Burkitt lymphoma, peripheral T-cell lymphoma-lymphoepitheliod variant)
- Classic Hodgkin lymphoma
- Toxoplasmosis

Necrotizing granulomas

- Mycobacterial infection (*Mycobacterium tuberculosis* and atypical mycobacterial lymphadenitis)
- Fungal lymphadenitis (eg, *Histoplasma* and *Coccidiomycosis* lymphadenitis)
- Bacterial lymphadenitis
- Cat-scratch lymphadenitis
- Lymphogranuloma venereum

Other entities with areas of necrosis

- Histiocytic necrotizing lymphadenitis (Kikuchi-Fujimoto disease)
- Systemic lupus lymphadenopathy
- Epstein-Barr virus lymphadenitis

Vascular proliferations

- Vascular transformation of sinuses
- Infections (eg, bacillary angiomatosis, mycobacterial spindle cell pseudotumor)
- Kaposi sarcoma

[a]Etiology is usually unclear.

[b]Plasma cell and multicentric variants usually show some follicles with hyaline-vascular lesions.

- *If the architecture is effaced, what is the pattern of effacement?*
- *Are there any other characteristic morphologic features (eg, areas of necrosis, abnormal collections of histiocytes, large atypical cells, increased eosinophils or plasma cells, etc.)?*
- *Is it reactive or neoplastic?*
- *What is the differential diagnosis?*

Many of these questions can be answered at low magnification (2× objective). The morphologic and cellular details are then appreciated at higher magnifications. After formulating a differential diagnosis, a targeted panel of immunohistochemical stains should be ordered. In cases where flow cytometry is available, differential diagnosis can be further narrowed such that few to no immunohistochemical stains are required in some cases.

As outlined in Table 1.1, there are several different histologic patterns in lymph node pathology. Each pattern is associated with a differential diagnosis; however, there is often overlap with several patterns seen in one lymph node. This table is by no means a comprehensive list of all possible entities but rather an overview of common, and some rare, diseases associated with each pattern. Occasional entities, such as nodular lymphocyte predominant B-cell lymphoma or mantle cell lymphoma, can have two or more different patterns. The two most common histologic patterns are nodular/follicular and diffuse (Figures 1.1 and 1.2). Entities associated with diffuse pattern are rarely benign, and this pattern is easily recognizable as the lymph node architecture is typically diffusely obliterated. The nodular/follicular pattern is more complex, as it includes a number of

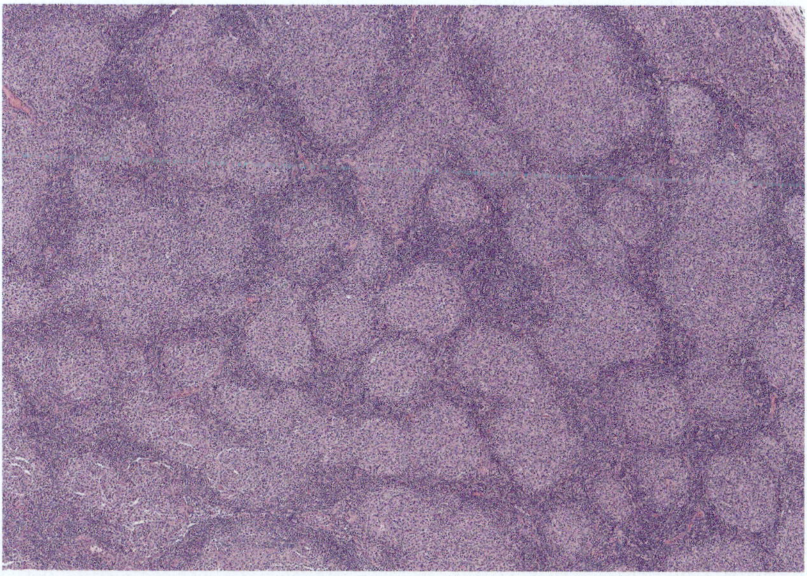

FIGURE 1.1 **Follicular pattern.** Follicular lymphoma is a typical example of follicular pattern with back-to-back neoplastic follicles.

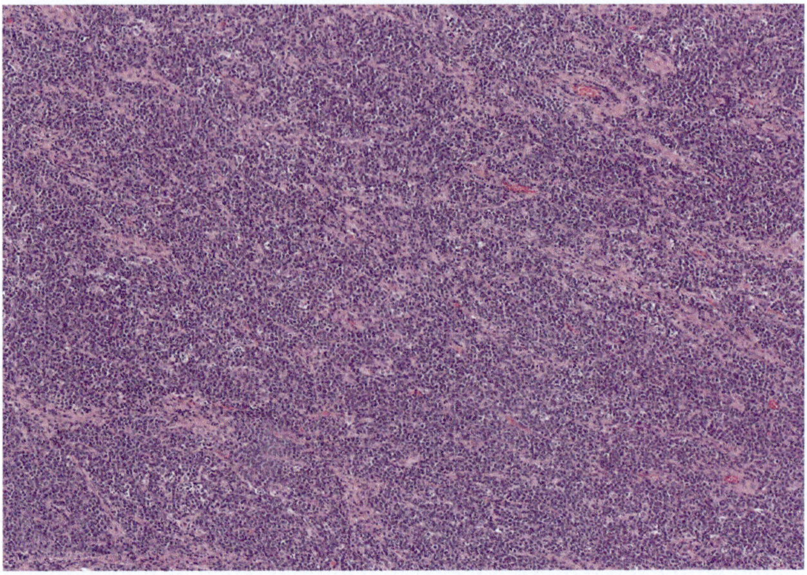

FIGURE 1.2 **Diffuse pattern.** Diffuse large B-cell lymphoma shows diffuse sheets of lymphoma cells.

benign and malignant entities, many of which overlap morphologically.[1,4-7] Within this pattern, other histologic clues can be utilized to narrow the differential diagnosis on H&E. These histologic details with their associated challenges and pitfalls are discussed throughout the book.

Finally, it is critical to incorporate clinical and radiologic information when making a diagnosis of hematologic diseases. In fact, some entities, such as posttransplant lymphoproliferative disorders, are primarily defined by clinical circumstances. Ideally, when evaluating a lymph node biopsy, a pathologist should know the following information:

- Patient's age and gender
- Sites of involvement (nodal or extranodal)
- If lymphadenopathy is present (if so, localized vs diffuse)
- Previous hematologic diseases
- History of autoimmunity
- History of primary or secondary immunosuppression (eg, HIV status, organ transplantation, immunomodulatory drugs)
- Complete blood count in some cases

NORMAL LYMPH NODE HISTOLOGY

Lymph nodes are part of the lymphoid system and are organized in groups throughout the body. They range in size from 2 to 20 mm and are normally not easily palpable in adults. They become prominent only when enlarged due to a reactive or neoplastic process. Their main role is to filter lymphatic fluid and trap foreign antigens. Furthermore, within the lymph node, the intricate microenvironment presents antigens to immune cells, which results in an adaptive immune response.[4,8] Solid knowledge of normal lymph node histology, different structures, compartments, and cell types is essential when evaluating lymph node biopsies.

Lymph nodes are surrounded by a thin fibrous capsule (Figure 1.3) that can be distorted (most commonly thickened) in reactive conditions and lymphomas, which can be a helpful clue in the diagnosis of these diseases (Figure 1.4). Lymph nodes are round to ovoid and (in a "perfect" histologic cut through the lymph node hilum) they appear slightly bean shaped with three distinct compartments–cortex, paracortex, and medulla (Figure 1.5). B cells stain with pan B-cell markers (ie, CD19, CD20, CD79a, PAX5) (Figure 1.6), while T cells stain with CD3 (Figure 1.7). However, in everyday practice, lymph nodes can be biopsied, embedded, and sectioned in many different planes, which sometimes makes it difficult to recognize different compartments and understand immunohistochemical staining patterns.

Cortex

The cortex is a B-cell compartment of the lymph node and contains lymphoid follicles, primary and secondary (Figure 1.8). The primary follicles contain naïve B lymphocytes that are small and round, with condensed chromatin and scant cytoplasm (Figure 1.9). These B cells express pan-B-cell markers

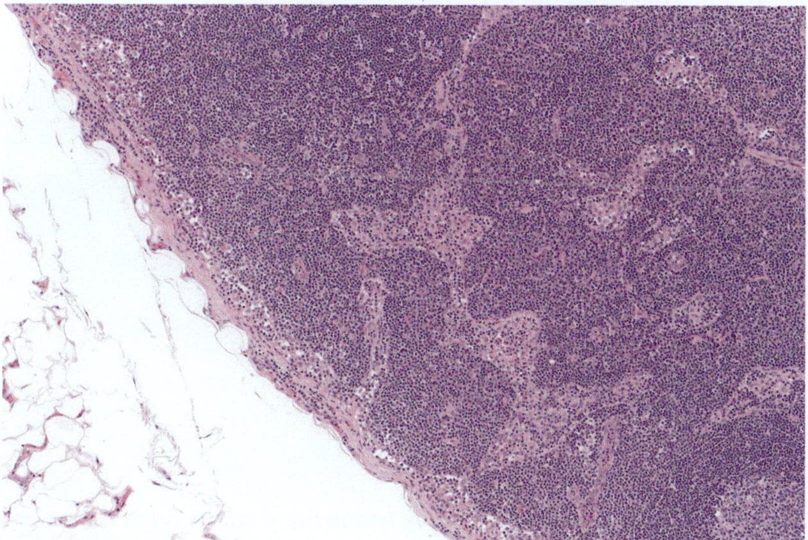

FIGURE 1.3 Unremarkable lymph node capsule is thin and delicate.

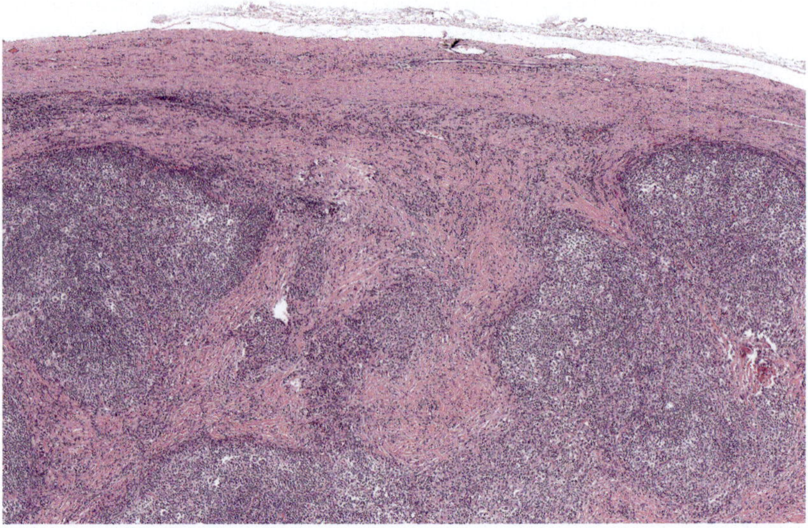

FIGURE 1.4 **Thickened lymph node capsule.** Classic Hodgkin lymphoma, nodular sclerosis subtype shows markedly thickened capsule, which is a helpful diagnostic clue and one of the morphologic criteria for diagnosis.

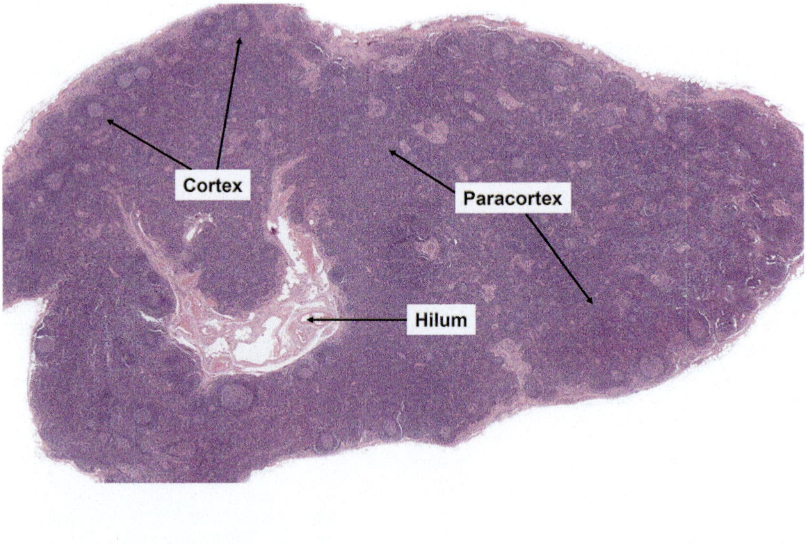

FIGURE 1.5 **Low-power view of a reactive lymph node cut through the hilum illustrates different histologic compartments.**

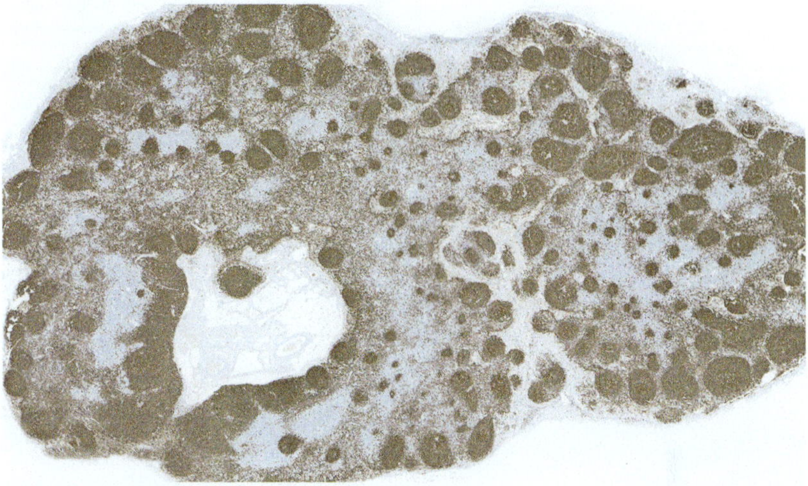

FIGURE 1.6 B-cell areas are highlighted by CD20 immunohistochemical stain.

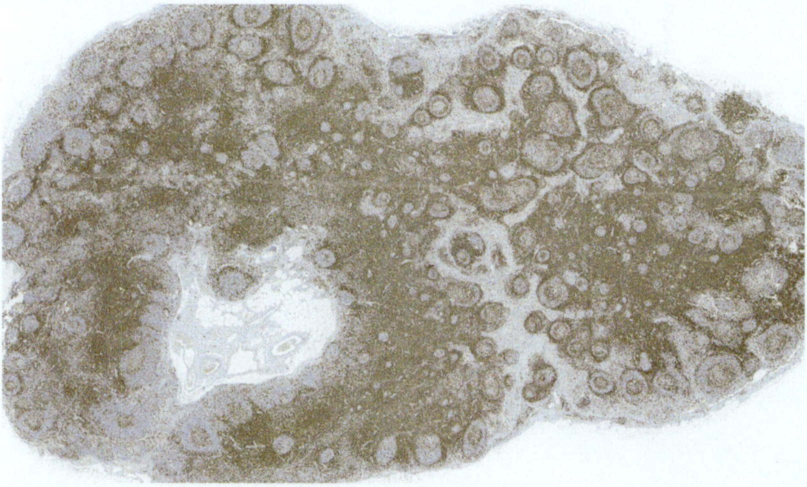

FIGURE 1.7 T cells are positive for CD3 immunohistochemical stain.

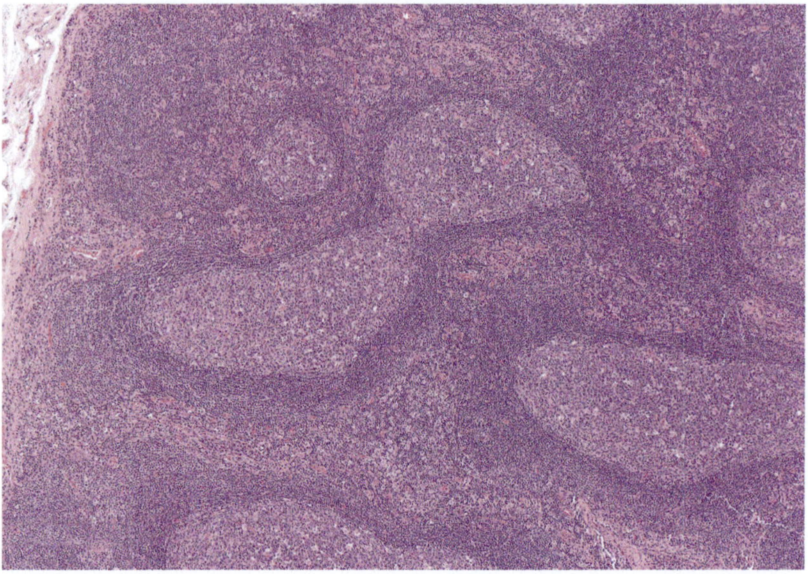

FIGURE 1.8 **Lymph node cortex.** Secondary follicles with reactive germinal centers in the cortical area.

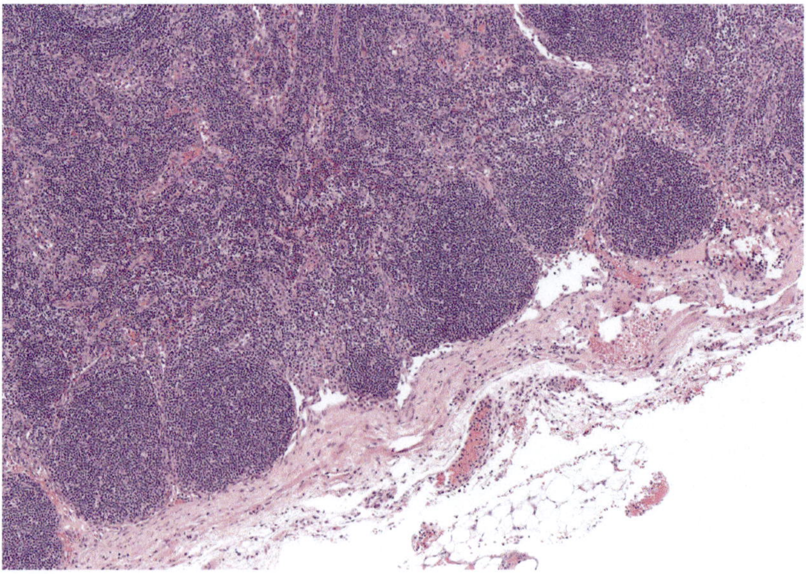

FIGURE 1.9 **Primary follicles are composed of small lymphocytes.**

and the anti-apoptotic protein BCL2, which is important for their survival in the primary follicles (Figure 1.10). Of note, a subset of primary follicle B cells normally express CD5 (Figure 1.11), which can occasionally be appreciated by immunohistochemical stains and should not be interpreted as aberrant expression that is seen in some B-cell lymphomas.[8-11] Upon antigenic stimulation, primary follicles become secondary (reactive) follicles. Secondary follicles are composed of several compartments including a central germinal center surrounded by a mantle zone, as well as an outer marginal zone (Figure 1.12). Similar to the primary follicles, the mantle zone is composed of small naïve B cells with scant cytoplasm that express BCL2, IgM, and IgD (Figures 1.13 and 1.14). The germinal center contains several cell types including B cells (centroblasts and centrocytes), follicular helper T cells, follicular dendritic cells, and histiocytes (tingible-body macrophages). As they pass through the germinal center, B cells undergo somatic hypermutation of the immunoglobulin variable region genes and heavy chain switching (from IgM to IgG or IgA). The B cells that are best fitted for a particular antigen are selected for proliferation, while the ineffective ones are promptly destroyed via programmed cell death, apoptosis. To allow for apoptosis, the antiapoptotic protein BCL2 is downregulated in normal germinal centers.[12-14] Scattered tingible-body macrophages with engulfed apoptotic debris are readily apparent in germinal centers. The reactive germinal centers appear polarized, that is, have a dark zone

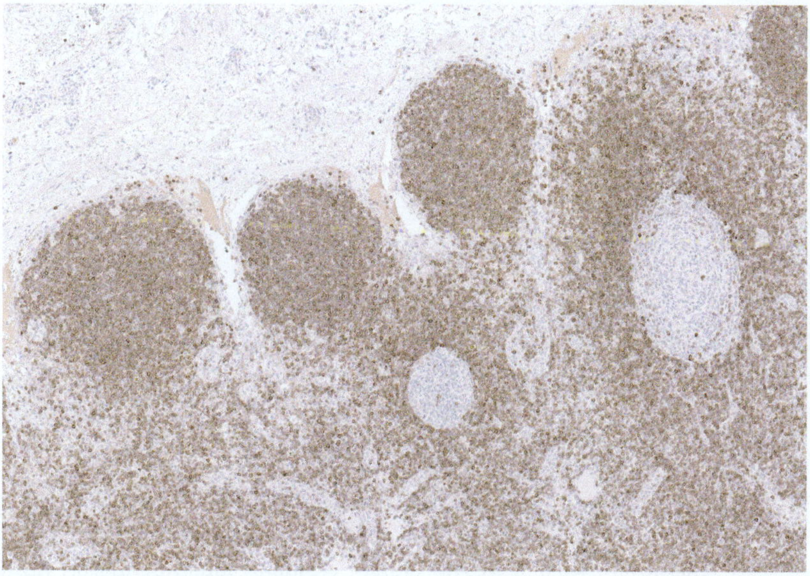

FIGURE 1.10 Immunohistochemical stain for BCL2 is positive in primary follicles and negative in germinal centers of secondary follicles.

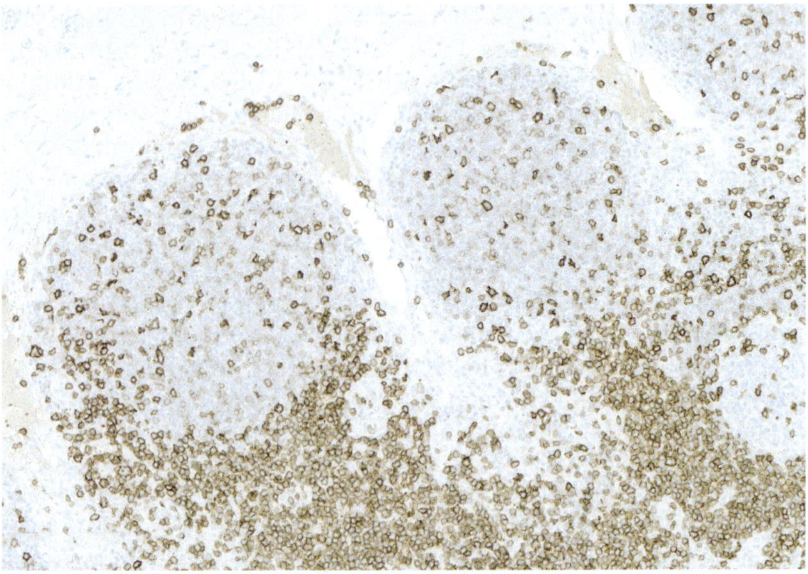

FIGURE 1.11 Subset of B cells in the primary follicles of reactive lymph node weakly stains with CD5 immunohistochemical stain.

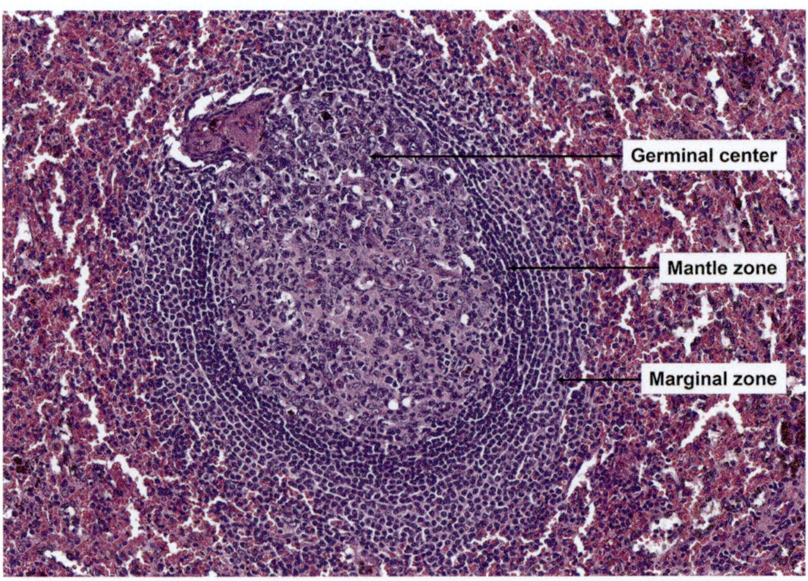

FIGURE 1.12 Secondary follicle in the spleen showing well-delineated germinal center, mantle, and marginal zone.

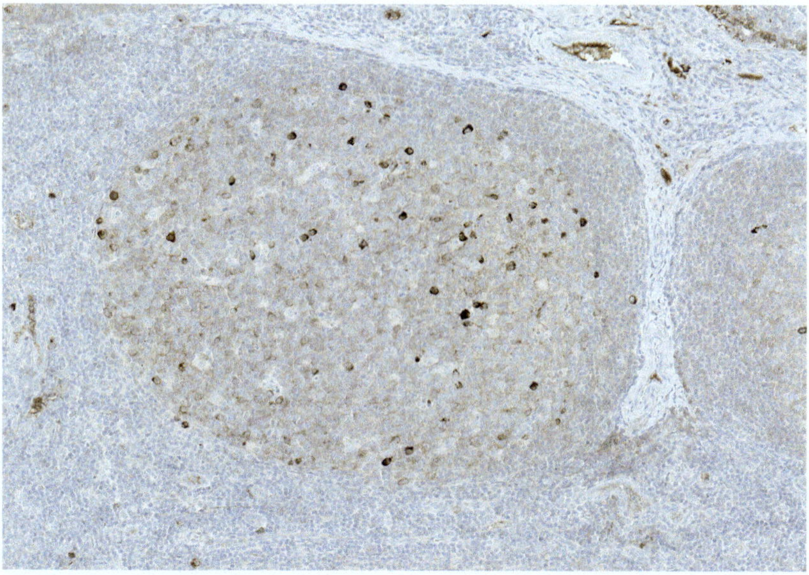

FIGURE 1.13 Immunohistochemical stain for IgM weakly stains B cells in the mantle zone as well as in the germinal center.

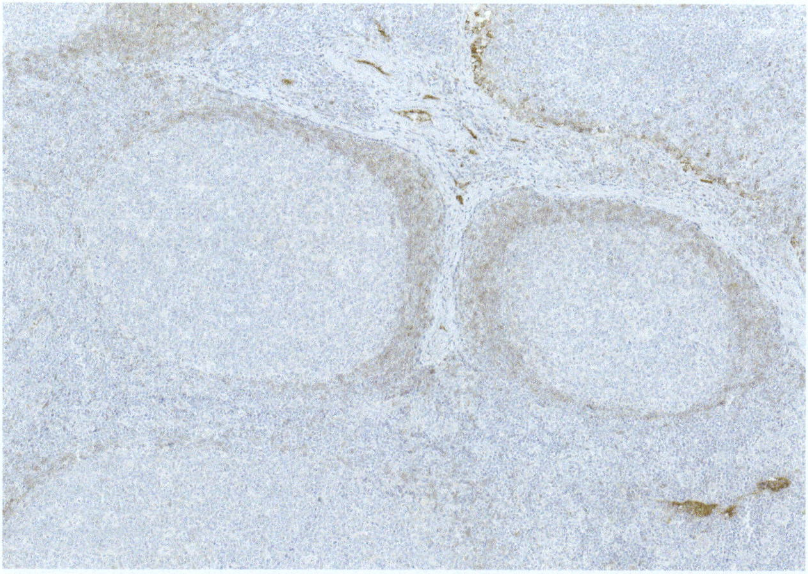

FIGURE 1.14 Mantle zone B cells are positive by IgD immunohistochemical stain.

composed predominantly of centroblasts and a light zone composed of centrocytes (Figure 1.15). Centroblasts are large cells with round nuclei, open chromatin, and several peripherally placed nucleoli. In contrast, centrocytes are smaller with irregular (and frequently cleaved) nuclei and condensed chromatin. B cells of the germinal center express CD10 and BCL6 and, as mentioned above, are negative for BCL2 (Figure 1.16A-C). Follicular dendritic cells (FDCs) serve as antigen-presenting cells to B lymphocytes and provide structural support in primary and secondary follicles. They have a distinct histologic appearance with large rectangular nuclei, open chromatin and central small eosinophilic nucleoli. Commonly, two nuclei are touching ("kissing"), which makes them easily recognizable (Figure 1.17).[15,16] It is important to be familiar with FDCs and not to mistake them for centroblasts when grading follicular lymphoma. Follicular dendritic cell meshworks are highlighted by CD21, CD23, and CD35 immunostains (Figure 1.18). Finally, germinal centers contain scattered follicular helper T cells, which assist B cells during T-cell-dependent immune responses. They express CD4, CD10, BCL6, PD1 (CD279), ICOS, and CXCL13. CD10 expression is usually brighter than on the background B cells (Figure 1.19).[17,18] The marginal zone surrounds the mantle zone and is best appreciated in the mesenteric lymph nodes and spleen (Figure 1.12). It is not usually visible in most reactive lymph nodes and is composed of memory B cells that have more abundant cytoplasm, imparting a paler appearance to the marginal zone compared with the mantle zone.[4]

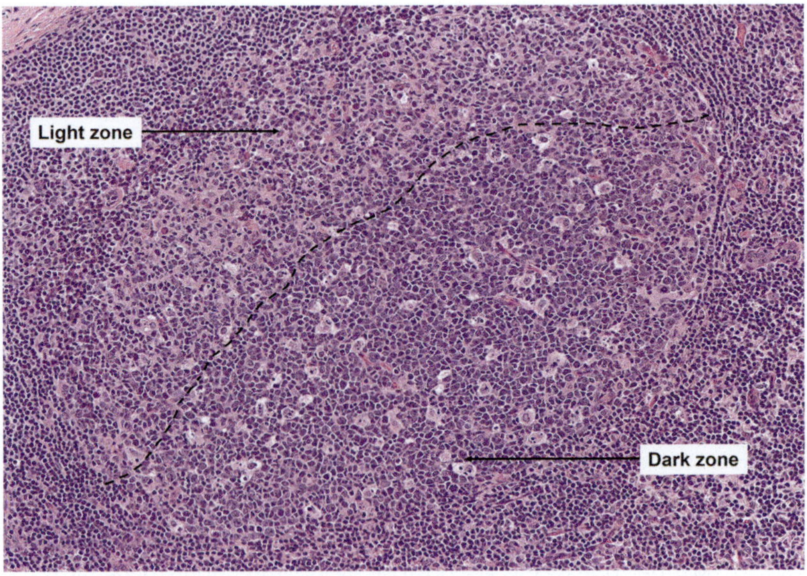

FIGURE 1.15 **Polarized germinal center.** The light zone is composed predominantly of small centrocytes, while the dark zone contains predominantly large centroblasts.

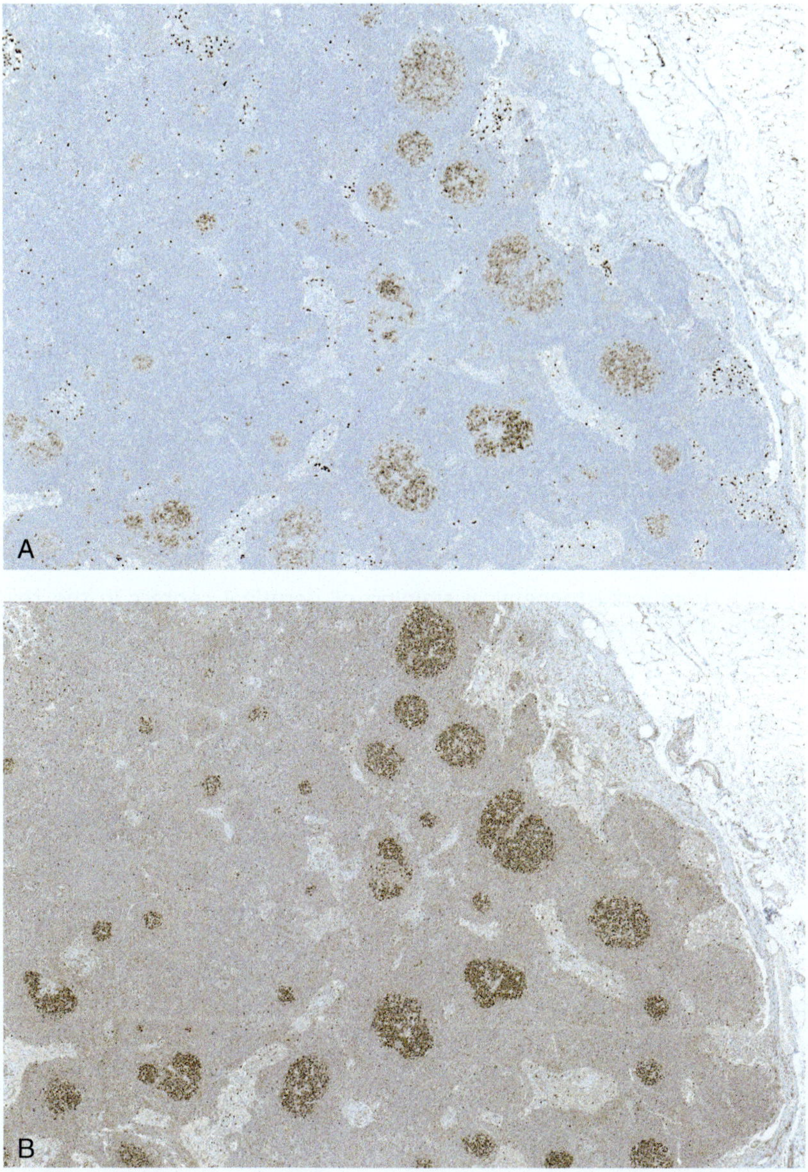

FIGURE 1.16 (*Continued*)

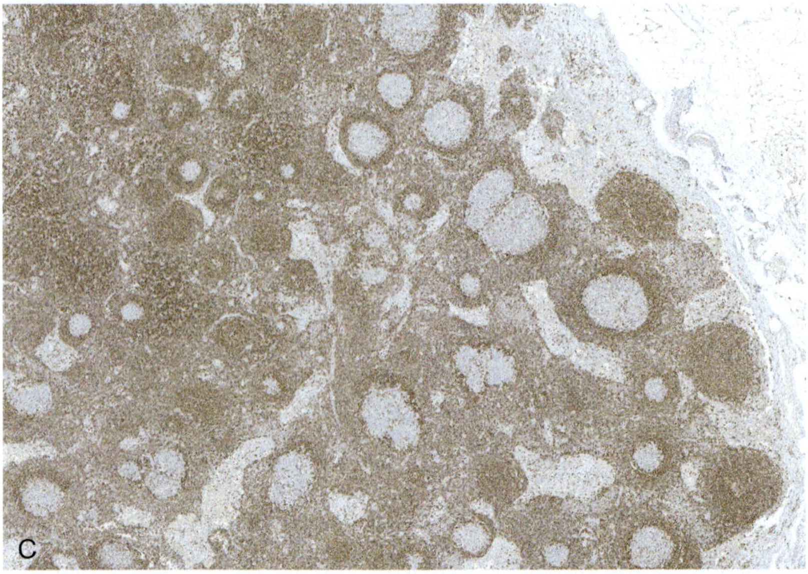

FIGURE 1.16 **Immunohistochemical staining of germinal centers in the reactive lymph node.** Germinal centers are positive for CD10 (A) and BCL6 (B), and are negative for BCL2 (C).

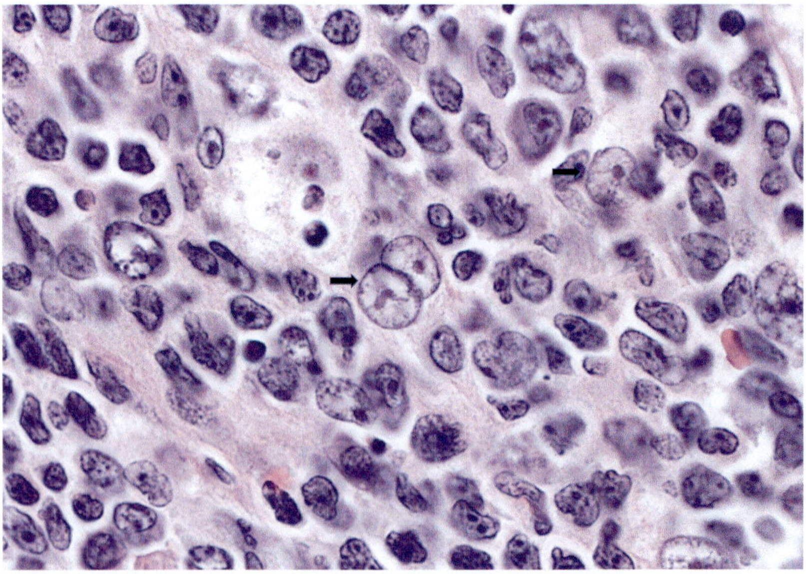

FIGURE 1.17 **Follicular dendritic cells in the germinal center (arrows).** They show large nuclei, open chromatin, and central eosinophilic nucleoli and can be seen singly or in pairs ("kissing" cells).

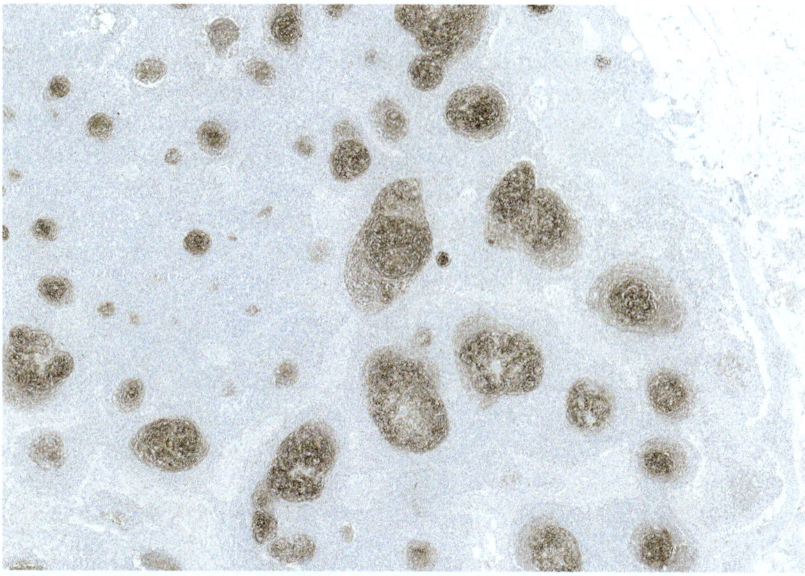

FIGURE 1.18 Tight follicular dendritic cell meshworks in the lymphoid follicles are highlighted with CD21 immunohistochemical stain.

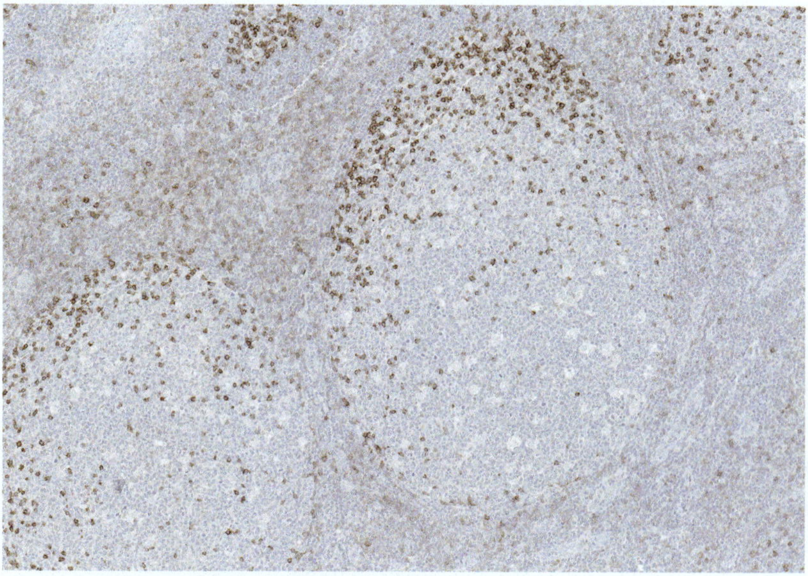

FIGURE 1.19 Follicular helper T cells in the germinal center are demonstrated with PD-1 immunohistochemical stain.

Paracortex

The paracortex is predominantly a T-cell compartment that is found under the cortex and in between the B-cell follicles. It contains predominantly small lymphocytes, admixed with some B and T immunoblasts (large cells with open chromatin and prominent central nucleoli), and scattered antigen-presenting cells including histiocytes, interdigitating dendritic cells, and Langerhans cells, which can be distinguished by immunohistochemical stains (Table 1.2; Figure 1.20).[8,19] The T cells express pan-T-cell

TABLE 1.2 Immunophenotype of Different Structures and Cells Found in Cortex, Paracortex, and Medulla

Structures/Cells of a Lymph Node	Antigens Expressed
Cortex	
Primary follicles (naïve B cells)	Pan-B-cell markers (CD19, CD20, CD22, CD79a), PAX5, CD5 (small subset+), BCL2, IgM, IgD, surface immunoglobulin (Ig) light chains (kappa:lambda = 2:1)
Secondary follicles	
Mantle zone (naïve B cells)	Pan-B-cell markers, PAX5, CD23, IgM, IgD, surface Ig light chains, BCL2
Germinal center	
B cells (centrocytes and centroblasts)	Pan-B-cell markers, PAX5, CD10, BCL6, surface Ig light chains
Follicular helper T cells	CD4, CD10, BCL6, PD1 (CD279), CXCL13
Follicular dendritic cells	CD21, CD23, CD35, clusterin
Histiocytes (tingible-body macrophages)	CD4, CD68, CD163
Marginal zone (memory B cells)	Pan-B-cell markers, PAX5, BCL2
Paracortex	
T cells	Pan-T-cell markers (CD2, sCD3, CD5, CD7), CD4:CD8 = 3-4:1; BCL2
NK cells	CD2, cCD3, CD56
Plasmacytoid dendritic cells	CD43, CD123, CD303
Langerhans cells	CD1a, S100, langerin
Interdigitating dendritic cells	S100
High endothelial venules	CD31, CD34, ERG
Medulla	
Plasma cells	CD138, MUM1, polytypic cytoplasmic Ig light chains

antigens (CD2, CD3, CD5, CD7) and BCL2, with occasional partial loss of CD7 in reactive conditions (Figure 1.7). CD4-positive T cells predominate over CD8-positive ones with an approximate CD4:CD8 ratio of 3-4:1. Plasmacytoid dendritic cells are another cell type that are seen in the paracortex, usually in small clusters in proximity to vessels. These cells secrete interferon gamma and are involved in viral immunity. They can be visualized with a CD123 immunohistochemical stain. In some diseases, such as hyaline vascular Castleman disease, the plasmacytoid dendritic cells are increased and frequently apparent on H&E sections.[4,20]

In addition, the paracortex contains distinct endothelial venules, which are lined by cuboidal endothelial cells and express lymphocyte homing receptors that recruit lymphocytes to the paracortex.[21]

Medulla

The medulla (or medullary cords) is the main site of plasma-cell proliferation and antibody production. In addition to mature plasma cells, the medullary cords contain small lymphocytes, plasmacytoid lymphocytes, and plasmablasts. Medullary cords are separated by medullary sinuses. Plasma cells express CD138, MUM1, and cytoplasmic light chains, kappa or lambda.[4,8]

The immunophenotypes of different structures and cells found in the cortex, paracortex, and medulla are summarized in Table 1.2.

A network of lymphatic sinuses, which are divided into subcapsular, cortical, and medullary, carry the lymph from the surface of the lymph

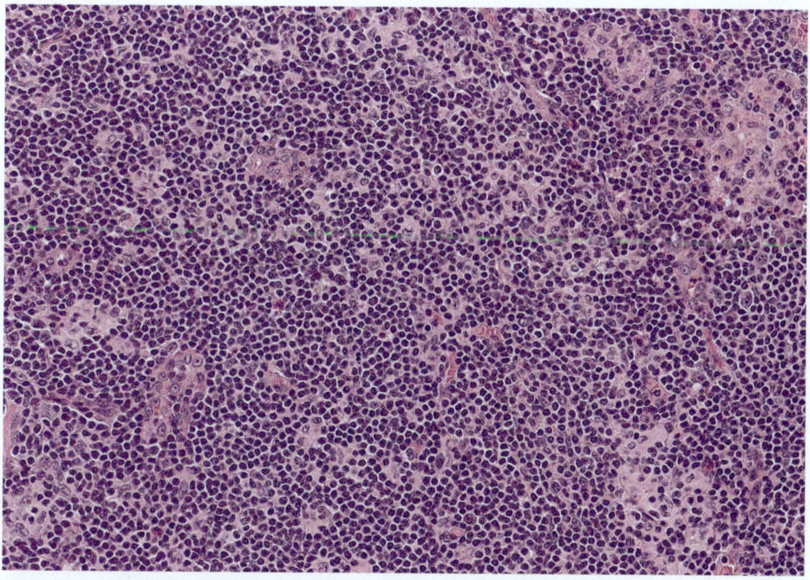

FIGURE 1.20 **Paracortex.** Small lymphocytes (mainly T cells) predominate in the paracortex, admixed with scattered immunoblasts and large cells with pale eosinophilic cytoplasm, which include histiocytes, interdigitating dendritic cells, and Langerhans cells.

node (where it enters via afferent lymphatics) through the lymph node parenchyma into the medulla and lymph node hilum, where it leaves the lymph node via efferent lymphatic vessels in the hilum. In a "normal" lymph node, as well as in many reactive conditions, lymph node sinuses (at least some of them) are open and are easily appreciated on H&E slides. They contain a mixture of cells, including numerous macrophages, small lymphocytes, immunoblasts, plasma cells, and neutrophils (Figure 1.21). In lymph nodes involved by lymphomas, sinuses are usually obliterated and not visible. In some conditions, such as Langerhans cell histiocytosis or sinus histiocytosis with massive lymphadenopathy (Rosai-Dorfman disease), sinuses are distended and filled by Langerhans cells and histiocytes, respectively (Figure 1.22). Lymph nodes receive blood supply from the arteries that enter through the lymph node hilum and branch out into capillary networks in the lymph node parenchyma. Similarly, veins exit the lymph node through the hilum.[4,8]

SMALL/NEEDLE CORE BIOPSY EVALUATION—CHALLENGES AND PITFALLS

Small/needle core lymph node biopsies have become increasingly more common in the workup of patients with lymphadenopathy and suspicion for lymphoma. This minimally invasive procedure is generally safe and well tolerated by patients and certainly preferred over open biopsy in deep seated lymph nodes found in sites such as the mediastinum, mesentery, and retroperitoneum. Furthermore, multiple studies have demonstrated

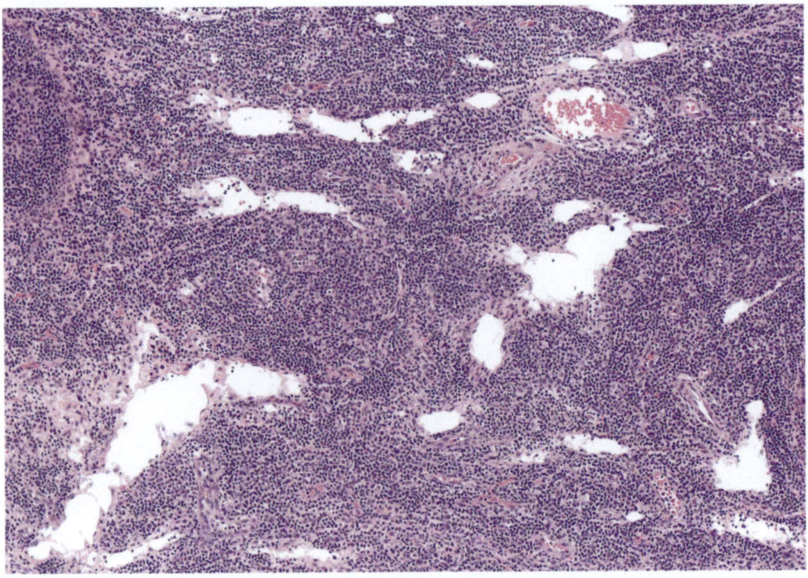

FIGURE 1.21 Widely open cortical sinuses in reactive lymph node.

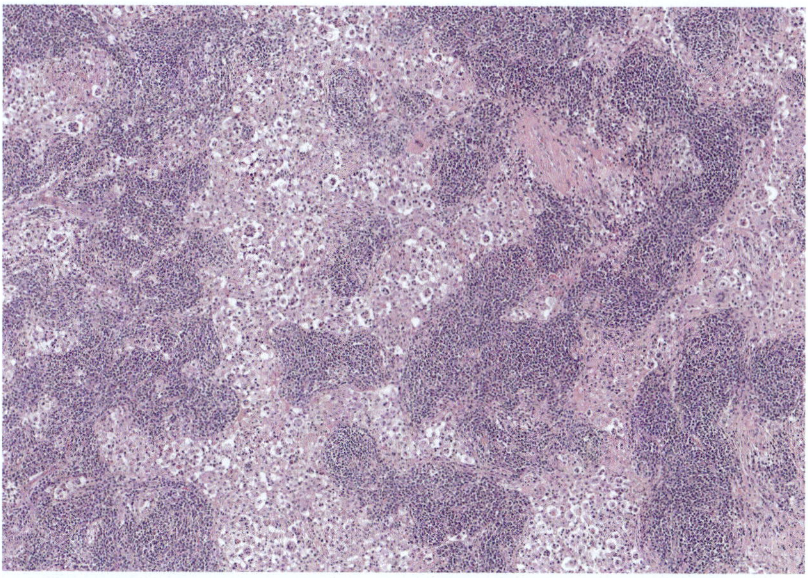

FIGURE 1.22 **Sinus histiocytosis with massive lymphadenopathy (Rosai-Dorfman disease).** Lymph node sinuses are markedly distended and filled with large atypical histiocytes that show emperipolesis.

satisfactory sampling in the majority of examined needle cores and diagnostic accuracy of over 80%.[22-27] In our experience, the correct diagnosis can usually be rendered in most small/needle core lymph node biopsies. It is advisable to take multiple core biopsies (eg, 5-10 if possible) to procure adequate material for morphologic evaluation and ancillary studies. However, it is critical for pathologists to be aware of the problems, pitfalls, and limitations when making a diagnosis using such limited tissue. It is important to remember that the same diagnostic criteria used to diagnose different entities in larger biopsies should be applied to small lymph node biopsies. However, trying to "push" the diagnosis in a limited specimen, when histologic criteria are not met, is hazardous and not in anyone's best interest. Some of the commonly encountered challenges when dealing with needle core biopsies are the following:

- Scant or inadequate tissue–There is no good answer to a question "how small is too small?", as this is case dependent. Nevertheless, assessment of morphology and interpretation of immunohistochemical stains should not be done on small specks of tissue, as this can lead to grave mistakes (Figure 1.23). For example, small fragments of reactive germinal centers can be mistaken for a large B-cell lymphoma if only centroblast-predominant areas are sampled. Furthermore, in some cases a limited specimen might be adequate to formulate a differential diagnosis on an H&E slide but too limited for further

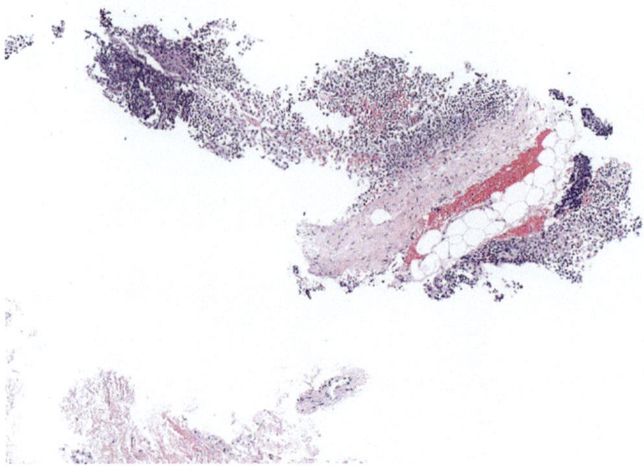

FIGURE 1.23 **Scant biopsy.** This biopsy shows less than 1 mm of lymphoid tissue with predominantly small lymphocytes and is an example of inadequate lymph node sampling.

immunophenotyping or other ancillary studies. Another common situation is core biopsies in which the tissue is completely necrotic. Although these frequently represent tumor necrosis, the lack of viable cells precludes further workup and diagnosis, and a repeat biopsy should be requested (Figure 1.24). In some instances, completely fibrotic cores with no lymphoma cells are obtained (Figure 1.25). In particular, mediastinal masses can have a very thick capsule and/or be very fibrotic, which can cause multiple biopsy attempts to be unsuccessful in procuring diagnostic tissue. Figure 1.26 illustrates how variation in needle core sampling of a fibrotic mediastinal lymph node can render adequate or inadequate specimen.

- Crush artifact–Significant crush artifact is a common problem in needle core biopsies and precludes pattern recognition and assessment of cellular details (Figure 1.27). Immunohistochemical stains can be performed on these specimens and, in many cases, it is possible to say whether the lesion is lymphoma or not. However, it is best to avoid a more specific classification if the morphology cannot be appreciated on H&E-stained sections.
- Difficulties in assessing morphology and pattern of infiltration–In some cases, because of poor fixation and suboptimal staining (frequently due to thick and overstained sections), it is very difficult to appreciate different lymph node compartments (Figure 1.28). Furthermore, in some needle core biopsies, the architecture and pattern of infiltration are difficult to assess due to the sampled area

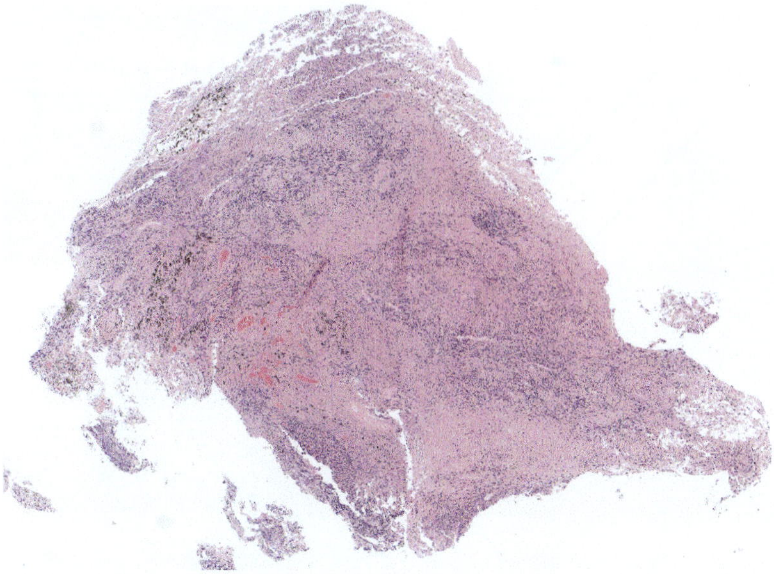

FIGURE 1.24 **Necrotic biopsy.** This is an example of completely necrotic biopsy in a patient with previous history of lymphoma, also inadequate for diagnostic purposes.

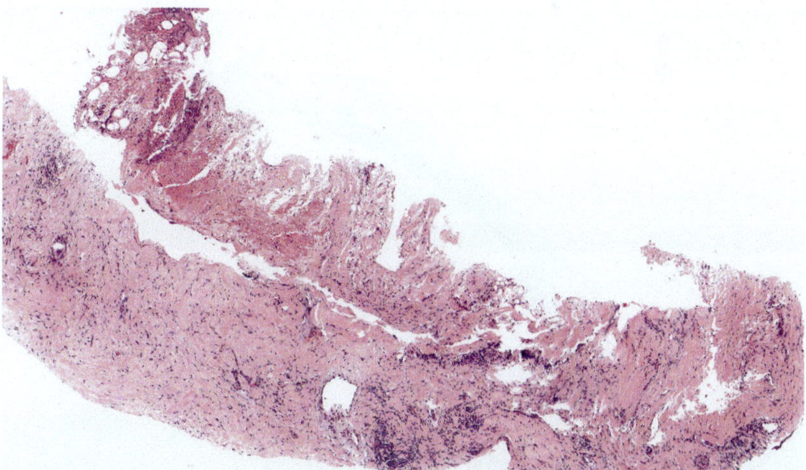

FIGURE 1.25 **Fibrotic biopsy.** This is a completely fibrotic biopsy of a large mediastinal mass. Repeated sampling revealed classic Hodgkin lymphoma.

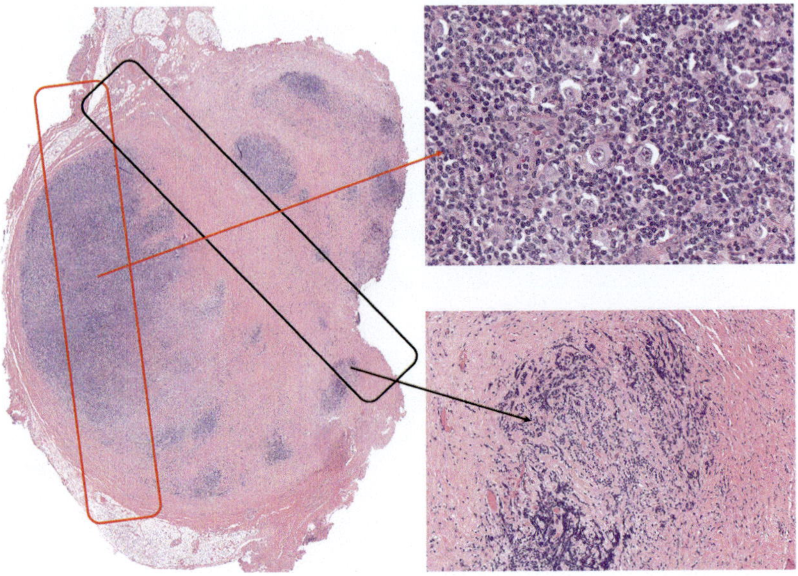

FIGURE 1.26 **Lymph node with classic Hodgkin lymphoma—variation in needle core sampling.** The figure demonstrates how two different core biopsy samples of markedly fibrotic lymph node can render a diagnostic biopsy (red core) and inadequate, largely fibrotic biopsy (black core).

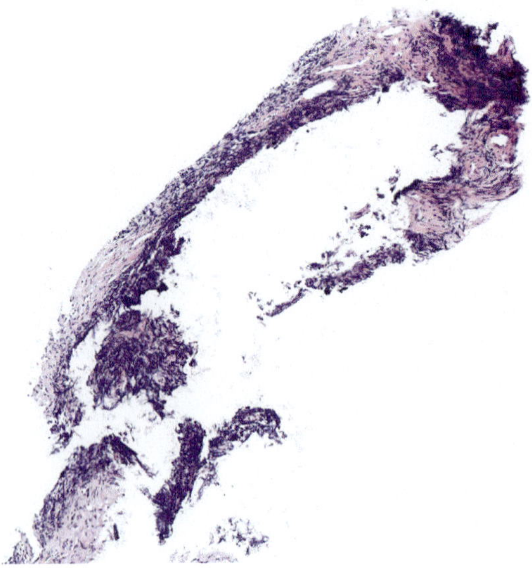

FIGURE 1.27 **Crush artifact.** Cells are completely crushed, precluding assessment of pattern or cellular details.

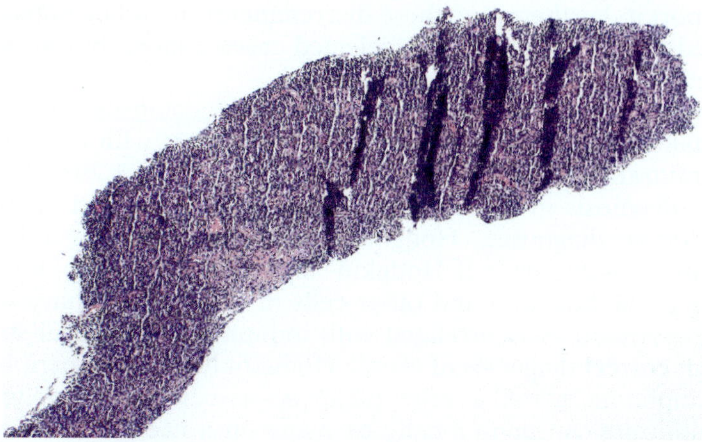

FIGURE 1.28 **Poorly fixed and thick-sectioned needle core biopsy.** In this reactive lymph node architecture cannot be appreciated due to suboptimal sectioning and staining.

being relatively small. This problem is more commonly encountered in lymphomas composed of smaller cells (such as low-grade B-cell lymphomas) than diffuse large B-cell lymphoma or high-grade B-cell lymphoma.[4,28] A brief panel of immunohistochemical stains (eg, CD20, CD3, CD5, CD10, BCL6, and BCL2) can be helpful in highlighting different lymph node compartments and/or pattern of infiltration. When performing immunohistochemical stains in a stepwise fashion, it is prudent to cut a number of unstained slides to be used later for additional stains, as repeated cutting of the block for ancillary studies can quickly exhaust the tissue.

- Discrepancy between flow cytometry and morphology–In some cases of needle core biopsies, a separate sample is submitted for flow cytometry. If a separate sample for flow cytometry is not taken, the cores should be submitted for morphologic examination, which is preferred in situations where tissue is limited. Flow cytometry is frequently a great ancillary tool that can narrow the differential diagnosis and guide the further workup of needle core biopsy. However, in some instances a clonal population is detected by flow cytometry but morphologic assessment does not reveal a lymphoma, or it reveals a completely different/unrelated lymphoma. This discrepancy could be due to several things, such as differences in lymph node sampling (eg, sample sent to flow cytometry was lymphoma and tissue biopsy sampled benign area). Alternatively, small clones detected by flow cytometry can originate from blood and not the sampled lymph node. It is important to remember that, in these "discrepant" cases, morphology remains the gold standard. In short, one should not diagnose a lymphoma based on flow cytometry if the morphology does not support it. Furthermore, these discrepancies should be noted and discussed in a comment, and, in selected cases, a larger biopsy could be recommended.

- Specimens with polymorphous infiltrate and Hodgkin-like cells–The most challenging of the core biopsies are the ones with a polymorphous infiltrate, including large, atypical cells (Figure 1.29). The differential diagnosis in these cases is frequently broad and includes, among other diagnoses, Hodgkin lymphoma, T-cell lymphoma, and benign conditions.[1,4] If Hodgkin- and Reed-Sternberg-like cells are present, architecture and other cells in the infiltrate have to be carefully assessed and correlated with immunohistochemical stains. Although correct diagnosis of classic Hodgkin lymphoma, peripheral T-cell lymphoma, as well as other diagnoses associated with polymorphous infiltrate can undoubtedly be made on a needle core biopsy, these cases frequently require considerable experience, extensive immunohistochemical stains, and possible molecular studies. If there is any doubt about the diagnosis, it is best to request a larger, excisional biopsy.
- Entities that are very difficult to diagnose on a needle core biopsy–Some entities are very difficult to reliably diagnose on a small biopsy.

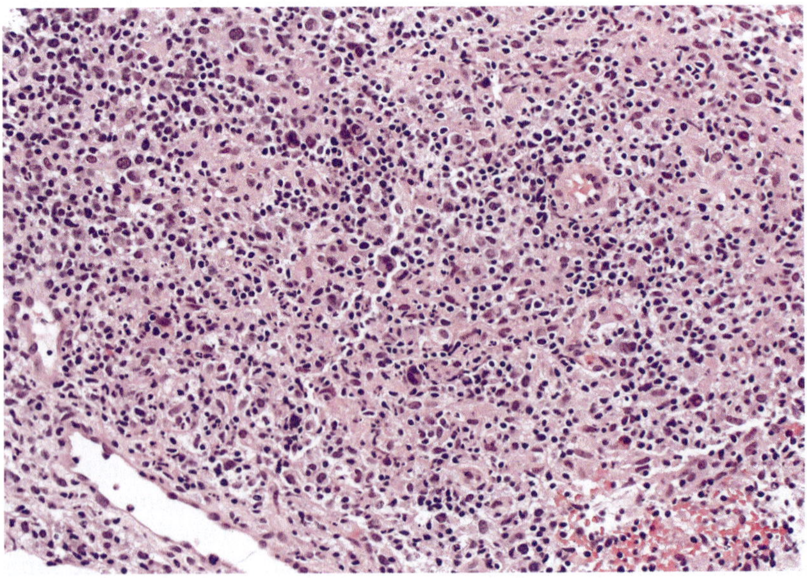

FIGURE 1.29 **Lymph node with polymorphous infiltrate.** The infiltrate is composed of small lymphocytes, plasma cells, histiocytes, and scattered large, Hodgkin-like cells.

The classic example is discerning a variant (diffuse) pattern of nodular lymphocyte-predominant B-cell lymphoma from T-cell/histiocyte-rich large B-cell lymphoma. Distinguishing between these two entities is not reliable or prudent on a needle core biopsy. This differential diagnosis is challenging even on a generous excisional biopsy and requires correlation with clinical and radiologic findings. Furthermore, T-cell lymphomas, as already mentioned above, are notoriously difficult to diagnose on a core biopsy, as are Epstein-Barr virus (EBV)-driven lymphoproliferative disorders. Also, reactive processes frequently cannot be fully described on a core. In these challenging situations, deferring to a larger biopsy (incisional/excisional) for a definitive diagnosis is strongly recommended.

NONHEMATOPOIETIC ENTITIES MIMICKING LYMPHOMA

Pathologists should always remember that other malignancies can mimic lymphomas. In the context of a lymph node biopsy, tumors most likely to mimic a lymphoid neoplasm include metastatic melanoma or metastatic carcinomas with a "small round blue cell" morphology. Table 1.3 summarizes nonhematopoietic tumors with different morphologic appearances that can mimic lymphomas.

TABLE 1.3 Nonhematopoietic Neoplasms That Metastasize to Lymph Nodes and Can Mimic Lymphoma

Nonhematopoietic Neoplasms
Small Round Blue Cell Tumors
Melanoma
Small cell carcinoma
Merkel cell carcinoma
Sarcomas (eg, rhabdomyosarcoma, poorly differentiated synovial sarcoma)
Tumors With Plasmacytoid Morphology
Melanoma
Plasmacytoid urothelial carcinoma
Tumors With Prominent Sclerosis and Inflammation
Well-differentiated liposarcoma (inflammatory/sclerosing variant)
Seminoma
Tumors With Epithelioid or Anaplastic Features
Melanoma
Carcinoma (different sites)

Small Round Blue Cell Tumors

Melanomas can mimic almost any tumor in the human body. Occasionally, they can have a high nuclear to cytoplasmic ratio (ie, "small cell" morphology), which can mimic a lymphoma, such as diffuse large B-cell lymphoma[29] (Figure 1.30). While CD138 is typically associated with plasma cell differentiation, it can also be positive in melanomas as well as carcinomas.[30] Melanomas also stain for MUM1.[31] Unlike lymphomas, melanomas are positive for SOX10, S100, HMB45, and Melan A.

Diffuse lymph node involvement by a small cell carcinoma can mimic a hematolymphoid neoplasm clinically, radiologically, and sometimes histologically.[32] Pan-lymphoid markers (eg, CD45) are typically negative in small cell carcinoma, although these tumors commonly express PAX5, a commonly used B-cell marker.[33] Small cell carcinoma stains for cytokeratin (eg, AE1/AE3, Cam 5.2) and neuroendocrine markers (eg, synaptophysin and chromogranin). Careful examination at higher power is necessary before dismissing stains as "negative" as expression can be quite focal and weak (ie, perinuclear dot-like pattern). Merkel cell carcinoma is a high-grade neuroendocrine carcinoma that arises in the skin and has a morphology very similar to small cell carcinoma in other parts of the body (Figure 1.31). It stains for neuroendocrine markers and cytokeratin, CK20 (in a dot-like pattern). This tumor occasionally stains for PAX5 and TdT, potentially masquerading a Merkel cell carcinoma as a lymphoblastic lymphoma to the unsuspecting pathologist.[34]

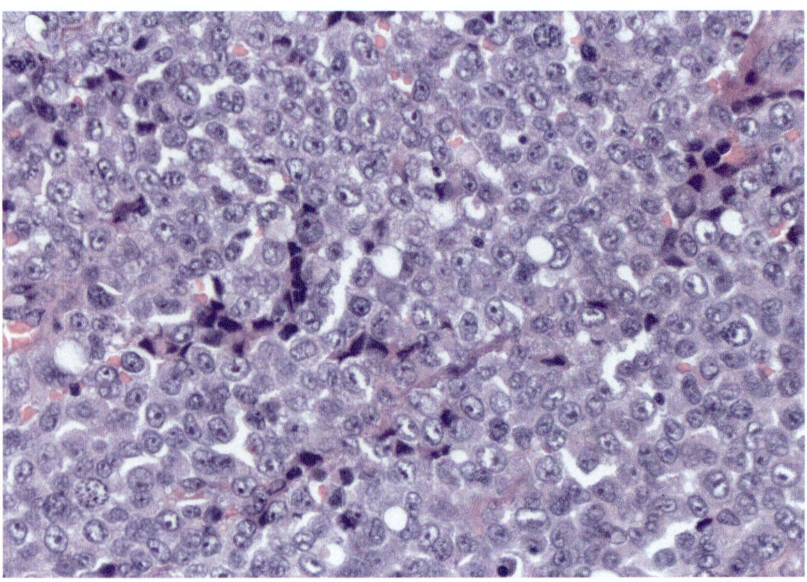

FIGURE 1.30 Melanoma with a high nuclear to cytoplasmic ratio that mimics a lymphoma.

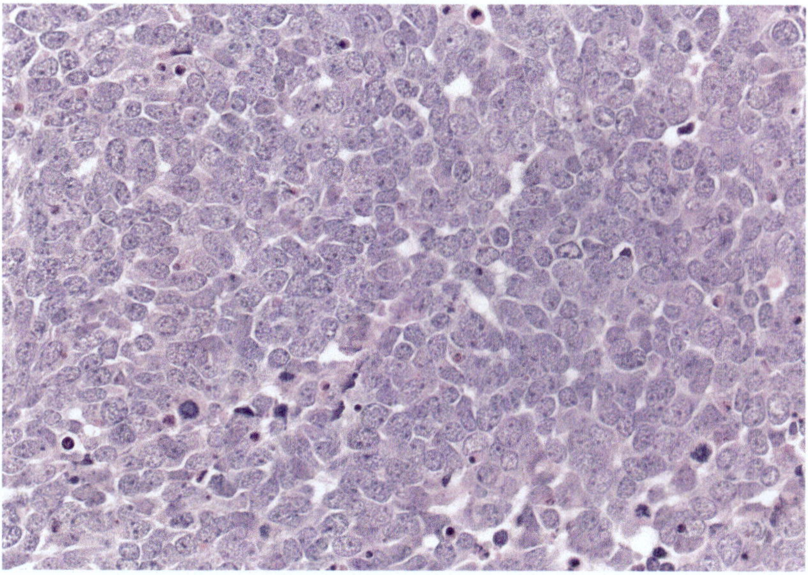

FIGURE 1.31 Merkel cell carcinoma shows histologic resemblance to a high-grade lymphoma.

Lymphomas can have morphologic overlap with small round blue cell sarcomas, such as Ewing sarcoma, desmoplastic round cell tumor (Figure 1.32), rhabdomyosarcoma (Figure 1.33), poorly differentiated synovial sarcoma, and undifferentiated round cell sarcoma, among other possibilities. While lymph node metastasis from a sarcoma is generally rare, vigilance is still paramount. Rhabdomyosarcoma and synovial sarcoma are two small round blue cell sarcomas that commonly metastasize to the lymph nodes.[35] Rhabdomyosarcoma exhibits a disproportional potential to metastasize to the lymph node.[36] Despite their skeletal muscle differentiation, the tumor cells in rhabdomyosarcomas (such as embryonal and alveolar) are typically quite immature and appear as small round blue cells with little cytoplasm. They are positive for desmin and are highlighted by MyoD1 and/or myogenin. Of note, alveolar rhabdomyosarcoma often stains for PAX5.[37] Although synovial sarcoma is typically associated with a "biphasic" morphology of spindled and "glandular-like" cells, the tumor can exhibit a poorly differentiated phenotype, which has a small round blue cell appearance. If metastatic to the lymph node, this appearance could emulate a high-grade lymphoma. These tumors are negative for lymphoid markers and will demonstrate either an *SYT-SSX1* or *SYT-SSX2* fusion transcript by sequencing.[38,39]

Tumors With Plasmacytoid Morphology

Melanoma, "the great mimicker," can also exhibit a plasmacytoid appearance that can emulate a plasma cell neoplasm or lymphoplasmacytic

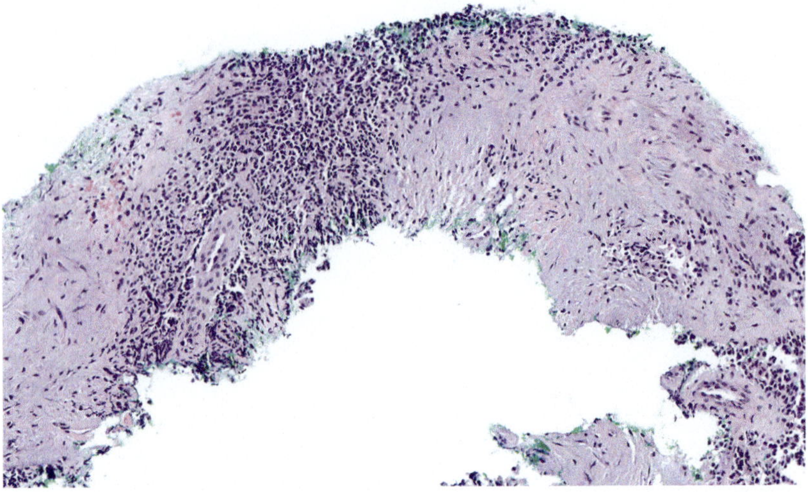

FIGURE 1.32 **Desmoplastic small round cell tumor metastatic to a lymph node mimics lymphoma.** The tumor shows prominent desmoplasia, a helpful diagnostic clue.

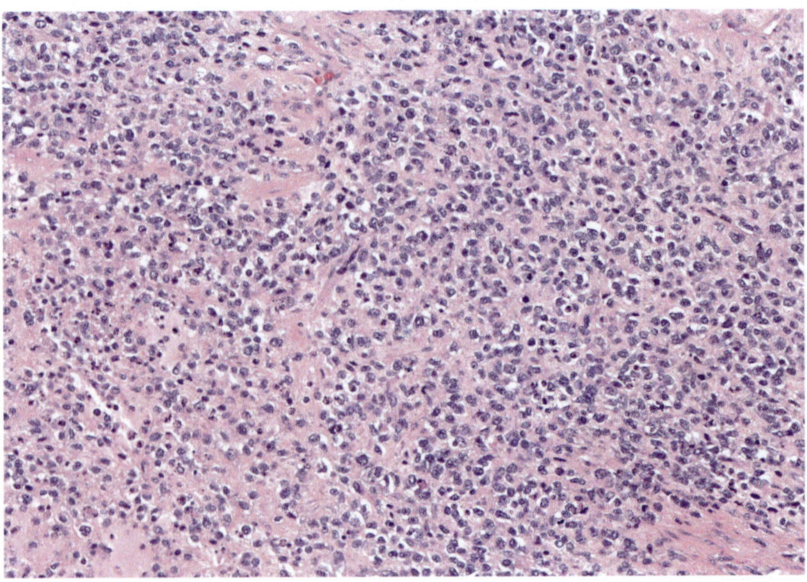

FIGURE 1.33 **Rhabdomyosarcoma with atypical large cells with little cytoplasm mimicking large cell lymphoma.**

morphology. While a clinical history will usually tip off the pathologist to confirm melanocytic differentiation, 3% to 4% of metastatic melanomas will be from an unknown primary site.[30]

Plasmacytoid urothelial carcinoma can also exhibit morphologic features that are eerily similar to plasma cells (Figures 1.34 and 1.35). While this subtype often extends along peritoneal surfaces, it can still metastasize to the lymph nodes and mimic a plasma cell neoplasm. CD138 can create further confusion as the urothelial carcinomas can be positive for this marker. Keratin markers are helpful in distinguishing this tumor from a plasma cell neoplasm.[30,40]

Tumors and Nonneoplastic Conditions With Prominent Sclerosis and Inflammation ("Sclerotic Pattern")

While this text primarily addresses tumors that can mimic a hematolymphoid neoplasm in a lymph node, it is often difficult for a pathologist or clinician to discern whether a sampled tissue is in fact a lymph node. This is particularly true in sclerosing/inflammatory conditions in which a dense fibrotic nodule in the retroperitoneum can mimic a lymph node on imaging. Such sclerosing/inflammatory processes that could morphologically mirror a hematolymphoid neoplasm include inflammatory/sclerosing variant of well-differentiated liposarcoma, IgG4-related disease, or metastatic tumor (such as seminoma) with prominent associated inflammation.

While well-differentiated liposarcoma is typically considered an "adipocytic tumor," this entity can attract such a prominent chronic

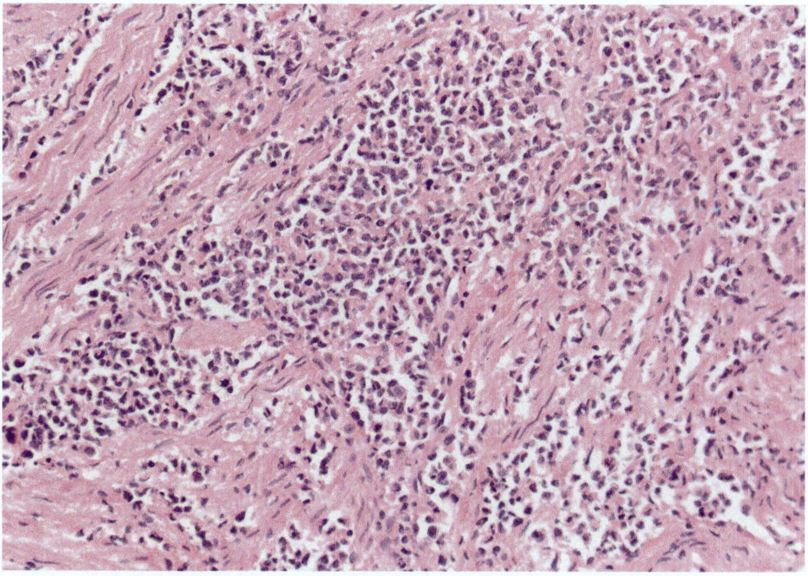

FIGURE 1.34 Plasmacytoid urothelial carcinoma exhibits a plasmacytoid morphology that mimics a lymphoma or plasma cell neoplasm.

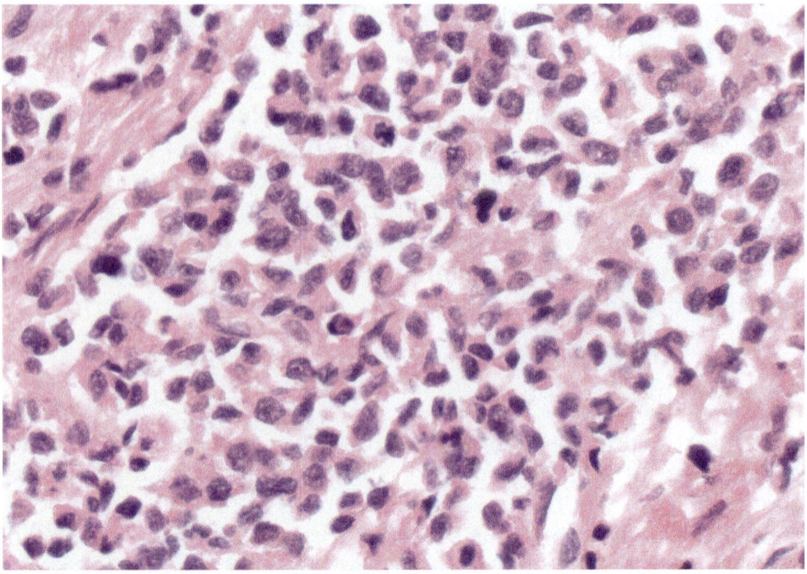

FIGURE 1.35 **Plasmacytoid urothelial carcinoma.** The tumor cells are highly discohesive and mimic plasmacytoid lymphocytes/plasma cells.

inflammatory response that it can mimic a lymph node on a needle core biopsy (Figure 1.36). Although well-differentiated liposarcoma contains atypical cells with enlarged and hyperchromatic nuclei, these cells can be obscured in the inflammatory variant. In fact, these malignant cells can sometimes exhibit features reminiscent of Hodgkin/Reed-Sternberg cells (Figure 1.37).[41,42] The lymphocytes in the liposarcoma will be predominantly small T-cell lymphocytes. Well-differentiated liposarcomas will typically show amplification of the *MDM2* gene by fluorescence in situ hybridization study, which is a necessary test to resolve this diagnostic dilemma.

IgG4-related disease includes a group of diseases that have been reported in diverse locations throughout the body. These are morphologically characterized by dense fibrosis, extensive lymphoplasmacytic inflammation and phlebitis. As this process can lead to the formation of mass-like lesions, patients are often suspected of having a malignancy.[43,44] Morphologically, this condition can mimic low-grade B-cell lymphoma. Increased IgG4 staining and an increased IgG4/IgG ratio are characteristically seen. However, correlation with clinical, laboratory, and radiologic findings is necessary for making a final diagnosis.

Tumors With Epithelioid or Anaplastic Morphology

Many of the entities previously covered, such as metastatic melanoma or carcinomas from various sites, can show epithelioid or anaplastic morphology and potentially mimic a primary hematolymphoid process. These

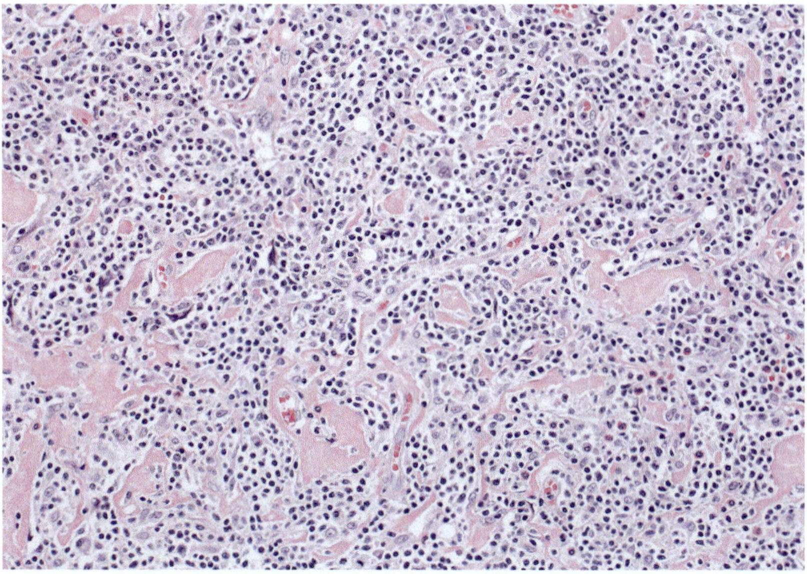

FIGURE 1.36 **Well-differentiated liposarcomas show a robust chronic inflammatory response that it can sometimes be mistaken for a lymphoma.**

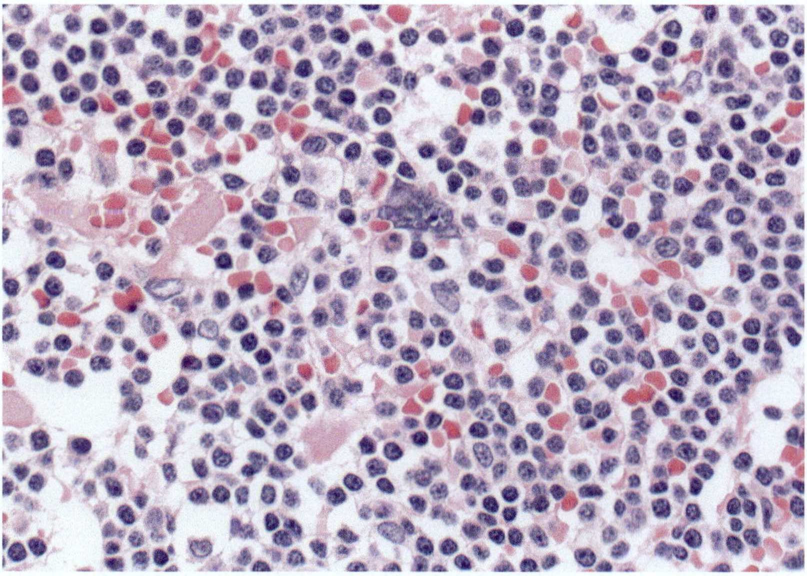

FIGURE 1.37 **Well-differentiated liposarcoma.** The multinucleated tumor cell seen in this higher-power microphotograph mimics a Reed-Sternberg cell.

are not as elusive as the appearance should prompt a pathologist to cast a wide net in determining tumor differentiation. Of note, it is important to remember that anaplastic large cell lymphoma can occasionally stain for keratin, which should not be misinterpreted as carcinoma.[11] When dealing with a metastatic tumor of unknown primary with "anaplastic" morphology, a proposed initial panel is the following: CD20, CD3, CD30, SOX10, AE1/AE3, SMA, and desmin.

REFERENCES

1. Swerdlow SH, Campo E, Harris NL, et al. *WHO Classification of Tumours of Haematopoietic and Lymphoid Tissues*. IARC; 2017.
2. Campo E, Jaffe ES, Cook JR, et al. The International Consensus Classification of Mature Lymphoid Neoplasms: a report from the Clinical Advisory Committee. *Blood*. 2022;140(11):1229-1253. doi:10.1182/blood.2022015851
3. Alaggio R, Amador C, Anagnostopoulos I, et al. The 5th edition of the World Health Organization Classification of Haematolymphoid Tumours: lymphoid neoplasms. *Leukemia*. 2022;36(7):1720-1748.
4. Medeiros LJ. *Ioachim's Lymph Node Pathology*. 5th ed. Wolters Kluwer Health; 2021.
5. Duffield AS, Venkataraman G, Song JY. *Atlas of Lymph Node Pathology. A Pattern-Based Approach*. Wolters Kluwer; 2021.
6. Tzankov A, Dirnhofer S. A pattern-based approach to reactive lymphadenopathies. *Semin Diagn Pathol*. 2018;35(1):4-19.
7. Slack GW. The pathology of reactive lymphadenopathies: a discussion of common reactive patterns and their malignant mimics. *Arch Pathol Lab Med*. 2016;140(9):881-892.
8. Mills S. *Histology for Pathologists*. 5th ed. Wolters Kluwer; 2020.
9. Willard-Mack CL. Normal structure, function, and histology of lymph nodes. *Toxicol Pathol*. 2006;34(5):409-424.
10. Gretz JE, Anderson AO, Shaw S. Cords, channels, corridors and conduits: critical architectural elements facilitating cell interactions in the lymph node cortex. *Immunol Rev*. 1997;156:11-24.
11. Jaffe ESAD, Campo E, Harris NL, Quintanilla-Martinez L. *Hematopathology*. 2nd ed. Elsevier; 2017.
12. Camacho SA, Kosco-Vilbois MH, Berek C. The dynamic structure of the germinal center. *Immunol Today*. 1998;19(11):511-514.
13. Klein U, Dalla-Favera R. Germinal centres: role in B-cell physiology and malignancy. *Nat Rev Immunol*. 2008;8(1):22-33.
14. Victora GD, Nussenzweig MC. Germinal centers. *Annu Rev Immunol*. 2012;30:429-457.
15. Pakalniskyte D, Schraml BU. Tissue-specific diversity and functions of conventional dendritic cells. *Adv Immunol*. 2017;134:89-135.
16. Kranich J, Krautler NJ. How follicular dendritic cells shape the B-cell antigenome. *Front Immunol*. 2016;7:225.
17. Ueno H, Banchereau J, Vinuesa CG. Pathophysiology of T follicular helper cells in humans and mice. *Nat Immunol*. 2015;16(2):142-152.
18. Mintz MA, Cyster JG. T follicular helper cells in germinal center B cell selection and lymphomagenesis. *Immunol Rev*. 2020;296(1):48-61.
19. Kaldjian EP, Gretz JE, Anderson AO, Shi Y, Shaw S. Spatial and molecular organization of lymph node T cell cortex: a labyrinthine cavity bounded by an epithelium-like monolayer of fibroblastic reticular cells anchored to basement membrane-like extracellular matrix. *Int Immunol*. 2001;13(10):1243-1253.

20. Swiecki M, Colonna M. The multifaceted biology of plasmacytoid dendritic cells. *Nat Rev Immunol.* 2015;15(8):471-485.
21. Mionnet C, Sanos SL, Mondor I, et al. High endothelial venules as traffic control points maintaining lymphocyte population homeostasis in lymph nodes. *Blood.* 2011;118(23):6115-6122.
22. Hu Q, Naushad H, Xie Q, Al-Howaidi I, Wang M, Fu K. Needle-core biopsy in the pathologic diagnosis of malignant lymphoma showing high reproducibility among pathologists. *Am J Clin Pathol.* 2013;140(2):238-247.
23. de Larrinoa AF, del Cura J, Zabala R, Fuertes E, Bilbao F, Lopez JI. Value of ultrasound-guided core biopsy in the diagnosis of malignant lymphoma. *J Clin Ultrasound.* 2007;35(6):295-301.
24. Nguyen BM, Halprin C, Olimpiadi Y, Traum P, Yeh JJ, Dauphine C. Core needle biopsy is a safe and accurate initial diagnostic procedure for suspected lymphoma. *Am J Surg.* 2014;208(6):1003-1008, discussion 1007-1008.
25. Cohen OC, Brodermann MH, Dervin A, et al. Lymph node core biopsies reliably permit diagnosis of lymphoproliferative diseases. Real-World Experience from 554 sequential core biopsies from a single centre. *Eur J Haematol.* 2021;106(2):267-272.
26. Wilczynski A, Gorg C, Timmesfeld N, et al. Value and diagnostic accuracy of ultrasound-guided full core needle biopsy in the diagnosis of lymphadenopathy: a retrospective evaluation of 793 cases. *J Ultrasound Med.* 2020;39(3):559-567.
27. Skelton E, Jewison A, Okpaluba C, et al. Image-guided core needle biopsy in the diagnosis of malignant lymphoma. *Eur J Surg Oncol.* 2015;41(7):852-858.
28. Ranheim EA. Pearls and pitfalls in the diagnostic workup of small lymph node biopsies. *Mod Pathol.* 2019;32(suppl 1):38-43.
29. Ronen S, Czaja RC, Ronen N, Pantazis CG, Iczkowski KA. Small cell variant of metastatic melanoma: a mimicker of lymphoblastic Leukemia/lymphoma. *Dermatopathology (Basel).* 2019;6(4):231-236.
30. Charfi S, Ellouze S, Mnif H, Amouri A, Khabir A, Sellami-Boudawara T. Plasmacytoid melanoma of the urinary bladder and lymph nodes with immunohistochemical expression of plasma cell markers revealing primary esophageal melanoma. *Case Rep Pathol.* 2012;2012:916256.
31. Ferenczi K, Lastra RR, Farkas T, et al. MUM-1 expression differentiates tumors in the PEComa family from clear cell sarcoma and melanoma. *Int J Surg Pathol.* 2012;20(1):29-36.
32. Politikos I, Sheikine Y. Small cell lung cancer mimicking high-grade lymphoma in a patient with concurrent B-cell lymphoproliferative disorder. *Blood.* 2015;126(8):1041.
33. Kanteti R, Nallasura V, Loganathan S, et al. PAX5 is expressed in small-cell lung cancer and positively regulates c-Met transcription. *Lab Invest.* 2009;89(3):301-314.
34. Kolhe R, Reid MD, Lee JR, Cohen C, Ramalingam P. Immunohistochemical expression of PAX5 and TdT by Merkel cell carcinoma and pulmonary small cell carcinoma: a potential diagnostic pitfall but useful discriminatory marker. *Int J Clin Exp Pathol.* 2013;6(2):142-147.
35. Fong Y, Coit DG, Woodruff JM, Brennan MF. Lymph node metastasis from soft tissue sarcoma in adults. Analysis of data from a prospective database of 1772 sarcoma patients. *Ann Surg.* 1993;217(1):72-77.
36. Gusho CA, Fice MP, O'Donoghue CM, Gitelis S, Blank AT. A population-based analysis of lymph node metastasis in extremity soft tissue sarcoma: an update. *J Surg Res.* 2021;262:121-129.
37. Morgenstern DA, Gibson S, Sebire NJ, Anderson J. PAX5 expression in rhabdomyosarcoma. *Am J Surg Pathol.* 2009;33(10):1575-1577.
38. Folpe AL, Schmidt RA, Chapman D, Gown AM. Poorly differentiated synovial sarcoma: immunohistochemical distinction from primitive neuroectodermal tumors and high-grade malignant peripheral nerve sheath tumors. *Am J Surg Pathol.* 1998;22(6):673-682.

39. Baranov E, McBride MJ, Bellizzi AM, et al. A novel SS18-SSX fusion-specific Antibody for the diagnosis of synovial sarcoma. *Am J Surg Pathol.* 2020;44(7):922-933.
40. Lopez-Beltran A, Requena MJ, Montironi R, Blanca A, Cheng L. Plasmacytoid urothelial carcinoma of the bladder. *Hum Pathol.* 2009;40(7):1023-1028.
41. Kraus MD, Guillou L, Fletcher CDM. Well-differentiated inflammatory liposarcoma: an uncommon and easily overlooked variant of a common sarcoma. *Am J Surg Pathol.* 1997;21(5):518-527.
42. Lim CS, Cooper CL, Delprado W, Kench J, McCarthy SW, Scolyer RA. Retroperitoneal inflammatory liposarcoma in a patient with non-Hodgkin lymphoma: a report highlighting diagnostic pitfalls. *Pathol Res Int.* 2010;2010:505436.
43. Liu Y, Xue F, Yang J, Zhang Y. Immunoglobulin G4-related disease mimicking lymphoma in a Chinese patient. *Rheumatol Int.* 2015;35(10):1749-1752.
44. Noh D, Park CK, Kwon SY. Immunoglobulin G4-related sclerosing disease invading the trachea and superior vena cava in mediastinum. *Eur J Cardiothorac Surg.* 2014;45(3):573-575.

2

DIAGNOSTIC METHODS AND ANCILLARY STUDIES

DANIEL S. MARTIG and REBECCA L. KING

PROCESSING OF THE LYMPH NODE BIOPSY SPECIMEN

One of the most important aspects to achieving the correct diagnosis is to obtain a sufficient quantity of tissue in the lymph node biopsy and to process the tissue in an optimal manner to allow for necessary studies to be performed.[1,2] Tissue should be sent fresh to pathology for optimal specimen management as this allows for appropriate triage and processing.[1] It is critical to understand the clinical situation and the question being interrogated, as the approach to processing the lymph node biopsy will vary greatly depending on what is being evaluated (Figure 2.1). From Chapter 1, ideal clinical information to have at the time of triage includes:

- Age and gender
- Sites of involvement (nodal or extranodal)
- If lymphadenopathy is present (if so, localized vs diffuse)
- Previous hematologic diseases
- History of autoimmunity
- History of primary or secondary immunosuppression (eg, HIV status, organ transplantation, immunomodulatory drugs)
- Complete blood count in some cases

If metastatic malignancy involving the lymph node is the specific clinical concern, a frozen section of the lymph node biopsy may be appropriate if it will change operative management at the time of the biopsy. Otherwise, frozen section has limited utility and should generally be discouraged, as it usually decreases the quality of permanent hematoxylin and eosin (H&E) sections. Depending on the situation, touch preparations can be made, and tissue can be divided for formalin fixation, flow cytometry (RPMI solution), cytogenetic studies, and potential snap freezing for molecular studies. If an infectious etiology is suspected,

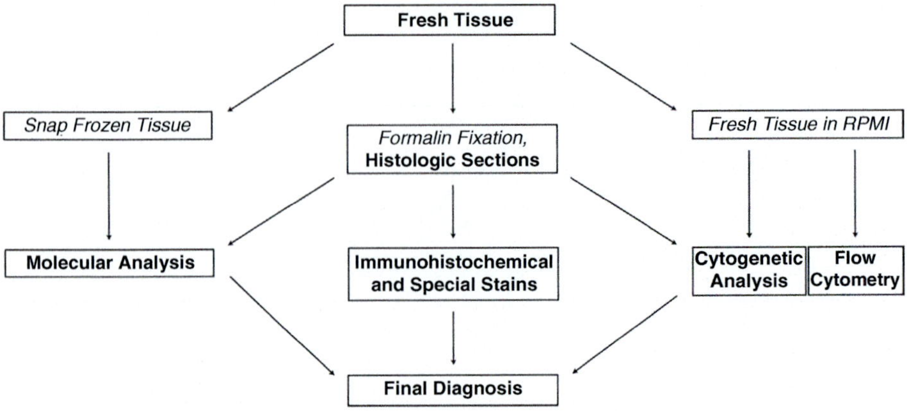

FIGURE 2.1 Flow chart for triaging a fresh lymph node biopsy.

a separate sample submitted in a sterile container directly to microbiology is recommended to prevent cross contamination in the gross room. A discussion with the oncologist and/or surgeon before or during biopsy procurement may be appropriate as certain steps (eg, sterile containers for microbiological studies) should be completed before the biopsy reaches the gross room. Importantly, histologic examination should take precedence if tissue is limited.

While there are several fixatives available, 10% neutral buffered formalin is widely available and is an appropriate fixative for the vast majority of studies needed for diagnosis on a lymph node biopsy. It is recommended that even small biopsies fix for at least 4 to 8 hours to ensure the quality of H&E histology.[1] Fixation should not exceed 24 hours though, as overfixation can result in interference with immunohistochemical stains and decreased yield if DNA or RNA extraction is attempted.[3-5] For routine H&E sections, the optimal thickness is 3 to 4 µm, which results in the most detailed cellular morphology.[6]

SPECIAL STAINS

One important special study that is useful in reactive and neoplastic lymph node settings is evaluating for Epstein-Barr virus (EBV). This is commonly accomplished by in situ hybridization (ISH) using a commercially available probe that assesses for the presence of EBV-encoded RNA (EBER) transcripts.[7] This study is important for reactive cases (ie, EBV lymphadenitis) and for a wide spectrum of lymphoproliferative disorders, such as EBV-positive lymphomas and posttransplant lymphoproliferative disorders. EBER-ISH (with appropriately staining positive and negative control slides) is the gold standard when evaluating for the presence of EBV as it captures all latency states of the virus.[8]

In addition, several special stains for infectious organisms are available, such as acid-fast bacteria stains for acid-fast organisms; periodic acid–Schiff, Fontana-Masson, or Grocott methenamine silver stains for fungal organisms; and Warthin-Starry stain and Brown and Brenn/Gram stain for other bacterial organisms. However, if there is strong consideration for an infectious cause, a separate specimen collected in a sterile container for culture is recommended for best evaluation for infectious organisms, especially if mycobacterial or fungal infection is suspected.[9,10]

Congo red staining can be performed on lymph node biopsies to assess for amyloid in the appropriate clinical setting. Other special stains (ie, Verhoeff-Van Gieson for elastic fibers, trichrome, reticulin) are of limited utility in the lymph node biopsy.

IMMUNOHISTOCHEMISTRY

Immunohistochemistry (IHC) is a powerful tool when interrogating lymph node specimens. IHC stains are typically done in panels to demonstrate a specific immunophenotype for an abnormal cell population. Suggestions for IHC panels are further described in later chapters, but a comprehensive IHC list with associated neoplastic hematologic entities is shown in Table 2.1. In addition, several IHC stains for microorganisms, including cytomegalovirus, Epstein-Barr virus, herpes simplex virus, *Treponema pallidum*, and varicella-zoster virus, are available.

FLOW CYTOMETRIC ANALYSIS

Flow cytometry is a critical tool for assessing the immunophenotype of cell populations. Since cells are queried singly during flow cytometric analysis, the methodology allows for simultaneous assessment of multiple surface or cytoplasmic markers for each cell as it passes through the flow cytometer. This allows for development of panels of multiple markers to determine if the sample is involved by an abnormal population.

As with any ancillary study, the morphologic assessment of the tissue sample should determine if flow cytometry is an appropriate analysis to perform. Laboratories generally develop B-cell, T-cell, and acute leukemia panels. However, correlation with morphologic findings should drive the decision of whether or not to perform flow cytometry. For example, while it is possible for some reference laboratories to assess for lymphomas with scattered neoplastic cells such as classic Hodgkin lymphoma,[21] this diagnosis can be made using morphology and an appropriate IHC panel. Thus, flow cytometry is generally not necessary for routine diagnosis of classic Hodgkin lymphoma.

For B-cell lymphomas, flow cytometry is often a principal methodology for demonstrating light chain restriction and an abnormal B-cell immunophenotype (Figure 2.2). Recently, the discovery of TRBC1 as a reliable indicator of T-cell clonality by flow cytometry[22,23] is significant as it

TABLE 2.1 Comprehensive List of IHC Stains Used in Assessment of Lymph Nodes

Marker	Comments	Associated Entities
CD2, CD3, CD7	Pan-T-cell markers	T-cell lymphomas
CD4, CD8	Helper and cytotoxic T-cell subsets, respectively	T-cell lymphomas
CD5	T-cell marker, aberrant CD5 expression in CLL/SLL, MCL, and subset of MZL, rarely positive in LPL and DLBCL[11]	B-cell lymphomas and T-cell lymphomas
CD19, CD20, CD22, CD79a, PAX5	B-cell markers	B-cell lymphomas
CD10	Germinal center marker, also expressed by follicular helper T cells and immature neoplasms	FL, DLBCL, T-cell lymphomas, immature B- and T-lymphoid neoplasms, and rare cases of LPL and HCL
CD11c*, CD25, CD103, CD123		B-cell lymphomas *CD11c also stains some myeloid and histiocytic neoplasms
CD15	Granulocytes and monocytes, activated B and T cells	CHL
CD21, CD23, CD35	Dendritic cell markers	Nonspecific, highlights follicular dendritic cell meshworks, CD21 most sensitive in AITL[12]
CD30	Activation marker	CHL, ALCL, DLBCL
CD43	T-cell marker	Aberrantly expressed in some B-cell lymphomas such as MZL, MCL, and CLL/SLL
CD45	General hematolymphoid marker	Nonspecific marker; notably absent in CHL
CD56	T/NK-cell marker	Expressed by some T-cell lymphomas, NK cell lymphomas, and some PCN
CD68	Histiocyte marker	Histiocytic neoplasms
CD163	More specific histiocytic marker	Histiocytic neoplasms
CD207 (Langerin), CD1a	Langerhans cell markers	Langerhans cell histiocytosis

TABLE 2.1 Comprehensive List of IHC Stains Used in Assessment of Lymph Nodes (Continued)

Marker	Comments	Associated Entities
Annexin A1	Most specific for HCL	HCL
BCL1 (cyclin D1)	Can show weak background staining in histiocytes and endothelial cells	HCL, MCL, PCN
BCL2	Nongerminal center B cells and T cells	FL, DLBCL
BCL6, LMO2*, GCET	Germinal center markers	FL *LMO2 also seen in immature T-cell neoplasms[13]
BRAF V600E	Positive when a BRAF V600E mutation is present	HCL, histiocytic neoplasms
IgD	Highlights mantle zone B cells	Nonspecific
IgM		B-cell lymphomas, LPL
IgG, IgG4		PCN, MZL, IgG4-related disease
IRTA1, MNDA*	Cell surface markers	MZL *MNDA particularly helpful when differential is FL vs MZL[14,15]
Kappa and lambda	Light chain restriction	B-cell lymphomas and PCN
LEF1	T cells, can be aberrantly expressed on B cells	CLL/SLL
Lysozyme	Positive in histiocytes, monocytes, and neutrophils	Myeloid neoplasms and histiocytic neoplasms
MAL, PD-L2 (CD273), CD23		PMBL[16-18]
MPO	Myeloid marker	Myeloid neoplasms and expressed in histiocytes of Kikuchi-Fujimoto disease
MUM1	Post–germinal center marker	DLBCL, strong expression in Hodgkin/Reed-Sternberg cells of CHL
OCT2*, BOB1	B-cell markers, stronger in germinal centers	NLPBL and CHL *Strong expression of OCT2 by LP cells of NLPBL; loss in CHL[11]

(Continued)

TABLE 2.1 **Comprehensive List of IHC Stains Used in Assessment of Lymph Nodes (Continued)**

Marker	Comments	Associated Entities
p53	Tumor suppressor	Nonspecific
p63	Tumor suppressor	ALCL
SOX11	Transcription factor	MCL, including cyclin D1-negative MCL
TCR beta F1/TCR delta	T-cell subsets	T-cell lymphomas
TdT	Immature cells	Lymphoblasts, can be seen aberrantly in high-grade lymphomas[19,20]
TIA1, granzyme B	Cytotoxic markers	T-cell lymphomas

AITL, angioimmunoblastic T-cell lymphoma; ALCL, anaplastic large cell lymphoma; CHL, classic Hodgkin lymphoma; CLL/SLL, chronic lymphocytic leukemia/small lymphocytic lymphoma; DLBCL, diffuse large B-cell lymphoma; FL, follicular lymphoma; HCL, hairy cell leukemia; LPL, lymphoplasmacytic lymphoma; MCL, mantle cell lymphoma; MZL, marginal zone lymphoma; NLPBL, nodular lymphocyte predominant B-cell lymphoma; PCN, plasma cell neoplasm; PMBL, primary mediastinal large B-cell lymphoma.

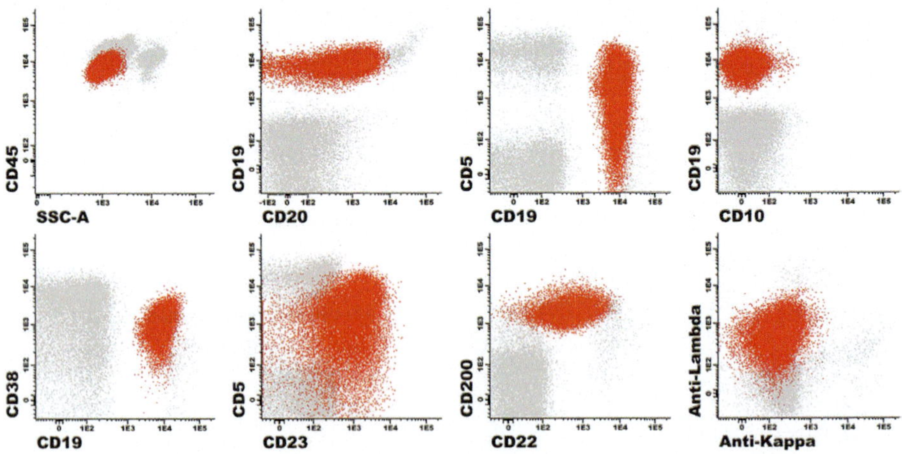

FIGURE 2.2 B-cell flow cytometry panel demonstrating an abnormal B-cell population with chronic lymphocytic leukemia/small lymphocytic lymphoma-like phenotype.

allows for a more definitive assessment of T cells, in addition to assessment for an abnormal T-cell phenotype.

Flow cytometry is a very sensitive method, and caution in interpretation of results is advised since small clonal populations can be detected in reactive settings.[24,25] As with all ancillary studies, flow cytometry results should always be interpreted in correlation with the morphologic impression. In addition, while B- and T-cell lymphomas make up the majority of lymph node flow cytometric analyses, immature lymphoid and myeloid neoplasms are known to involve tissue sites as well, and flow cytometry is often very helpful in characterizing immature-appearing/blastoid cells.

FISH AND OTHER CYTOGENETIC ANALYSES

Fluorescence in situ hybridization (FISH) is a method that allows for investigation of specific chromosomal abnormalities. As highlighted in its name, FISH employs fluorescent DNA probes that are complementary to a target DNA sequence that includes a chromosomal abnormality of interest.[26] If a chromosomal abnormality is present, the fluorescent probe can hybridize to the target DNA sequence, which allows for visualization of the specific abnormality. FISH can be performed on metaphase or interphase chromosomes. FISH studies can be performed on fresh or formalin-fixed, paraffin-embedded (FFPE) tissue. The most common approaches are dual-color, dual-fusion (DC/DF) and breakapart probes (BAP). DC/DF FISH is that in which two gene regions are colored with different probes (usually red and green) and a fusion (yellow) signal is formed if the regions colocalize in a rearrangement. BAP FISH involves probes in two colors (red and green) placed on either side of a gene breakpoint. If there is a rearrangement involving that gene the signal pattern goes from two normal fusions (yellow) to one fusion and one each of red and green signals (Figure 2.3).

Array comparative genomic hybridization or array CGH (aCGH) is a useful tool for identifying unbalanced chromosomal abnormalities, which result in a net gain or loss of genetic material.[27] This method uses patient DNA and control DNA, which are differentially labeled with fluorescent dyes. A microarray is employed, which contains small target sequences of DNA arranged in an organized way. Both the patient and control DNA

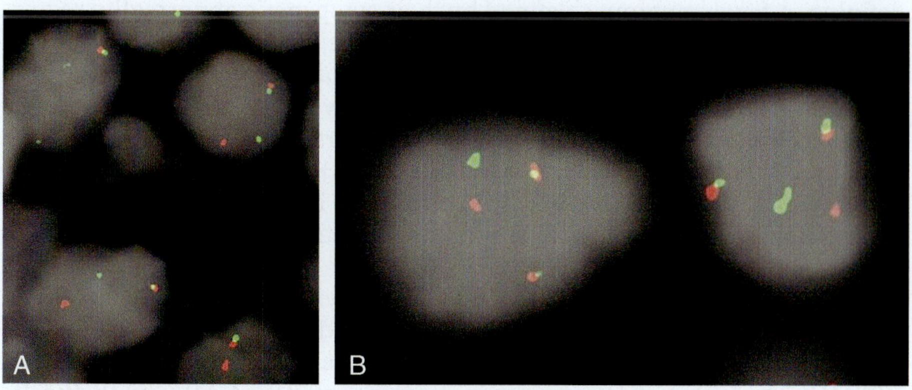

FIGURE 2.3 Examples of (A) breakapart probe FISH showing a broken MYC signal and (B) positive dual-color, dual-fusion showing a MYC-IGH translocation.

are applied to the microarray, and the relative intensity of fluorescence is captured by a digital imaging system. Using the control DNA as a normal reference, the patient DNA can again be assessed for increase or decrease in genetic material at different positions along the genome. aCGH can be done on fresh or FFPE tissue.

An exhaustive list of lymphomas with recurrent cytogenetic abnormalities is beyond the scope of this chapter. Below are a few examples of diseases in which cytogenetic studies can be useful in the diagnostic workup. Other examples are discussed in the corresponding chapters.

Small B-cell Lymphomas

Many small B-cell lymphomas have well-known, recurrent cytogenetic abnormalities. The vast majority of mantle cell lymphomas (>95%) demonstrate a translocation between *CCND1* (cyclin D1) and an IGH gene (t(11;14)(q13;q32)).[11] This abnormality can be queried if needed by using a DC/DF *CCND1*-IGH probe set, although this is rarely needed if a cyclin D1 immunohistochemical stain can be performed. Meanwhile, follicular lymphoma is associated with a translocation between *BCL2* and IGH genes (t(14;18)(q32;q21)).[11] Either a DC/DF probe set or a *BCL2* BAP probe can be used. Chronic lymphocytic leukemia/small lymphocytic lymphoma (CLL/SLL) does not have any specific genetic markers, but the vast majority of cases demonstrate a cytogenetic abnormality by FISH or copy-number arrays. The most common aberration present is deletion 13q14.3, which is present in ~50% of cases, and is followed by trisomy 12 or partial trisomy 12q13, present in ~20% of cases. Lower-frequency abnormalities include deletion in 11q22-23, 17p13, or 6q21.[11] Panels of probes assessing these abnormalities are commonly performed for prognosis in CLL/SLL.

Large/High-grade B-cell Lymphomas

For large and high-grade B-cell lymphomas, there are a variety of structural chromosomal abnormalities, which for the most part are not diagnosis defining. A few lymphomas defined by their cytogenetic abnormality require FISH for appropriate classification. In the majority of cases these FISH studies can be done on FFPE. High-grade and large B-cell lymphomas that demonstrate a *MYC* translocation and also show *BCL2* or *BCL6* rearrangement meet criteria for the diagnosis of "high-grade B-cell lymphoma with *MYC* and *BCL2* rearrangement" or "high-grade B-cell lymphoma with *BCL6* rearrangement" (ie, "double-hit" and "triple-hit" lymphomas), which tend to be aggressive.[11,28] FISH studies should be prioritized on a limited biopsy as rearrangement status may affect the treatment approach. *MYC* BAP and *MYC*-IGH DC/DF are often performed along with *BCL2* and *BCL6* BAPs. *MYC* rearrangement status also is critical if Burkitt lymphoma (BL) is in the differential. The common abnormality in BL is a *MYC*-IGH rearrangement (t(8;14)(q24;q32)), but less common rearrangements of *MYC* with the IG kappa (t(2;8)) or lambda locus (t(8;22)) can occur.[11]

Other cytogenetic considerations for large B-cell lymphomas include *IRF4*- rearrangement status (assessed by *IRF4* BAP) when considering the diagnosis of large B-cell lymphoma with *IRF4* 6p25.3 rearrangement, and *ALK* translocation status (assessed by *ALK* BAP) in challenging cases of ALK-positive large B-cell lymphoma if the IHC is equivocal.

T-cell Lymphomas

T-cell prolymphocytic leukemia (T-PLL) is a neoplasm characterized by inversion of chromosome 14 (inv(14)(q11q32)) in the majority of cases (80%), with an additional 10% harboring a t(14;14)(q11;q32) abnormality.[11] These involve the *TCL1A* and TRAD loci. A smaller subset of cases harbor a t(X;14)(q28;q11) translocation involving *MTCP1*.

FISH for *ALK* translocation can be performed in cases of ALK-positive anaplastic large-cell lymphoma, but it is not mandatory for correct diagnosis provided the ALK stain is positive. In addition, *DUSP22* and *TP63* assays are important prognostic tests in cases of ALK-negative anaplastic large cell lymphoma.[29]

MOLECULAR ANALYSIS

Infectious Agents

Given that separate samples are frequently collected for microbiological studies if an infectious cause is suspected and immunohistochemical stains are available for several infectious organisms, the instances in which infectious disease molecular testing on FFPE is required for a lymph node biopsy diagnosis are limited.

One notable exception is polymerase chain reaction (PCR) testing for *Bartonella henselae* in suspected cases of cat-scratch disease (CSD). Microbiological cultures for *B. henselae* are generally not reliable as the organism is quite fastidious and slow growing, which may make identification difficult in routine laboratory settings.[30] While serological testing is widely available for detecting the organism, the results may be unavailable to the pathologist; thus, PCR testing on FFPE can be pursued given the correct morphological pattern for CSD. PCR testing has somewhat low reported sensitivity (43%-76%), but very high specificity (100%), and a positive test provides a definitive result to aid in the correct diagnosis.[31,32]

In very limited settings, broad-range PCR and next-generation molecular microbiological analysis to query numerous microbes on a single sample can be considered in the correct clinical setting. A discussion with the clinical team prior to biopsy is prudent in these situations to ensure proper and timely handling of the specimen in order to maximize the chance of proper study. While these tests are possible from FFPE tissue, fresh tissue is preferable.

Immunoglobulin/T-cell Receptor Gene Rearrangements

Clonality studies for immunoglobulin (B-cell) or T-cell receptor (T-cell) gene rearrangements can be powerful tools allowing one to prove a clonal origin of an abnormal population. DNA is extracted from fresh, frozen, or paraffin-embedded tissue and multiplex PCRs to multiple immunoglobulin (IG kappa, IG lambda, and IG heavy chain) or T-cell receptor (TCR beta, TCR gamma, and TCR delta) targets are analyzed. Each amplified locus is assessed for gene rearrangement patterns, which allows for determination of clonality (Figures 2.4 and 2.5). Methods such as the BIOMED-2 (EuroClonality) strategy have been thoroughly substantiated and allow for standardized protocols and interpretation of clonality.[33]

These studies can be performed in addition to flow cytometric analysis, or without it if no fresh tissue is available. Without a morphologic correlate, it is not advisable to make a diagnosis of lymphoma as prior studies have shown that identifying a morphologic correlate is key even if a clonality study is positive.[34]

Molecular assays to query single gene mutations can be powerful tools in several different lymph node entities. DNA is extracted from the neoplastic cell population, and primers that allow for detection of the

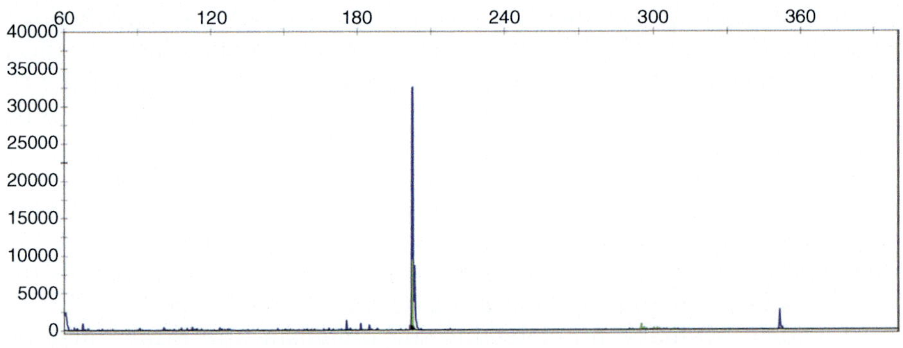

FIGURE 2.4 Example of positive T-cell receptor gene rearrangement study.

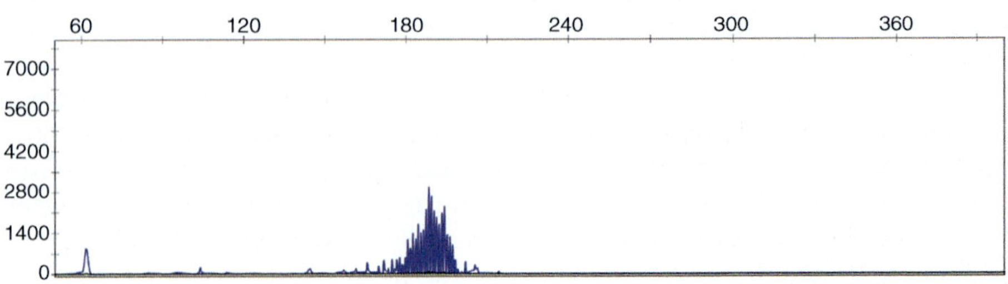

FIGURE 2.5 Example of negative T-cell receptor gene rearrangement study.

specific genetic aberration are used in a PCR reaction. These tests can be performed on FFPE or fresh/frozen tissue. Notably, *MYD88* mutations are present in approximately 90% of cases of lymphoplasmacytic lymphoma (LPL).[35] This can be a helpful confirmatory test, although *MYD88* is not strictly specific for LPL. In addition, *BRAF* V600E mutations are detectable in essentially all cases of hairy cell leukemia and are also observed frequently in histiocytic neoplasms such as Langerhans cell histiocytosis.[36] *BRAF* V600E is the therapeutic target for vemurafenib, a recently approved inhibitor chemotherapy agent; thus, this mutation may be important to demonstrate in some cases.

Lymphoid Next-generation Sequencing Assays

Continuous advances in sequencing technologies including lower costs of equipment and reagents, as well as more accurate and efficient analytical software tools, have allowed for increased clinical use of next-generation sequencing (NGS) assays.[37] Regarding NGS for lymphomas, more literature outlining the genetic profiles of both B-cell and T-cell lymphomas is emerging,[38,39] but the utility of NGS lymphoma panels has yet to be established as a standard of care in routine clinical settings. However, evidence is gathering NGS may be a powerful tool in the future. As an example, a recent study investigating lymphoid NGS in low-grade lymphoproliferative disorders demonstrated that NGS was able to help resolve the diagnosis in greater than 60% of challenging cases after a standard workup.[40] Proponents of this technology believe its implementation is on the horizon and will likely become a cornerstone for lymphoma classification, stratification, and targetable biomarker identification.

REFERENCES

1. Loo E, Siddiqi IN. Processing the lymph node biopsy. In: Day CE, ed. *Histopathology: Methods and Protocols, Methods in Molecular Biology*. Vol 1180. Humana Press; 2014:271-282.
2. Warnke RA, Rouse RV. Limitations encountered in the application of tissue section immunodiagnosis to the study of lymphomas and related disorders. *Hum Pathol.* 1985;16(4):326-331. PMID: 2579887.
3. Greer CE, Lund JK, Manos MM. PCR amplification from paraffin-embedded tissues: recommendations on fixatives for long-term storage and prospective studies. *PCR Methods Appl.* 1991;1(1):46-50. PMID: 1842921.
4. Greer CE, Wheeler CM, Manos MM. Sample preparation and PCR amplification from paraffin-embedded tissues. *PCR Methods Appl.* 1994;3(6):S113-S122. PMID: 7920232.
5. Greer CE, Peterson SL, Kiviat NB, et al. PCR amplification from paraffin-embedded tissues. Effects of fixative and fixation time. *Am J Clin Pathol.* 1991;95(2):117-124. PMID: 1846996.
6. Beard C, Nabers K, Bowling MC, et al. Achieving technical excellence in lymph node specimens: an update. *Lab Med.* 1985;16(8):468-475.
7. Loughrey M, Trivett M, Lade S, et al. Diagnostic application of Epstein-Barr virus-encoded RNA in situ hybridisation. *Pathology.* 2004;36(4):301-308. PMID: 15370127.

8. Herbert KM, Pimienta G. Consideration of Epstein-Barr virus-encoded noncoding RNAs EBER1 and EBER2 as a functional backup of viral oncoprotein latent membrane protein 1. *mBio*. 2016;7(1):e01926-e02015. PMID: 26787829.
9. Roberts FJ, Linsey S. The value of microbial cultures in diagnostic lymph-node biopsy. *J Infect Dis*. 1984;149(2):162-165. PMID: 6199435.
10. Freidig EE, McClure SP, Wilson WR, et al. Clinical-histologic-microbiologic analysis of 419 lymph node biopsy specimens. *Rev Infect Dis*. 1986;8(3):322-328. PMID: 3726392.
11. Swerdlow SH, Campo E, Harris NL, et al, eds. *WHO Classification of Tumours of Haematopoietic and Lymphoid Tissues*: IARC; 2017.
12. Troxell ML, Schwartz EJ, van de Rijn M, et al. Follicular dendritic cell immunohistochemical markers in angioimmunoblastic T-cell lymphoma. *Appl Immunohistochem Mol Morphol*. 2005;13(4):297-303. PMID: 16280657.
13. Jevremovic D, Roden AC, Ketterling RP, et al. LMO2 is a specific marker of T-lymphoblastic leukemia/lymphoma. *Am J Clin Pathol*. 2016;145(2):180-190. PMID: 26796495.
14. Kanellis G, Roncador G, Arribas A, et al. Identification of MNDA as a new marker for nodal marginal zone lymphoma. *Leukemia*. 2009;23(10):1847-1857. PMID: 19474799.
15. Wang Z, Cook JR. IRTA1 and MNDA expression in marginal zone lymphoma: utility in differential diagnosis and implications for classification. *Am J Clin Pathol*. 2019;151(3):337-343. PMID: 30346478.
16. Pileri SA, Gaidano G, Zinzani PL, et al. Primary mediastinal B-cell lymphoma: high frequency of BCL-6 mutations and consistent expression of the transcription factors OCT-2, BOB.1, and PU.1 in the absence of immunoglobulins. *Am J Pathol*. 2003;162(1):243-253. PMID: 12507907.
17. Jacquier A, Syrykh C, Bedgedjian I, et al. Immunohistochemistry with anti-MAL antibody and RNAscope with MAL probes are complementary techniques for diagnosis of primary mediastinal large B-cell lymphoma. *J Clin Pathol*. 2020;74(6):396-399. PMID: 32839159.
18. Bledsoe JR, Redd RA, Hasserjian RP, et al. The immunophenotypic spectrum of primary mediastinal large B-cell lymphoma reveals prognostic biomarkers associated with outcome. *Am J Hematol*. 2016;91(10):E436-E441. PMID: 27419920.
19. Moench L, Sachs Z, Aasen G, et al. Double- and triple-hit lymphomas can present with features suggestive of immaturity, including TdT expression, and create diagnostic challenges. *Leuk Lymphoma*. 2016;57(11):2626-2635. PMID: 26892631.
20. Ok CY, Medeiros LJ, Thakral B, et al. High-grade B-cell lymphomas with TdT expression: a diagnostic and classification dilemma. *Mod Pathol*. 2019;32(1):48-58. PMID: 30181564.
21. Martig DS, Fromm JR. A comparison and review of the flow cytometric findings in classic Hodgkin lymphoma, nodular lymphocyte predominant Hodgkin lymphoma, T cell/histiocyte rich large B cell lymphoma, and primary mediastinal large B cell lymphoma. *Cytometry B Clin Cytom*. 2022;102(1):14-25. PMID: 34878224.
22. Horna P, Shi M, Olteanu H, et al. Emerging role of T-cell receptor constant β chain-1 (TRBC1) expression in the flow cytometric diagnosis of T-cell malignancies. *Int J Mol Sci*. 2021;22(4):1817. PMID: 33673033.
23. Shi M, Jevremovic D, Otteson GE, et al. Single antibody detection of T-cell receptor αβ clonality by flow cytometry rapidly identifies mature T-cell neoplasms and monotypic small CD8-positive subsets of uncertain significance. *Cytometry B Clin Cytom*. 2020;98(1):99-107. PMID: 30972977.
24. Cozzolino I, Nappa S, Picardi M, et al. Clonal B-cell population in a reactive lymph node in acquired immunodeficiency syndrome. *Diagn Cytopathol*. 2009;37(12):910-914. PMID: 19582804.

25. Kussick SJ, Kalnoski M, Braziel RM, et al. Prominent clonal B-cell populations identified by flow cytometry in histologically reactive lymphoid proliferations. *Am J Clin Pathol.* 2004;121(4):464-472. PMID: 15080297.
26. O'Connor C. Fluorescence in situ hybridization (FISH). *Nature Education.* 2008;1(1):171. Accessed March 14, 2022. https://www.nature.com/scitable/topicpage/fluorescence-in-situ-hybridization-fish-327/
27. Theisen A. Microarray-based comparative genomic hybridization (aCGH). *Nature Education.* 2008;1(1):45. Accessed March 14, 2022. https://www.nature.com/scitable/topicpage/microarray-based-comparative-genomic-hybridization-acgh-45432/
28. Campo E, Jaffe ES, Cook JR, et al. The International Consensus Classification of Mature Lymphoid Neoplasms: a report from the Clinical Advisory Committee. *Blood.* 2022;40(11):1229-1253. doi:10.1182/blood.2022015851
29. Pedersen MB, Hamilton-Dutoit SJ, Bendix K, et al. DUSP22 and TP63 rearrangements predict outcome of ALK-negative anaplastic large cell lymphoma: a Danish Cohort Study. *Blood.* 2017;130(4):554-557. PMID: 28522440.
30. Lamps LW, Scott MA. Cat-scratch disease: historic, clinical, and pathologic perspectives. *Am J Clin Pathol.* 2004;121 suppl:S71-S80. PMID: 15298152.
31. Shin OR, Kim YR, Ban TH, et al. A case report of seronegative cat scratch disease, emphasizing the histopathologic point of view. *Diagn Pathol.* 2014;9:62. PMID: 24641870.
32. Hansmann Y, DeMartino S, Piémont Y, et al. Diagnosis of cat scratch disease with detection of Bartonella henselae by PCR: a study of patients with lymph node enlargement. *J Clin Microbiol.* 2005;43(8):3800-3806. PMID: 16081914.
33. Langerak AW, Groenen PJ, Brüggemann M, et al. EuroClonality/BIOMED-2 guidelines for interpretation and reporting of Ig/TCR clonality testing in suspected lymphoproliferations. *Leukemia.* 2012;26(10):2159-2171. PMID: 22918122.
34. Mendoza H, Tormey CA, Siddon AJ. Evaluation of positive B- and T-cell gene rearrangement studies in patients with negative morphology, flow cytometry, and Immunohistochemistry. *Arch Pathol Lab Med.* 2021;145(2):227-230. PMID: 32886749.
35. Yu X, Li W, Deng Q, et al. MYD88 L265P mutation in lymphoid malignancies. *Cancer Res.* 2018;78(10):2457-2462. PMID: 29703722.
36. Loo E, Khalili P, Beuhler K, et al. BRAF V600E mutation across multiple tumor types: correlation between DNA-based sequencing and mutation-specific immunohistochemistry. *Appl Immunohistochem Mol Morphol.* 2018;26(10):709-713. PMID: 29271794.
37. Ohgami RS, Rosenwald A, Bagg A. Next-generation sequencing for lymphomas: perfecting a pipeline for personalized pathobiologic and prognostic predictions. *J Mol Diagn.* 2018;20(2):163-165. PMID: 29355824.
38. Bogusz AM, Bagg A. Genetic aberrations in small B-cell lymphomas and leukemias: molecular pathology, clinical relevance and therapeutic targets. *Leuk Lymphoma.* 2016;57(9):1991-2013. PMID: 27121112.
39. Sandell RF, Boddicker RL, Feldman AL. Genetic landscape and classification of peripheral T cell lymphomas. *Curr Oncol Rep.* 2017;19(4):28. PMID: 28303495.
40. Jajosky AN, Havens NP, Sadri N, et al. Clinical utility of targeted next-generation sequencing in the evaluation of low-grade lymphoproliferative disorders. *Am J Clin Pathol.* 2021;156(3):433-444. PMID: 33712839.

3

BENIGN DISEASES INVOLVING LYMPH NODE

LAUREN B. SMITH and ANNA B. OWCZARCZYK

One of the most important jobs for the pathologist is to differentiate between benign and neoplastic conditions. Once that has been accomplished, it may be possible to formulate a diagnosis based on the morphologic findings in benign cases. Diagnosing benign entities is challenging on a small biopsy, since the lymph node architecture is frequently difficult to appreciate, and characteristic findings may not have been sampled. If some of the suggestive features are seen, a larger biopsy and/or additional laboratory studies, such as cultures and serologies, or in some cases universal polymerase chain reaction (PCR), could be performed to help confirm the possible etiologic agent.

FOLLICULAR AND PARACORTICAL HYPERPLASIA

Lymph nodes that become enlarged may show either follicular hyperplasia (FH), paracortical hyperplasia (PCH), or frequently a combination of both. The etiology of lymphoid hyperplasia is often unknown, but it may be secondary to bacterial infections, viruses, autoimmune diseases, drugs, or other conditions. Florid follicular hyperplasia (FFH) is less common in adults but is frequently seen in children with viral or bacterial infections. In adult patients with FFH, human immunodeficiency virus (HIV) infection should be considered.

FH is defined as an increased number of lymphoid follicles containing germinal centers. These follicles may be closely spaced, of variable size and shape, and often have germinal centers containing tingible body macrophages. Polarization of the follicles with dark and light zones, and distinct mantle zones, is typically evident. In FFH, the follicles may be so closely spaced that the germinal centers obscure the mantle zones (Figure 3.1). It is important on small biopsies not to mistake FFH for diffuse large B-cell lymphoma (DLBCL) or Burkitt lymphoma. In FFH, CD20 and CD3 will demonstrate nodularity, and Bcl-2 will be negative in the germinal center

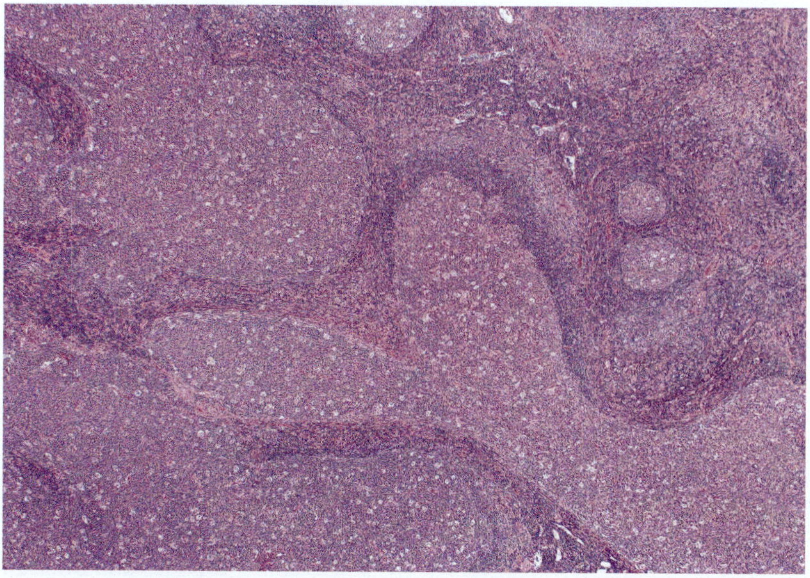

FIGURE 3.1 **Florid follicular hyperplasia.** Expanded follicles of varying size and shape, often seen in children with viral infections.

B cells. Furthermore, CD21 will highlight dense, intact follicular dendritic cell meshworks in the follicles. Reactive follicles must be distinguished from the neoplastic follicles of follicular lymphoma (FL). Table 3.1 summarizes the main differences in pathologic features between FH and FL. On a core biopsy, it can be very difficult to differentiate between FH and Bcl-2-negative FL. Recognizing abnormal follicles on hematoxylin & eosin (H&E)-stained sections becomes of paramount importance, as it is often possible to discern whether the follicle has reactive features. If the follicle is composed of homogeneous small centrocytes, it is unlikely to be reactive; however, follicles in grade 2 FL can be challenging, as they are more likely to resemble reactive follicles. Primary follicles can also be a pitfall and appear homogeneous, but CD10 and BCL6 are helpful, as these immunohistochemical stains should be negative in primary follicles. Small biopsies may also result in discordance between morphology and flow cytometric findings. Small, CD10-positive B-cell clones in a polyclonal background can be detected by flow cytometry in cases of FH.[1] However, true B-cell clones may be seen with reactive histology if there is partial nodal involvement by lymphoma or differences in sampling. Therefore, in cases with clones identified by flow cytometry but no evidence of lymphoma in a small/needle core biopsy, it is prudent to request an excisional/larger biopsy.

PCH is an expansion of the lymph node tissue that is between the follicles, an area composed predominantly of T cells. There are often admixed primary or secondary follicles that can be appreciated on core biopsy, although they will be more widely spaced than in FH (Figure 3.2). The

TABLE 3.1 **Differences in Pathologic Features Between Follicular Hyperplasia and Follicular Lymphoma**

Pathologic Features	Follicular Hyperplasia	Follicular Lymphoma
Shape and distribution of follicles	Large, can be irregular, usually spaced apart	Round, similar size and shape, frequently back-to-back
Perinodal involvement	Absent	Can be present
Polarity of follicles	Present	Absent
Mantle zones	Present	Absent or attenuated
Cellular composition	Polymorphous, many centroblasts	Monotonous, predominantly centrocytes in most cases
Tingible body macrophages	Present	Absent
CD10/BCL6 stain	Positive in germinal centers	Positive in neoplastic follicles and often in interfollicular areas
BCL2 stain	Negative in germinal centers	Positive in neoplastic follicles in the majority of cases
B-cell clonality studies	Polyclonal	Clonal in the majority of cases
FISH for *BCL2* and *BCL6*	Negative	*BCL2* rearranged in the majority of cases; *BCL6* in 5%-15%

lymphocytes in PCH are predominantly small and have clumped chromatin. Admixed plasma cells and scattered immunoblasts are frequently seen. CD20 and CD3 will show a predominance of small T cells over B cells, which can be reassuring on small core biopsies. Paracortical expansion can be seen in a variety of benign conditions, as well as lymphomas, which are discussed throughout this book. The T cells in lymphoma will be atypical, including variable size and atypical nuclear features, such as open chromatin or nuclear contour irregularity. Moreover, lymphomas typically show architectural effacement rather than limited paracortical involvement.[2,3]

SINUS HISTIOCYTOSIS

Sinus histiocytosis is another reactive finding in lymph nodes. This is a nonspecific finding, but it can be seen in lymph nodes draining malignancy.[4] The sinuses are distended by a proliferation of bland-appearing histiocytes in a background of normal lymph node architecture (Figure 3.3). This is a

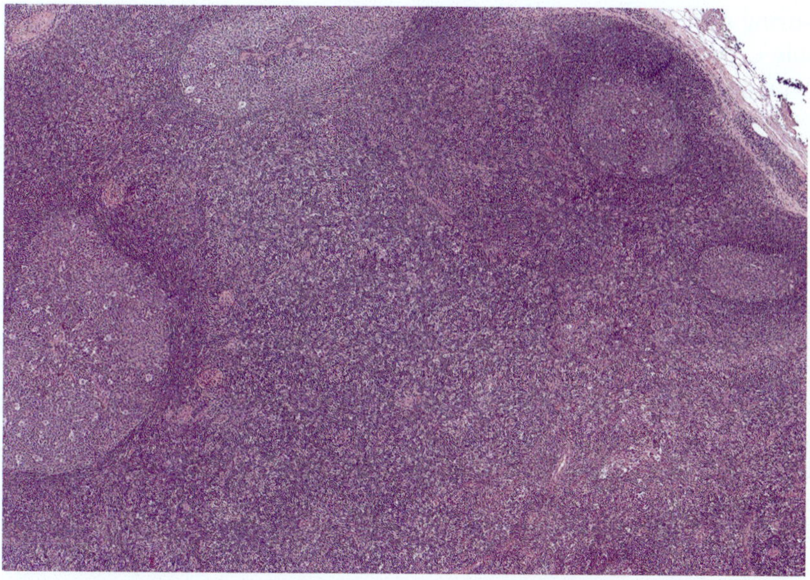

FIGURE 3.2 Paracortical hyperplasia with expansion of interfollicular areas.

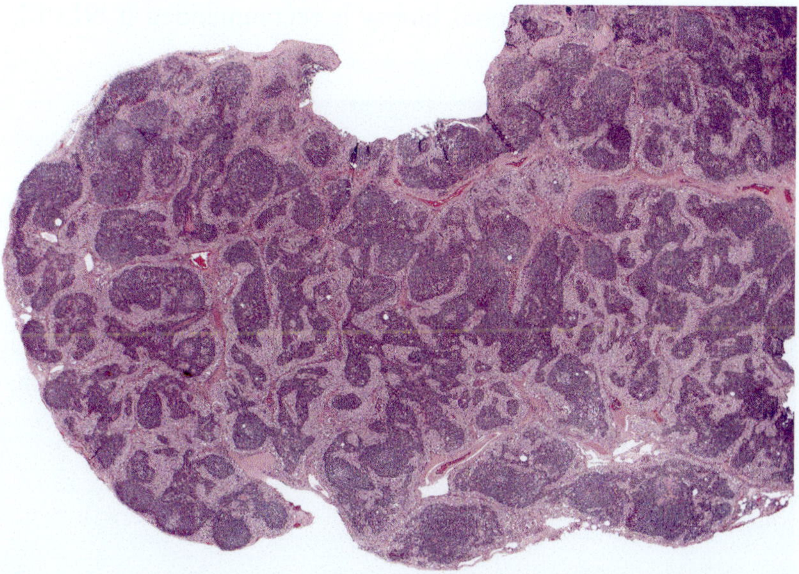

FIGURE 3.3 **Sinus histiocytosis.** Intact lymph node architecture with open sinuses filled with histiocytes.

reassuring sign on a small core biopsy, as most types of lymphoma (with the notable exceptions of lymphoplasmacytic lymphoma and angioimmunoblastic T-cell lymphoma) should not have open sinuses. This condition should not be confused with Rosai-Dorfman disease, in which the abnormal histiocytes have prominent emperipolesis and characteristic atypical nuclear features.

PROGRESSIVE TRANSFORMATION OF GERMINAL CENTERS

Progressive transformation of germinal centers (PTGC) is a descriptor for the finding of large follicles that have thickened mantle zones that "infiltrate" and disrupt/replace germinal centers. These follicles are typically interspersed in a background of normal-appearing secondary follicles. Lymph nodes containing PTGC are more commonly seen in children than adults, but this condition can also occur in older patients, including in IgG4 disease–related lymphadenopathy. Cervical lymph nodes are most commonly involved, but other lymph node groups can be affected. PTGC can recur, especially in children, and often in the same lymph node group. Different patterns have been described in PTGC from follicle lysis to complete absence of the germinal center (Figure 3.4).[3,5] Regardless, it is a benign finding that may be difficult to appreciate on a core biopsy. As there can be overlap morphologically with nodular lymphocyte predominant B-cell lymphoma (NLPBL), excisional biopsy is recommended if NLPBL is in

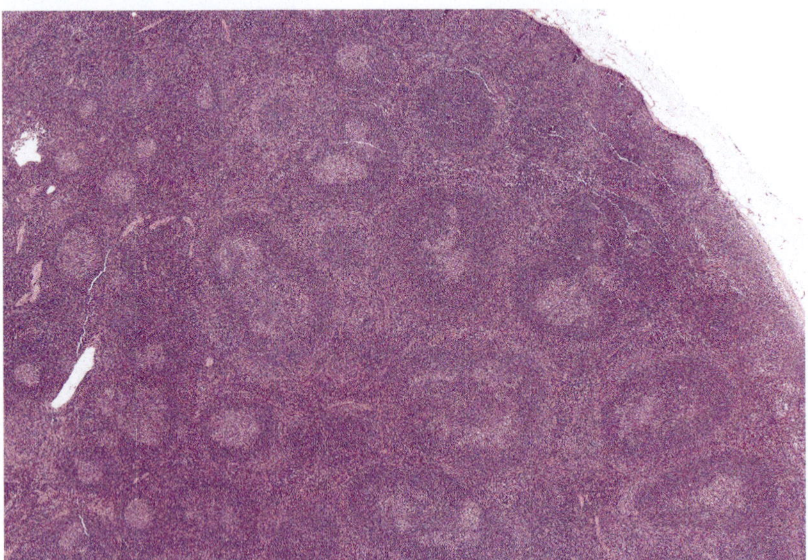

FIGURE 3.4 **Follicular hyperplasia with progressive transformation of germinal centers (PTGC).** Various stages of PTGC are shown, from follicle lysis to complete replacement by mantle zone cells.

the differential diagnosis.[6] Lymph nodes with NLPBL may show areas of PTGC, although PTGC alone is not considered a risk factor for NLPBL.[7] The differential diagnosis also includes the floral variant of FL, which can be negative for Bcl-2, and can be a pitfall.[3] Lymph nodes with PTGC in adults may have increased numbers of IgG4-positive plasma cells, and this is one of the recognized patterns seen in IgG4-related lymphadenopathy.[8] However, increased IgG4-positive plasma cells in a lymph node may also be a nonspecific finding, and correlation with other signs/symptoms of IgG4-related disease (eg, mesenteric/retroperitoneal fibrosis, pancreatitis, etc) and serologic findings is required for definitive diagnosis.

VIRAL LYMPHADENITIS

Viruses are a common cause of lymphadenitis, especially in children and young adults. While it may not always be possible to identify the etiology, some viruses have characteristic morphologic features that can be identified on lymph node biopsies. These diseases are also critically important, as they can be mistaken for lymphoma on the basis of their morphologic and clinical features. The entities that will be discussed here include Epstein-Barr virus (EBV), HIV, cytomegalovirus (CMV), and herpes simplex virus (HSV) lymphadenitis.

Epstein-Barr Virus Lymphadenitis (Infectious Mononucleosis)

EBV lymphadenitis can be suspected, both clinically and morphologically, in young patients with a viral syndrome and lymphadenopathy. EBV is a human herpesvirus 4 (HHV4) that is spread by bodily fluids, typically saliva. The virus infects B cells and epithelial cells in the nasopharynx, and elicits a CD8-positive cytotoxic T-cell response. Infectious mononucleosis (IM) is an acute manifestation of EBV infection, and patients often present with fever, fatigue, pharyngitis, and enlarged lymph nodes. Hepatosplenomegaly and/or thrombocytopenia may be present in some cases. In young children, the infection is often asymptomatic. Resolution typically occurs in a matter of weeks, although the infection persists in the body for life, and is controlled by the immune system. In resource-rich countries, the infection occurs later in childhood than in the resource-poor areas.[9]

Morphologically, the lymph node shows retained, but distorted, architecture including variably prominent follicles and typically a pronounced paracortical proliferation of mononuclear cells with vesicular chromatin and central basophilic nucleoli, consistent with reactive immunoblasts (Figures 3.5 and 3.6). Admixed plasma cells, eosinophils, histiocytes, and foci of necrosis may also be seen (Figure 3.7). Frequently, scattered Hodgkin-like and Reed-Sternberg (R-S)-like cells are seen, a common finding in all EBV-driven lymphoid proliferations (Figure 3.8). As this proliferation can cause alarm, it is essential not to misdiagnose these lymph nodes as classic Hodgkin lymphoma (CHL) or DLBCL. In comparison with CHL, the architecture is retained, and there is a spectrum

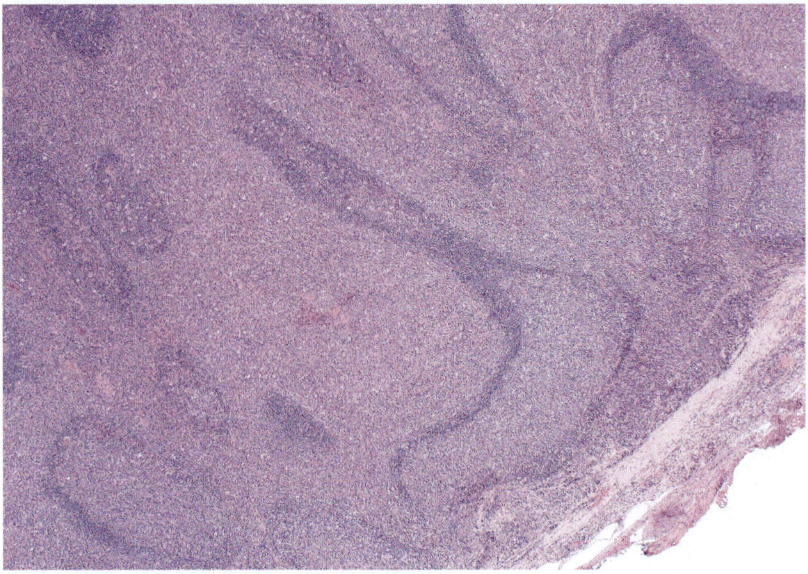

FIGURE 3.5 **Infectious mononucleosis.** Lymph node architecture distorted by a paracortical expansion in Epstein-Barr virus lymphadenitis.

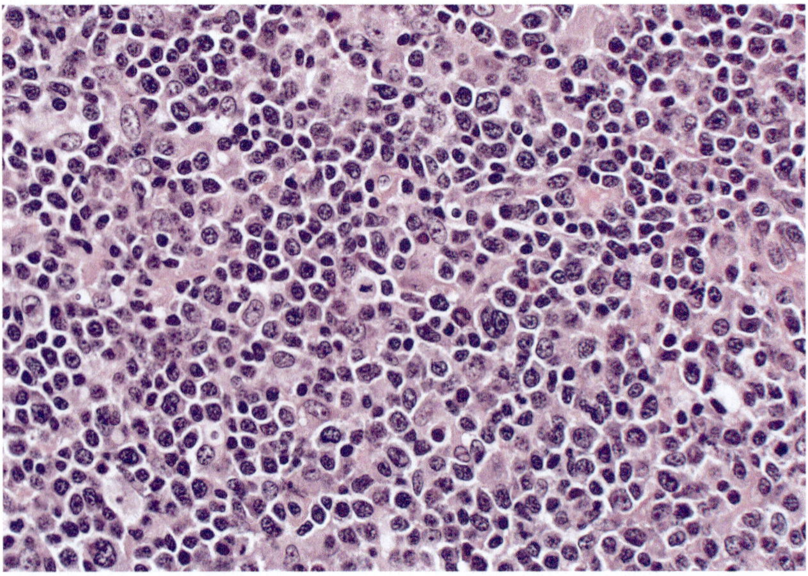

FIGURE 3.6 **Paracortical areas in EBV lymphadenitis show a proliferation of immunoblasts.**

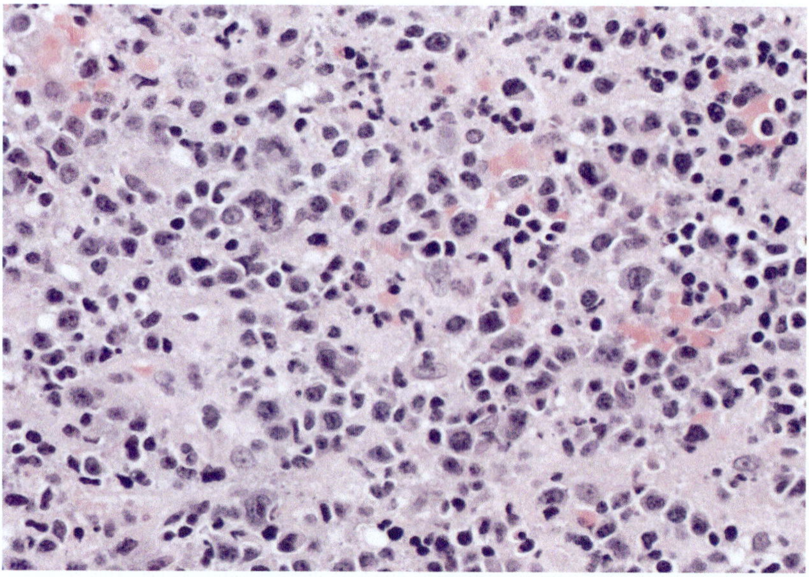

FIGURE 3.7 Areas with necrosis and increased plasma cells in EBV lymphadenitis.

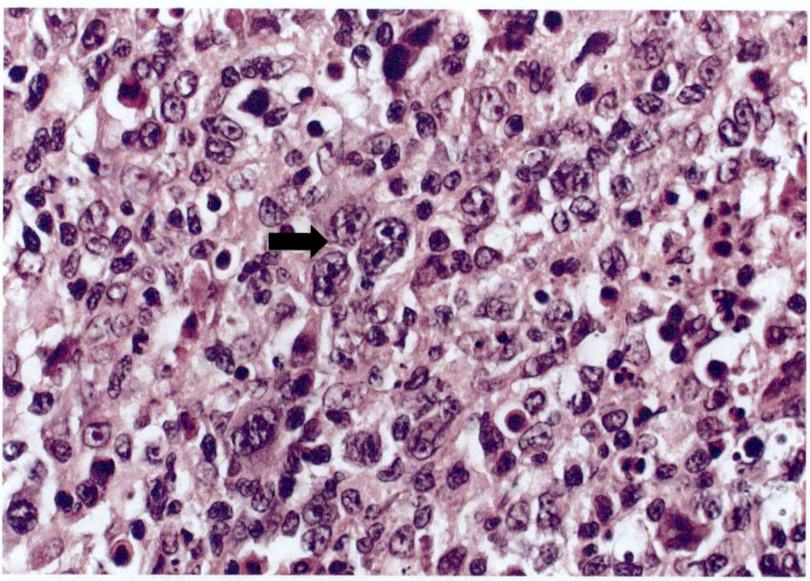

FIGURE 3.8 Increased immunoblasts, which may mimic Reed-Sternberg cells in EBV lymphadenitis (arrow).

of reactive cells including small lymphocytes, immunoblasts, R-S-like cells, and plasma cells. Immunohistochemistry is helpful in this differential diagnosis. While many of the immunoblasts may be positive for CD30, a subset will also express CD20, and some may express CD3. CD15 is negative, and CD45 (LCA) will be more variable than in CHL. Epstein-Barr virus-encoded RNA (EBER) in situ hybridization will mark numerous immunoblasts, as well as small lymphocytes, rather than the single scattered large cells, as seen in CHL (Figure 3.9). LMP1 and EBNA2 are also positive (viral latency III), in contrast to CHL, which has a latency II pattern (negative for EBNA2). The differential diagnosis and approach to these cases will heavily depend on the age and immunologic status of the patient. In young, immunocompetent individuals, primary EBV infection (IM) is the main consideration. If IM is not considered clinically early in the course of disease, the presence of lymphadenopathy may trigger an unnecessary lymph node biopsy and other workup for lymphoma. These biopsies, in turn, can be diagnostically challenging, as outlined above. It is of paramount importance not to interpret the immunoblastic proliferation as lymphoma, even if numerous CD30-positive cells are present.[10] While it can be difficult to appreciate architecture on a small biopsy, the diffuse EBV positivity in small and large cells, the age of the patient, and clinical presentation should all be helpful in recommending the monospot, a latex agglutination test. However, monospot can sometimes give false-negative results, especially in very young patients, and EBV serologies may be necessary for confirmation of acute infection. If a complete blood count is

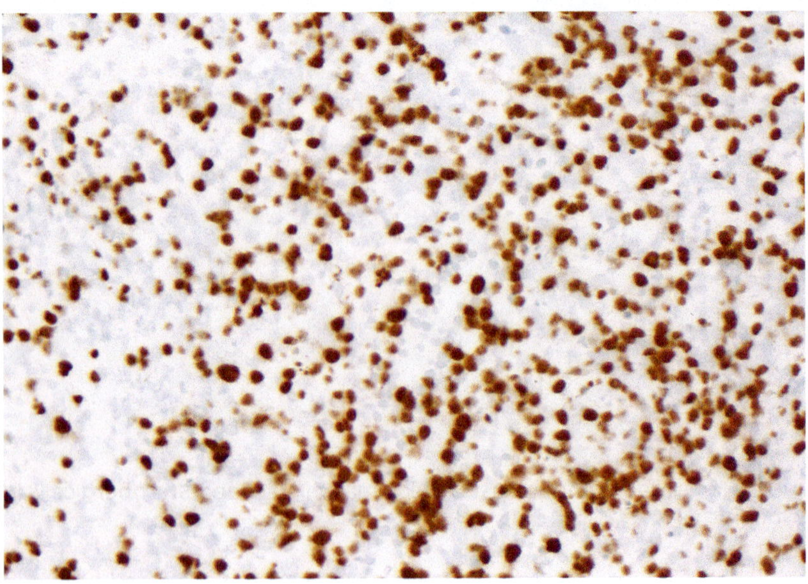

FIGURE 3.9 **Infectious mononucleosis.** In situ hybridization for Epstein-Barr virus–encoded RNA showing numerous positive cells.

performed, this can also be helpful, as patients often have an absolute lymphocytosis with reactive lymphocytes exhibiting deep blue cytoplasm or granular cytoplasm (large granular lymphocytes).

The differential diagnosis is broad in older and immunocompromised individuals (eg, patients on immunosuppressive drugs) who are more likely to have reactivation of EBV in the context of a lymphoproliferative disorder rather primary EBV infection. Some entities to consider in the differential diagnosis include EBV-positive DLBCL and polymorphic EBV-positive proliferations resembling posttransplant lymphoproliferative disorders.

Cytomegalovirus Lymphadenitis

CMV is another type of human herpesvirus 5 (HHV5). CMV infection occurs with exposure to body fluids including saliva, urine, blood, and breast milk. Clinically, infection in immunocompetent patients often occurs in childhood, and patients may be asymptomatic or may present with symptoms similar to those of EBV infection such as fatigue, lymphadenopathy, and night sweats. The infection tends to be severe in newborns and immunocompromised patients, such as organ transplant patients or HIV-positive individuals, in which it is an acquired immune deficiency syndrome (AIDS)-defining illness.[11]

Histologically, the features overlap with other causes of reactive lymphadenitis. CMV lymphadenitis may be difficult to distinguish from EBV infection, and other viral causes, unless characteristic large inclusions in CMV-infected cells are seen. Morphologic findings are nonspecific and include retained architecture with FH or PCH, an immunoblastic proliferation, increased histiocytes, and variable numbers of plasma cells.[12,13] Collections of monocytoid B cells are often present (Figure 3.10A and B). The characteristic large CMV inclusions, eosinophilic round nuclear inclusion surrounded by a clear halos, as well as cytoplasmic inclusions, can sometimes be found, and will be present within the monocytoid B-cell areas (Figure 3.11A). The peripheral blood may show reactive lymphocytes similar to the ones seen in EBV lymphadenitis.

Immunohistochemical confirmation with anti-CMV antibodies should be performed (Figure 3.11B). The infected cells may be very infrequent and could easily be absent from even large excisional biopsies. Serologies for CMV will likely identify the cause.

The primary differential diagnosis includes other nonspecific viral infections, as well as toxoplasma lymphadenitis, which may have very similar clinical and morphologic features, with the exception of the large intranuclear inclusions. Other pitfalls can include CHL, as the cells with viral inclusions may be positive for CD15.[14]

Herpes Simplex Virus Lymphadenitis

Two types of herpes simplex viruses, HSV-1 and HSV-2, infect humans and spread by direct contact with infected secretions. Primary infection is often asymptomatic, and lymphadenopathy is usually seen in the setting of virus reactivation. Patients may have regional lymphadenopathy (such

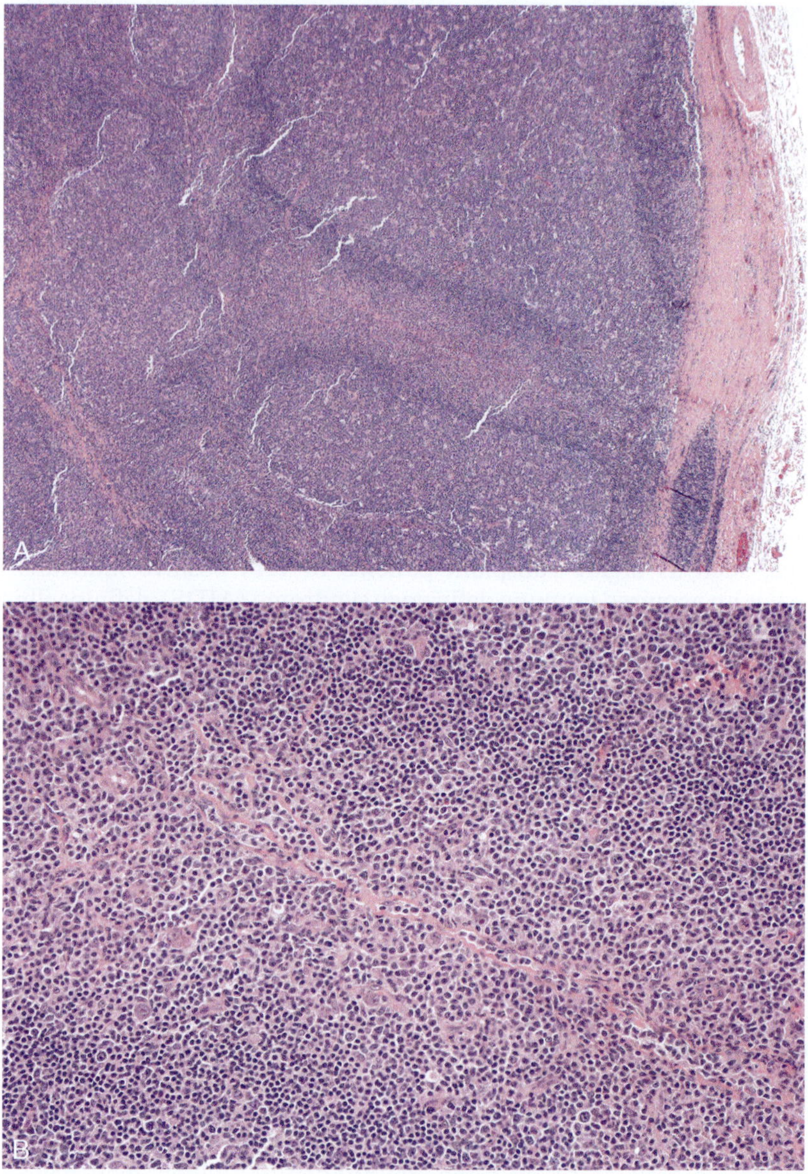

FIGURE 3.10 **Cytomegalovirus lymphadenitis.** Retained lymph node architecture with florid follicular hyperplasia (A) and sheets of monocytoid B cells (B).

as inguinal), or widespread disease, frequently due to an immunocompromised state (eg, HIV infection) or hematologic neoplasm.[15]

HSV lymphadenitis has similar histopathologic features as EBV and CMV lymphadenitis, in that there is often FH, sheets of monocytoid B cells, and/or paracortical expansion with frequent immunoblasts and occasional R-S- and Hodgkin-like cells. Cases show well-demarcated/abrupt areas of necrosis (Figure 3.12) with debris and ghosts of cells that

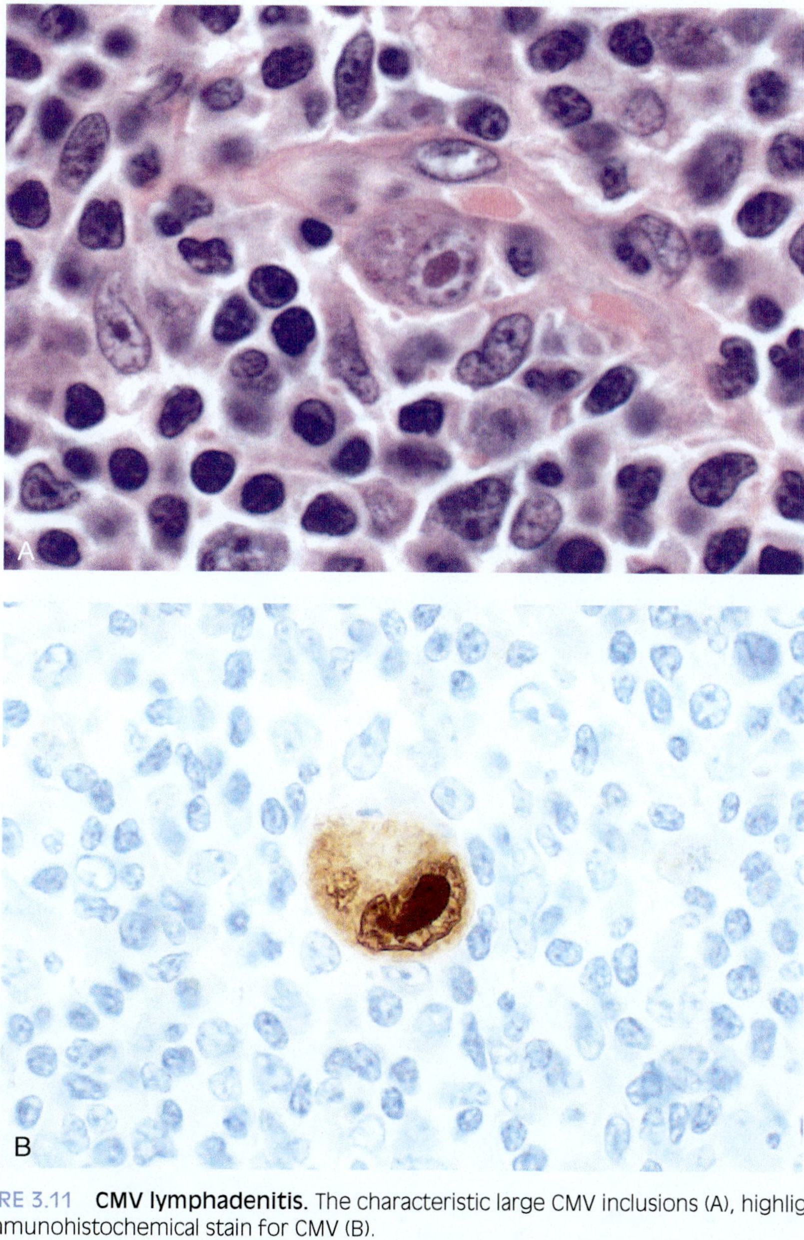

FIGURE 3.11 **CMV lymphadenitis.** The characteristic large CMV inclusions (A), highlighted by immunohistochemical stain for CMV (B).

contain viral inclusions (Figure 3.13). Typically, multinucleated giant cells with intranuclear inclusions, imparting a "ground-glass" appearance, are seen. Moreover, eosinophilic intranuclear and intracytoplasmic inclusions with clear halos can also be seen (Cowdry type A inclusions).

While HSV lymphadenitis may be seen in immunocompetent patients, lymph nodes are more often biopsied in patients with hematologic

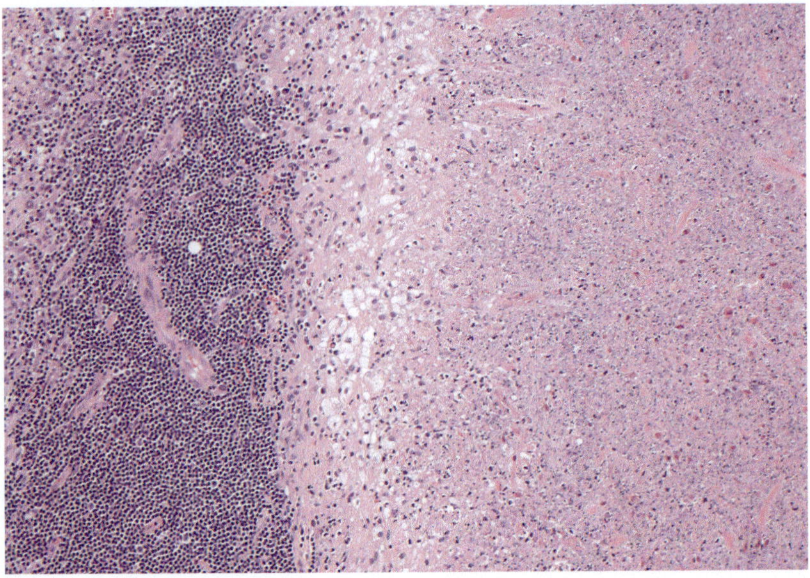

FIGURE 3.12 **Herpes simplex virus (HSV) lymphadenitis.** The biopsy from a patient with chronic lymphocytic leukemia/small lymphocytic lymphoma showing an abrupt transition from the lymphoma to the necrosis containing HSV inclusions.

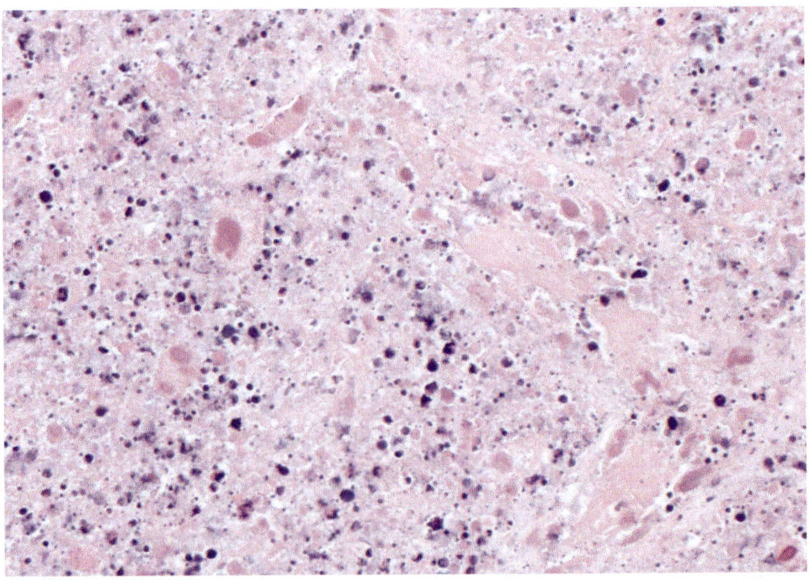

FIGURE 3.13 **HSV lymphadenitis.** Necrotic area where the characteristic viral inclusions are visible.

malignancies, such as chronic lymphocytic leukemia/small lymphocytic lymphoma (CLL/SLL), who are frequently immunocompromised. These patients undergo biopsy because there is clinical suspicion of transformation to DLBCL.[16,17] The biopsies in these cases characteristically show CLL/SLL with an abrupt transition to an area of necrosis, with cells containing characteristic inclusions, as described above. The diagnosis can be confirmed with immunohistochemistry for HSV-1 and/or HSV-2 (Figure 3.14).

Other than EBV and CMV, the differential diagnosis includes necrotic lymphomas and histiocytic necrotizing lymphadenitis (Kikuchi-Fujimoto lymphadenitis and systemic lupus erythematosus [SLE]). However, the viral inclusions are typically readily apparent in HSV, even in areas of prominent necrosis, and abrupt geographic necrosis in lymphoma is rare.

Human Immunodeficiency Virus Lymphadenitis

AIDS was first described in the early 1980s, and the HIV was soon thereafter discovered as the causative infectious agent. HIV infection quickly spread, causing a worldwide pandemic. Two strains of HIV exist (HIV-1 and HIV-2), with HIV-1 being the dominant strain around the world, while HIV-2 is largely restricted to Africa. HIV-1 is a retrovirus, spread by exposure to blood and body secretions of infected individuals. Clinically, three stages of HIV infection are recognized (acute, chronic/asymptomatic, and AIDS). HIV lymphadenitis can be seen at any stage during the disease. In the weeks after infection (acute phase), the patient usually has flu-like symptoms with lymphadenopathy. Enlarged lymph nodes can persist, while other acute

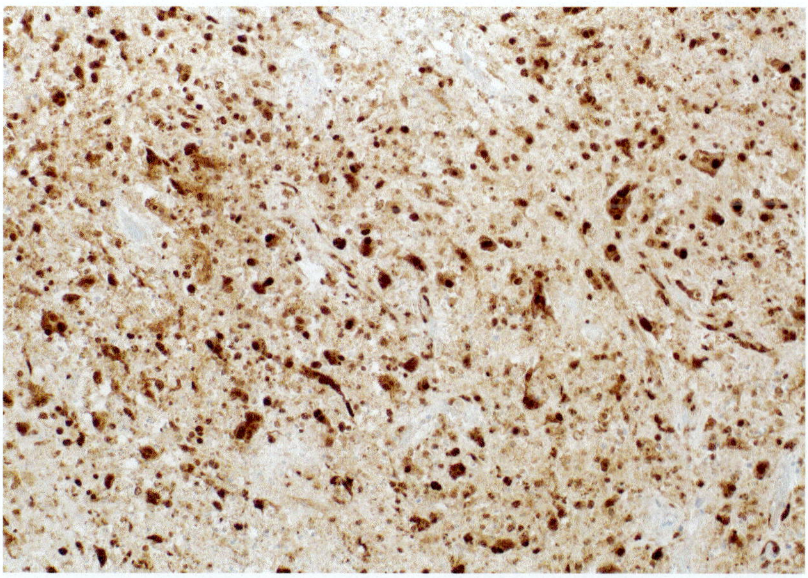

FIGURE 3.14 Immunohistochemical stain for HSV-1/HSV-2 showing numerous positive inclusions.

symptoms resolve. Patients with HIV may be biopsied because the infection has not been diagnosed, and the patient has unexplained lymphadenopathy. Once the diagnosis of HIV has been established, any new lymphadenopathy may be biopsied due to concern for lymphoma. HIV-positive individuals are at risk for high-grade lymphomas such as Burkitt lymphoma and DLBCL. In these cases, excluding lymphoma on a small biopsy is more important than recognizing the hallmarks of infection or the stage of the disease.

Morphologically, in the acute phase, the lymph node shows FFH. The follicles are often large and may be nearly confluent, with numerous tingible body macrophages and attenuated mantle zones. These have been termed "geographic" follicles due to their resemblance to land masses on a map. Follicles may be disrupted by small lymphocytes, so-called follicle lysis (Figure 3.15). Areas with monocytoid B cells may also be present. Acute and subacute/chronic phases may have large, multinucleated cells consistent with Warthin-Finkeldey-type giant cells (polykaryocytes), which are also seen in measles infection and Kimura disease.[12] The next stage of infection is considered the chronic phase, which may last years. In this phase, the follicles become more widely spaced and show involuted germinal centers. As the disease progresses, there is depletion of small lymphocytes, while plasma cells and blood vessels become more prominent (subacute stage) (Figure 3.16). In the later stages of disease, there is usually complete involution and hyalinization of the follicles. The lymphocytes are sparse, and vascular proliferation, as well as fibrosis, are prominent. Subacute and advanced stages of disease can histologically overlap with hyaline-vascular Castleman disease (CD) (Figure 3.17).[12] People with HIV infection can

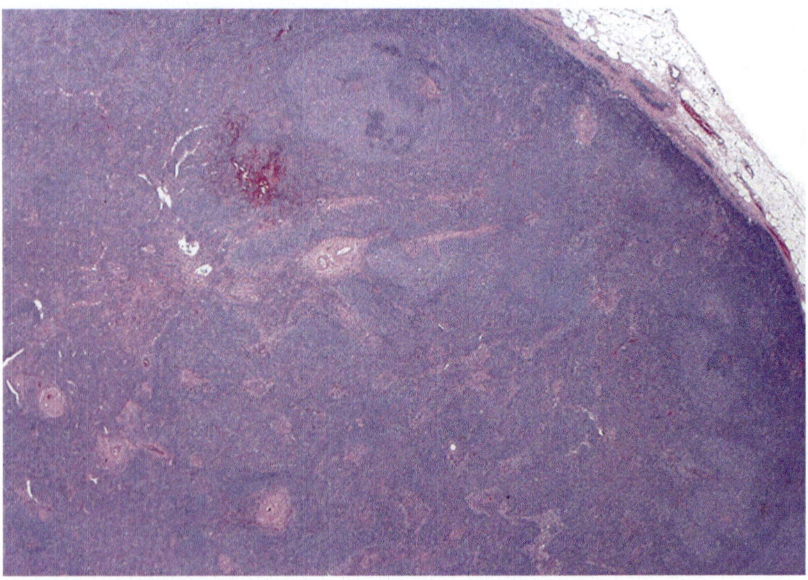

FIGURE 3.15 Acute HIV lymphadenitis showing follicle lysis.

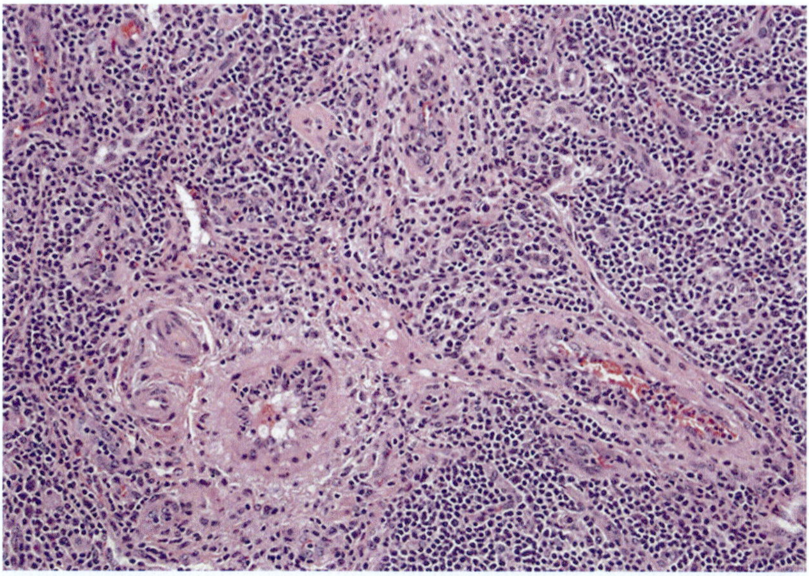

FIGURE 3.16 Subacute/chronic HIV lymphadenitis with increased vascularity and fibrosis.

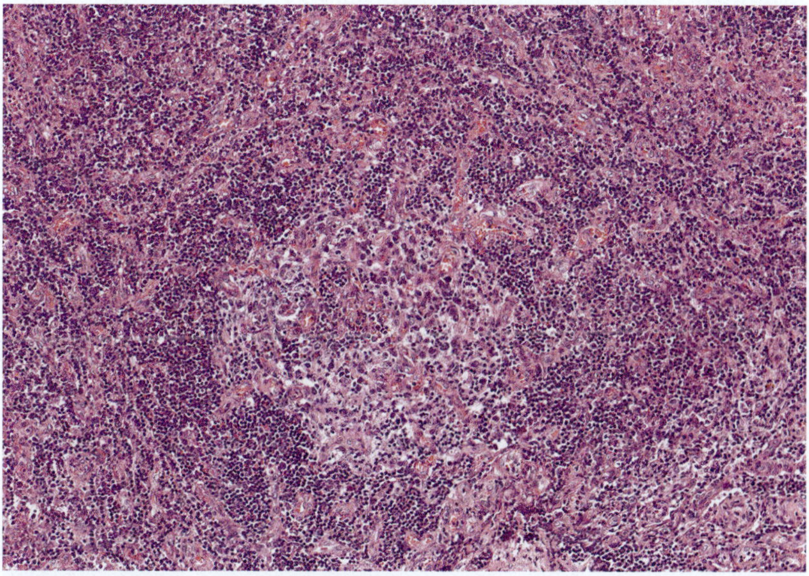

FIGURE 3.17 Subacute/chronic HIV lymphadenitis showing Castleman-like changes with markedly increased vascularity.

also develop multicentric CD, which will show HHV8-positive cells. Acute HIV lymphadenitis can histologically overlap with other viruses, such as EBV and CMV. It is important not to misdiagnose acute HIV infection as lymphoma on a small biopsy, as the large, nearly confluent germinal centers could be mistaken for DLBCL.

BACTERIAL LYMPHADENITIS

Cat-scratch Disease and Other Causes of Suppurative Lymphadenitis

Cat-scratch disease (CSD) is a zoonosis that occurs most commonly in young patients who have suffered a scratch or bite by a cat. The etiologic agent in this infection is *Bartonella henselae*, a gram-negative bacillus, which is also the culprit in bacillary angiomatosis (BA). CSD manifests as a skin lesion at the scratch site, followed by regional lymphadenopathy (usually cervical or axillary) several weeks later. In immunocompetent people, CSD is a self-limited illness that resolves in 6 to 12 weeks. However, immunocompromised patients can develop severe multisystemic illness.

Morphologically, the lymph nodes will typically show FH and foci of suppurative necrosis, circumscribed areas with sheets of neutrophils surrounded by a rim of organized histiocytes, which creates a stellate appearance (termed stellate microabscesses) (Figures 3.18 and 3.19).[12] Different morphologic stages exist, with small abscesses at the periphery progressing into larger ones occurring throughout the parenchyma.

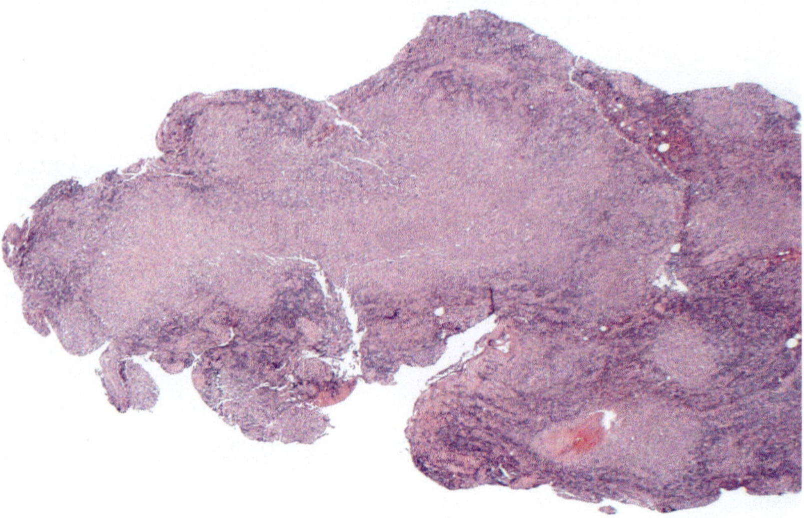

FIGURE 3.18 **Cat-scratch disease.** Geographic areas of necrosis can be seen on low magnification.

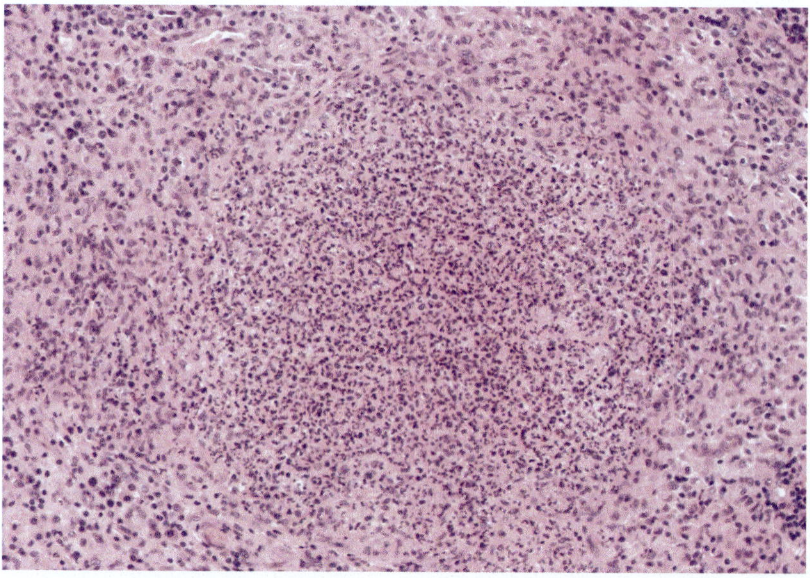

FIGURE 3.19 A characteristic abscess in cat-scratch disease containing neutrophils surrounded by a rim of histiocytes.

As the morphologic findings are not entirely specific for *B henselae*, confirmatory studies, such as serologies and PCR (the most sensitive modality), are often recommended. Immunohistochemical stain for *B henselae* will highlight the bacilli (Figure 3.20). Warthin-Starry silver stain can also be done, but it is notoriously difficult to interpret owing to high background staining.[18-20]

Suppurative lymphadenitis can be seen in other bacterial infections including lymphogranuloma venereum and *Campylobacter* infection. Lymphogranuloma venereum is caused by *Chlamydia trachomatis* and is more often seen in the inguinal lymph nodes from sexual transmission. Tularemia, a zoonosis caused by gram-negative coccobacillus *Francisella tularensis*, can show similar morphologic findings in lymph nodes. Perhaps one of the most important differential diagnoses of suppurative lymphadenitis is histiocytic necrotizing lymphadenitis (Kikuchi-Fujimoto disease [KFD]), which is characterized by necrosis with nuclear debris but distinctly lacking neutrophils.

Bacillary Angiomatosis

BA is caused by *B henselae*, the same gram-negative bacillus seen in CSD. It is an infection most commonly seen in HIV-positive patients and rarely other immunocompromised patients (eg, patients with chronic lymphocytic leukemia).[21] It is important to recognize this disease, as it can be treated with macrolide antibiotics, but may be fatal if overlooked. Clinically, BA

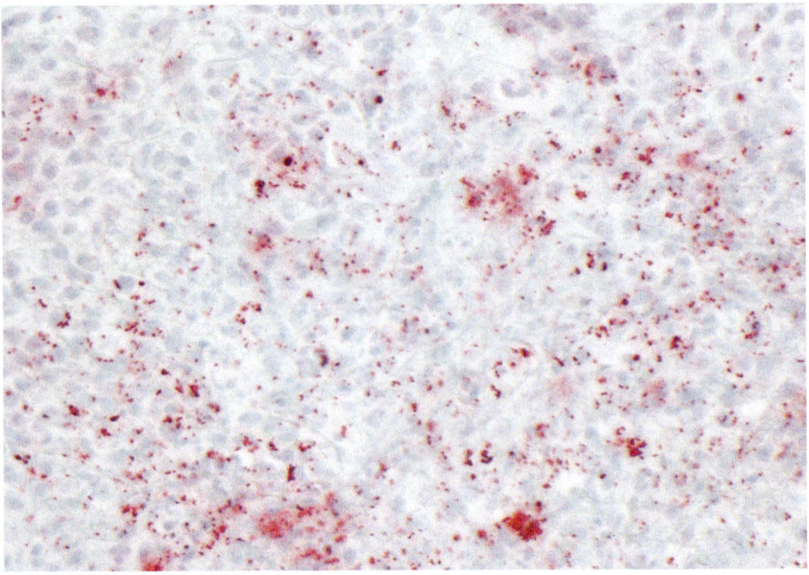

FIGURE 3.20 Immunohistochemical stain for *Bartonella henselae* showing numerous positive organisms in cat-scratch disease.

typically involves skin, but other sites such as lymph nodes (typically those draining the skin lesions) and internal organs can be involved.

Morphologically, this infection effaces lymph node parenchyma by a proliferation of small blood vessels. Eosinophilic granular material containing bacilli can be seen between the vessels (Figures 3.21 and 3.22). Scattered inflammatory cells, with a predominance of neutrophils, is seen, although clusters of plasma cells can also be present. BA is histologically distinguished from Kaposi sarcoma (KS) by the prominence of rounder, patent blood vessels and a relative lack of spindled epithelial cells and slit-like spaces, which are characteristic of KS. The endothelial cells in BA are plump and may obscure the vessel lumens. Numerous red blood cells are seen within the small vessels as well as extravasated ones. As it is rare and difficult to recognize morphologically, BA may be mistaken for a vascular tumor (such as angiosarcoma), especially if endothelial cells show some atypia. Immunohistochemistry for *B henselae* can be used for confirmation and will highlight numerous clustered bacilli (Figure 3.23).

Syphilitic (Luetic) Lymphadenitis

Syphilis (caused by spirochete *Treponema pallidum*) has made a resurgence as a cause of lymphadenitis in the United States, partly due to its frequent co-occurrence with HIV infection.[22] Clinically, three stages of syphilis are recognized, as well as latent stages that occur between the primary and secondary stages and after the resolution of the secondary stage.

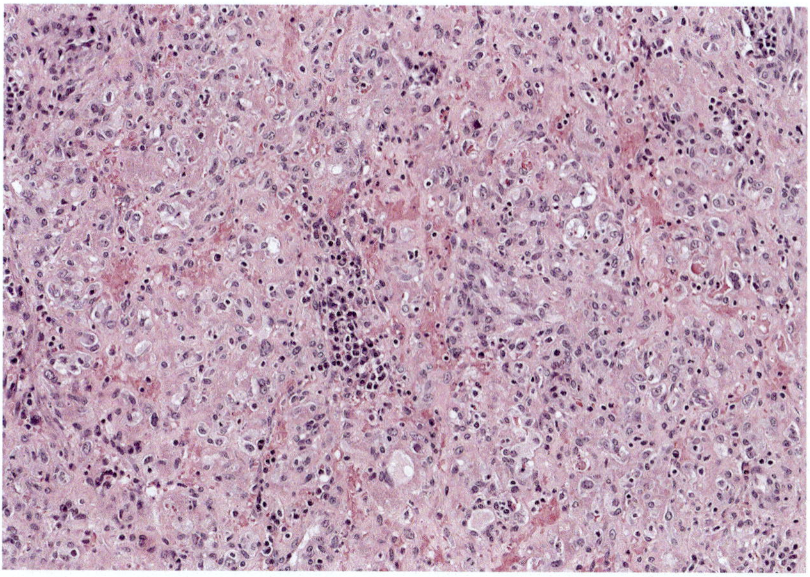

FIGURE 3.21 **Bacillary angiomatosis.** Proliferation of small vessels lined by plump endothelial cells containing red blood cells.

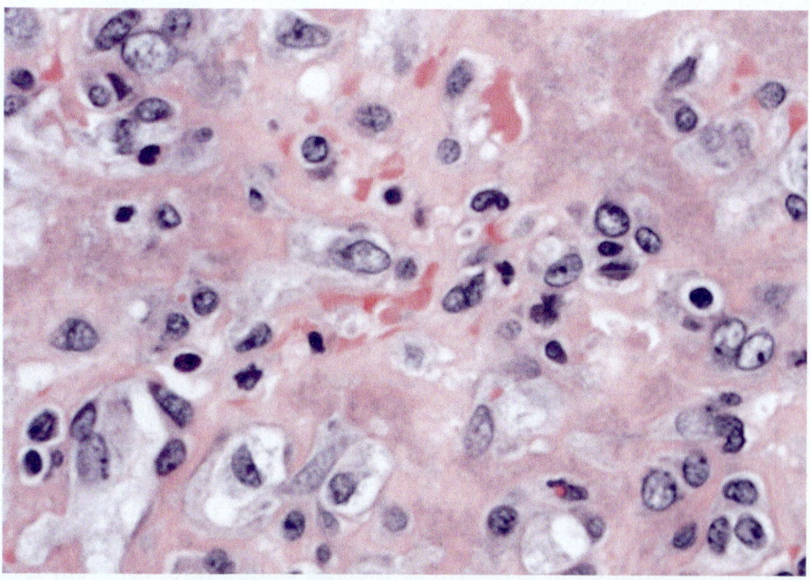

FIGURE 3.22 **Bacillary angiomatosis.** High magnification showing granular material between the vessels, corresponding to clusters of *Bartonella henselae* microorganisms.

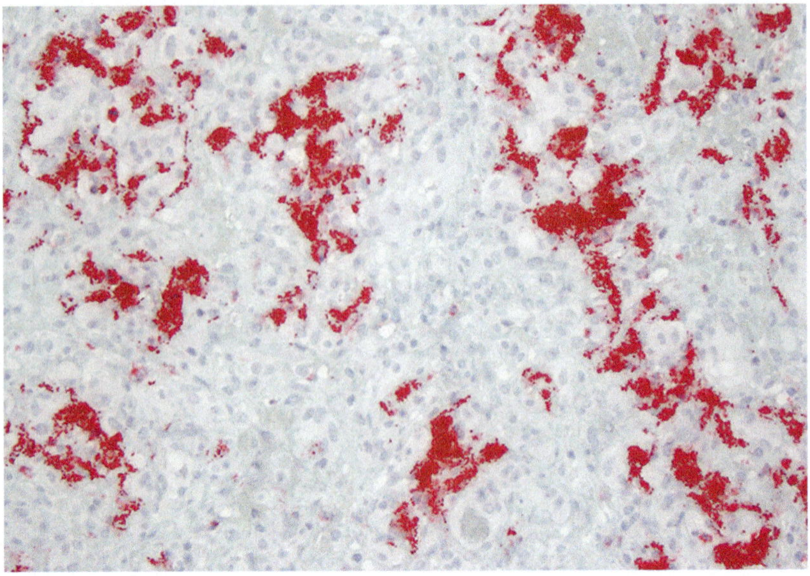

FIGURE 3.23 Immunohistochemical stain for *Bartonella henselae* showing clusters of organisms.

Lymph node involvement can be seen in either the primary or secondary stage of disease. Spirochetes spread to the lymph nodes within weeks to a month of the primary lesion (chancre) formation. Inguinal lymph nodes are the most frequent location, although it can also occur in lymph nodes draining the head and neck region. In the secondary stage of disease, there is usually widespread lymphadenopathy.

Many of the lymph node findings in syphilis are nonspecific and include features seen in other reactive conditions, including FH, which may be florid, as well as PCH.[23] More characteristic features include capsular thickening (often prominent) (Figure 3.24A) with sheets of plasma cells and lymphocytes, and with arteritis and phlebitis with neutrophils in the capsule and pericapsular tissues, as well as small intranodal vessels (Figure 3.24B). Paracortical areas sometimes show loose collections of epithelioid histiocytes/poorly formed granulomas.[24,25]

In suspected cases, spirochete immunohistochemistry is easy to interpret (Figure 3.25); however, it is not specific for *T. pallidum* and cross reacts with other spirochetes. Warthin-Starry stain will also be positive but is more challenging to interpret. PCR can be performed on the tissue section. Confirmation with serologies on the patient can also be done including nontreponemal tests–rapid plasma reagin and Venereal Disease Research Laboratory test. The positive nontreponemal tests can be confirmed with a more specific treponemal test.

Diagnosis of syphilis in a lymph node biopsy is frequently challenging and requires a great deal of suspicion. Characteristic histologic

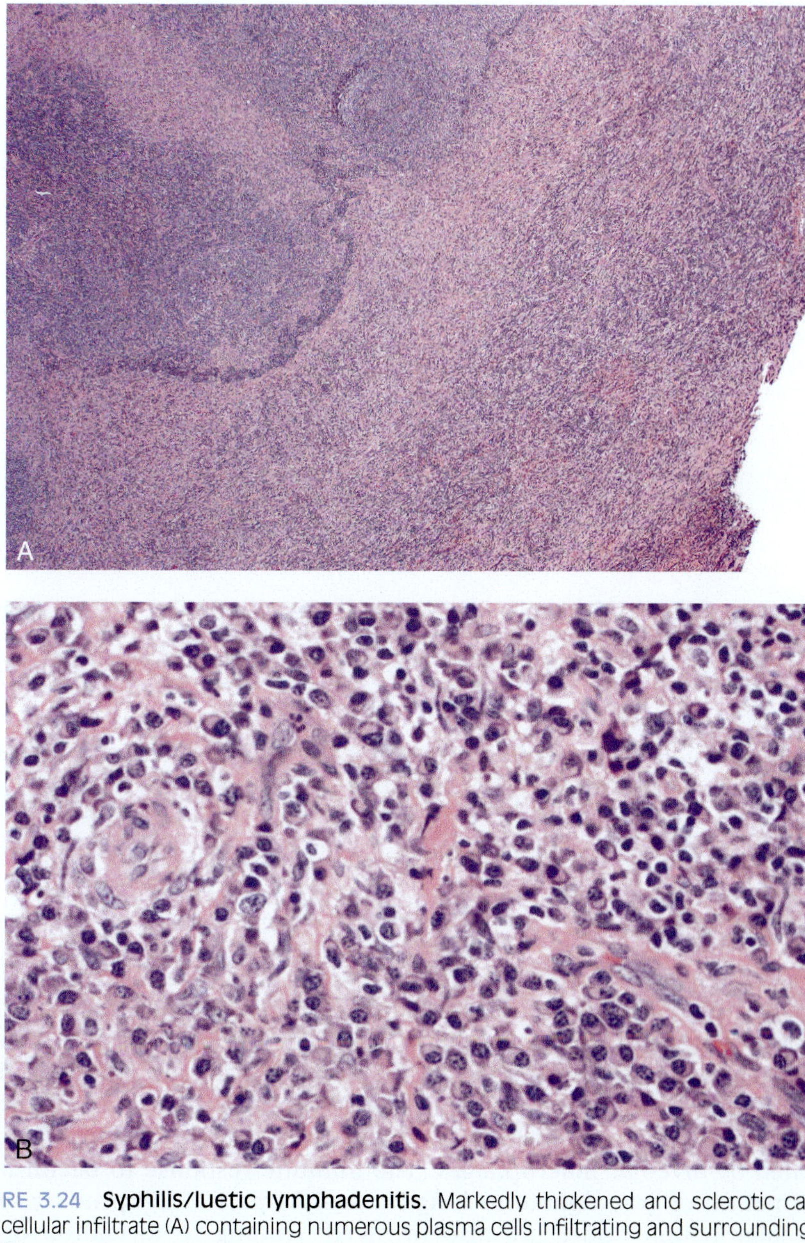

FIGURE 3.24 **Syphilis/luetic lymphadenitis.** Markedly thickened and sclerotic capsule with cellular infiltrate (A) containing numerous plasma cells infiltrating and surrounding vessels (B).

features might not be easily appreciated on a small/needle core biopsy. As outlined above, histologic findings can overlap with other reactive conditions that result in FH. Lymph nodes are usually biopsied due to suspicion for lymphoma or other entities, and syphilis is not clinically suspected. The thickened lymph node capsule can mimic classic Hodgkin lymphoma

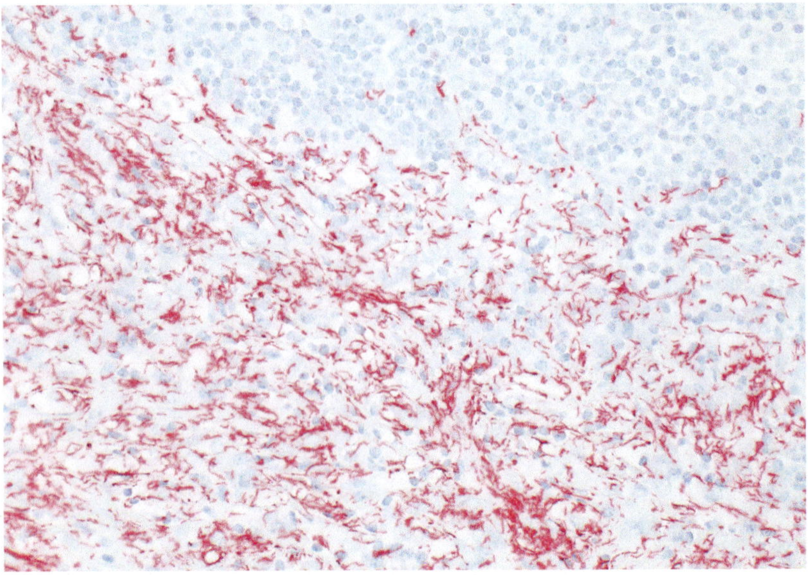

FIGURE 3.25 Spirochete immunohistochemical stain showing numerous positive organisms in luetic lymphadenitis.

(CHL), although plasma cells are not typically seen in the capsule of CHL. Furthermore, cases of CHL should not show marked FH.

MYCOBACTERIAL LYMPHADENITIS (*MYCOBACTERIUM TUBERCULOSIS* AND NONTUBERCULOUS MYCOBACTERIA)

Mycobacterium tuberculosis lymphadenitis is more common in resource-poor than in resource-rich countries. In the resource-poor areas, tuberculosis is one of the most common infectious causes of death. As with syphilis, tuberculosis reemerged in the United States as HIV infections rose.[26] Transmission occurs through aerosolized droplets of individuals with active infection. In primary infection, bacilli travel to lungs and are engulfed by alveolar macrophages. The immune response to bacilli leads to formation of granulomatous lung lesions. As part of the primary infection, hilar lymph nodes are also involved, leading to formation of the so-called Ghon complex (lung lesion and ipsilateral hilar lymphadenopathy). In most individuals, the Ghon complex will heal and calcify. Some patients can develop secondary tuberculosis, most commonly as a result of reactivation of the primary infection, where granulomatous inflammation involves lung parenchyma (typically the apex of the lung) and can lead to formation of a cavity. Furthermore, bacilli can spread into the lung or disseminate to other organs and lymph nodes through the lymphatics or hematogenous spread. Disseminated tuberculosis is most commonly seen in people with compromised immunity, such as in HIV infection, or may occur in the elderly or other immunocompromised populations. Lymph node involvement is most often seen in children and young adults, and the nodes in the head and neck region are the most commonly involved (so-called scrofula). Patients may present with systemic symptoms or be asymptomatic, and the lymph nodes are typically painless.

Mycobacterial infection, caused by *M tuberculosis,* presents with caseating/necrotizing granulomatous inflammation. Granulomas show central coagulative necrosis (eosinophilic and amorphous), surrounded by palisading epithelioid histiocytes, lymphocytes, and occasional giant cells (Figure 3.26). Mycobacterial lymphadenitis must be distinguished from fungal infections, which also present with necrotizing granulomatous inflammation. Another key differential diagnosis is sarcoidosis, which is typically not necrotic but may be hyalinized, usually with small, well-formed granulomas.[27] As the infectious organisms can be sparse, infection must always be excluded clinically before a diagnosis of sarcoidosis is made.

Histologic confirmation can be done with special stains including Fite-Faraco, Kinyoun, and Ziehl-Neelsen stains on paraffin-embedded tissue or auramine O fluorescent stain on fresh samples. On paraffin-embedded sections, *M. tuberculosis* appears as slender, beaded, red acid-fast bacilli. As it can be labor intensive to scour these tissues and the sensitivity is limited, PCR, a more sensitive method, may also be a helpful adjunct. Clinical

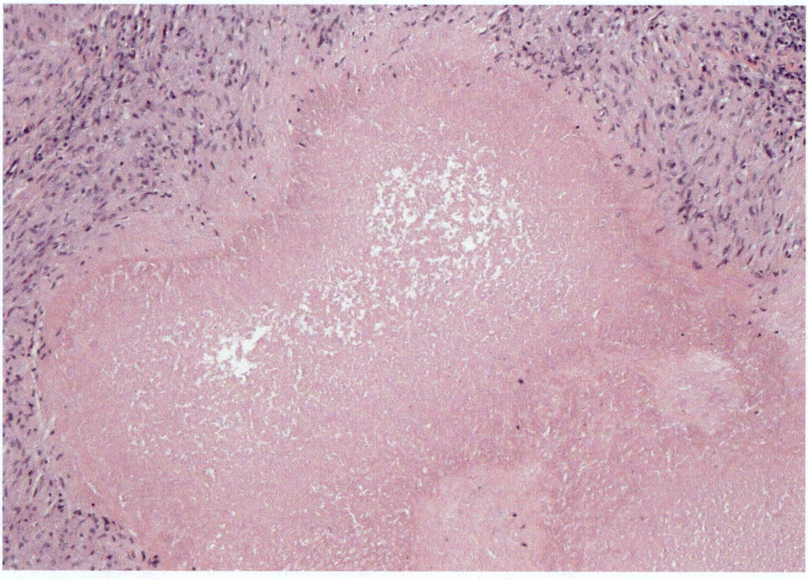

FIGURE 3.26 ***Mycobacterium tuberculosis* lymphadenitis.** Granuloma with central necrosis surrounded by palisading histiocytes.

testing of the patient with laboratory-based assays including culture (which takes weeks), skin testing, or other tests can also be done.[12]

A number of nontuberculous mycobacteria can cause disease in humans, but severe illness (ie, disseminated infection) usually occurs only in immunocompromised individuals, such as people with AIDS. *M. avium-intracellulare* (MAI) is one of the common causes of lymphadenitis and disseminated infection in patients with AIDS. Histologically, the lymph node architecture is effaced by sheets of pale foamy histiocytes (Figure 3.27A). In some cases, poorly formed granulomas can be seen. Ziehl-Neelsen and Fite stains can be used to demonstrate numerous acid-fast bacilli packing the histiocytes (Figure 3.27B). Whipple disease is an important differential diagnosis of MAI infection. Storage diseases may also be considered such as Gaucher disease or Niemann-Pick disease.[28,29]

FUNGAL LYMPHADENITIS

Histoplasma Lymphadenitis

Histoplasma infection is the most common fungal infection in the United States, most prevalent around the Ohio and Mississippi River Valleys.[30] *Histoplasma capsulatum*, a dimorphic fungus, is transmitted by inhalation of spores from contaminated soil (from bird and bat droppings). At body temperature, *Histoplasma* germinates into the yeast form within lung macrophages and spreads to regional lymph nodes. Similar to infection with *M tuberculosis*, the primary site of granulomatous infection is in the lungs, and affected lymph nodes become fibrotic and calcified. While the infection is typically controlled in immunocompetent individuals, it can reactivate if the person infected becomes immunocompromised. Clinical presentations of histoplasmosis include the acute pulmonary form (in people exposed to a large number of spores), chronic pulmonary disease, and disseminated histoplasmosis, which is typically seen in severely immunocompromised individuals, such as patients with AIDS, people undergoing chemotherapy, or solid organ transplant recipients. The fungus disseminates via the reticuloendothelial system and most commonly involves lymph nodes, bone marrow, liver, and spleen.[12]

Morphologically, lymph nodes show necrotizing granulomas surrounded by epithelioid histiocytes and giant cells (Figure 3.28A). The organisms can be seen as tiny vacuoles within the cytoplasm of histiocytes, and also in extracellular areas. Older lesions may have fibrosis and calcification, which can cause confusion with sarcoidosis. Confirmation requires Grocott methenamine silver (GMS) or periodic acid–Schiff stain. The GMS stain will demonstrate small yeast forms (2-4 µm), which have narrow-based budding (Figure 3.28B) and may be seen in clusters within macrophages. As it is ill-advised to provide definitive subclassification on morphology alone, confirmation can be done clinically with *H. capsulatum* antigen tests from blood or urine. In small biopsies, the organisms may be too infrequent to be seen with special stains.[31,32]

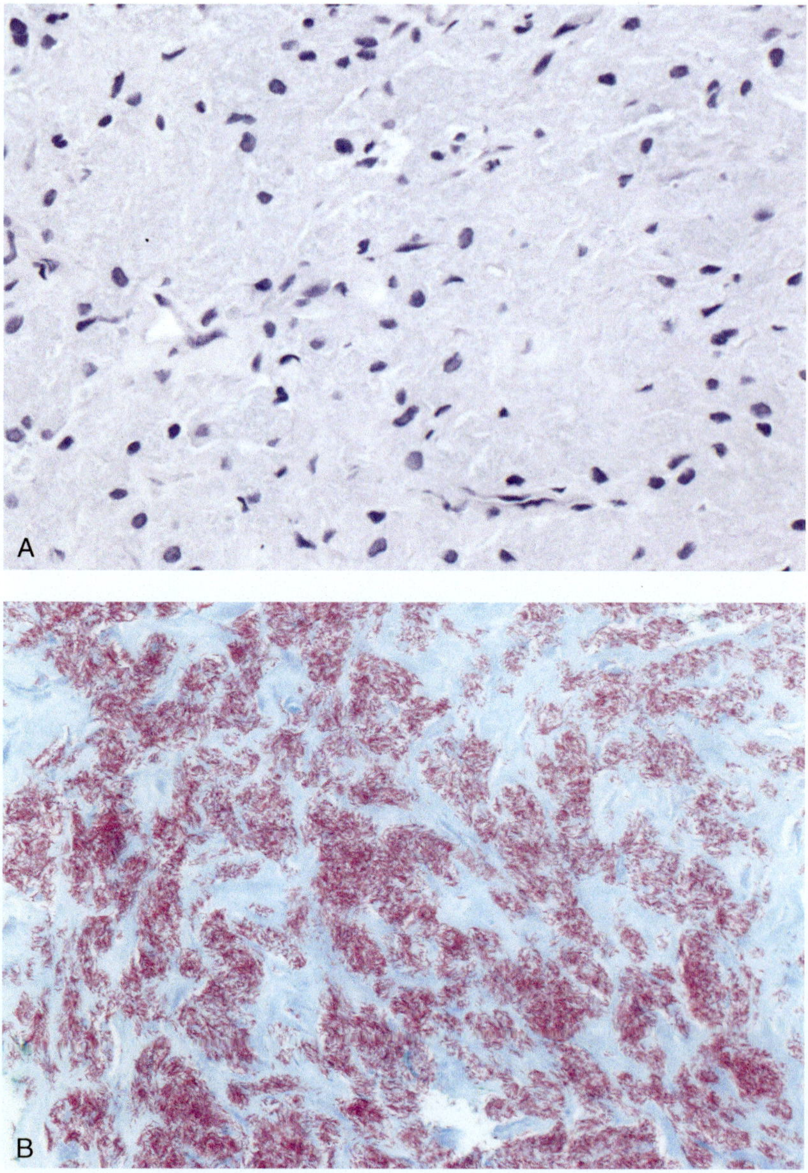

FIGURE 3.27 ***Mycobacterium-avium-intracellulare* lymphadenitis.** Sheets of foamy pale histiocytes containing numerous organisms (A). Special stain for acid-fast bacilli (Ziehl-Neelsen) showing histiocytes filled with acid-fast bacilli (B).

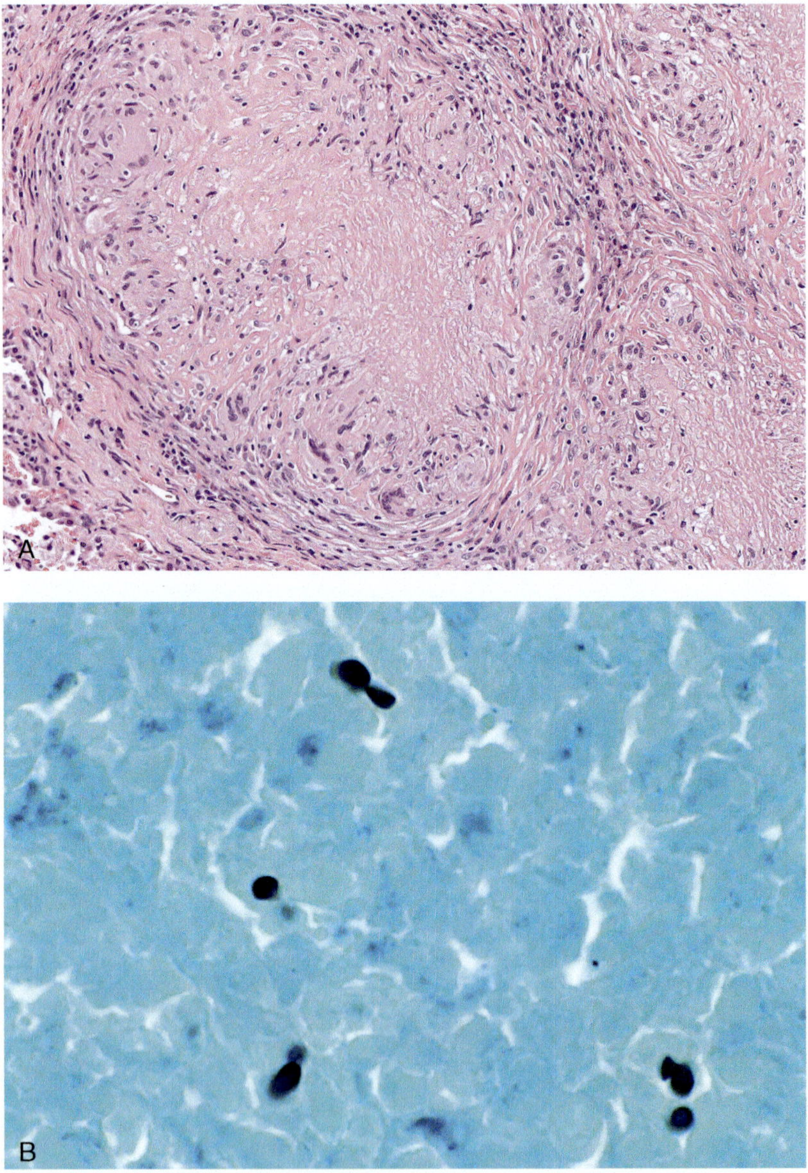

FIGURE 3.28 **Histoplasma lymphadenitis.** Granuloma with palisading histiocytes including occasional giant cells and central necrosis (A). Grocott methenamine silver stain shows small yeast with narrow-based budding (B).

Coccidiomycosis Lymphadenitis

Coccidiomycosis is caused by the dimorphic fungus *Coccidioides immitis*. The southwestern part of the United States is an endemic region for this infection, which occurs by inhalation of arthroconidia (the mycelial form) from the soil. In immunocompetent individuals, infection is frequently asymptomatic, or it causes a mild flu-like illness called San Joaquin valley fever. Lungs and local lymph nodes (hilar and mediastinal) are typically involved. Immunocompromised individuals, such as patients with AIDS, can develop severe disseminated illness with systemic lymphadenopathy.

Histologically, lymph nodes show granulomatous inflammation, frequently with necrosis. Fungal organisms (sporangia) are scattered in the granulomatous background and are easily appreciated on H&E-stained sections (Figure 3.29A). Sporangia can be immature or mature (up to 60 μm) and filled with endospores, which are released. The GMS stain highlights the organisms (Figure 3.29B). Diagnosis can be confirmed with serological tests.[12]

PROTOZOAL LYMPHADENITIS

Toxoplasma Lymphadenitis

Toxoplasmosis is an infection caused by *Toxoplasma gondii*, a protozoan parasite that infects warm-blooded animals and humans. The complex life cycle of *T. gondii* is beyond the scope of this book; however, the definitive host (where sexual reproduction occurs) is a cat, while humans and other animals are intermediate hosts. Humans can become infected by ingesting food or water contaminated by a cat's feces, incidentally ingesting cat feces containing oocysts by cleaning a litter box, for example, or by eating undercooked meat of animals that are intermediate hosts. Other modes of transmission include blood transfusion, organ transplantation, or transplacental from mother to fetus. In most people (80%-90%), infection remains asymptomatic. In symptomatic, immunocompetent individuals, toxoplasmosis manifests with lymphadenopathy (most commonly cervical), frequently accompanied by fever and myalgia. In immunosuppressed individuals (eg, patients with AIDS), *T. gondii* causes disseminated life-threatening infection. Congenital toxoplasmosis is also a severe systemic illness.

The architecture of the lymph node is often distorted but overall is preserved (Figure 3.30). The morphologic features in affected lymph nodes include the classic "triad" of FH, increased epithelioid histiocytes (frequently in clusters) encroaching on germinal centers, and collections of monocytoid B cells (Figure 3.31).[33] Additional histologic studies are typically not helpful, as the organisms (tachyzoites) will not usually be seen in lymph nodes of immunocompetent patients. Immunohistochemistry for *T. gondii* may find organisms in immunocompromised patients. PCR on tissue has the same limitations in immunocompetent patients and will also frequently be negative.[12]

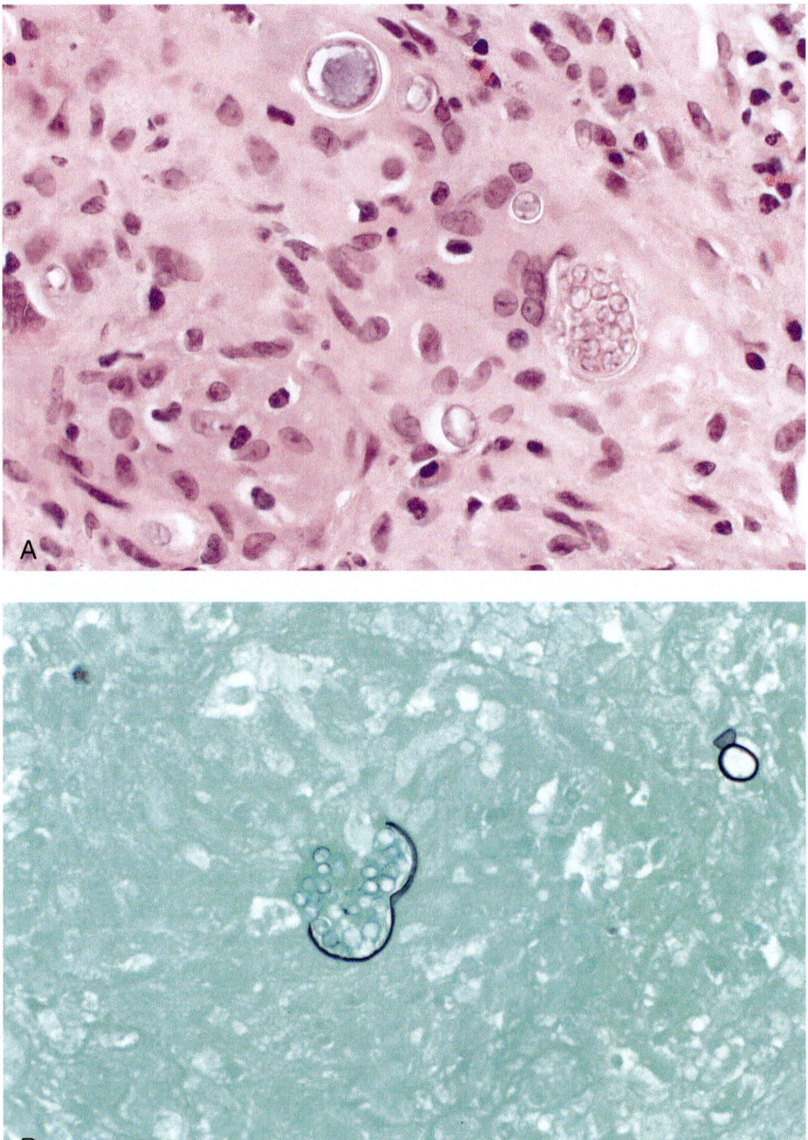

FIGURE 3.29 **Coccidiomycosis lymphadenitis.** Sporangia in different maturational stages in a background of granulomatous inflammation (A). The GMS stain is positive for organisms (B).

Confirmation typically requires serologic antibody titers, which may be negative in the setting of immunodeficiency. In cases exhibiting the described histologic triad (which may be difficult to appreciate on small core biopsies), this etiology is best suggested rather than unequivocally diagnosed, as other etiologies can manifest similar histologic features.

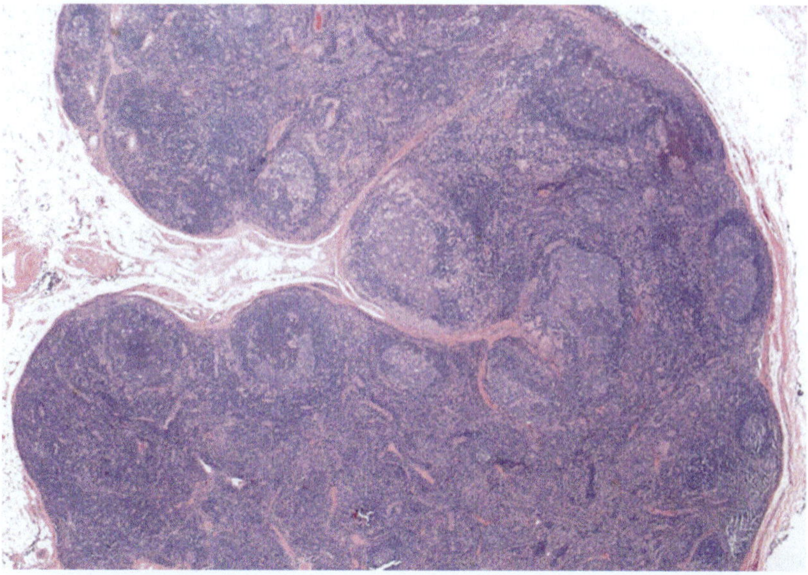

FIGURE 3.30 **Toxoplasma lymphadenitis.** Lymph node with intact architecture showing follicular hyperplasia.

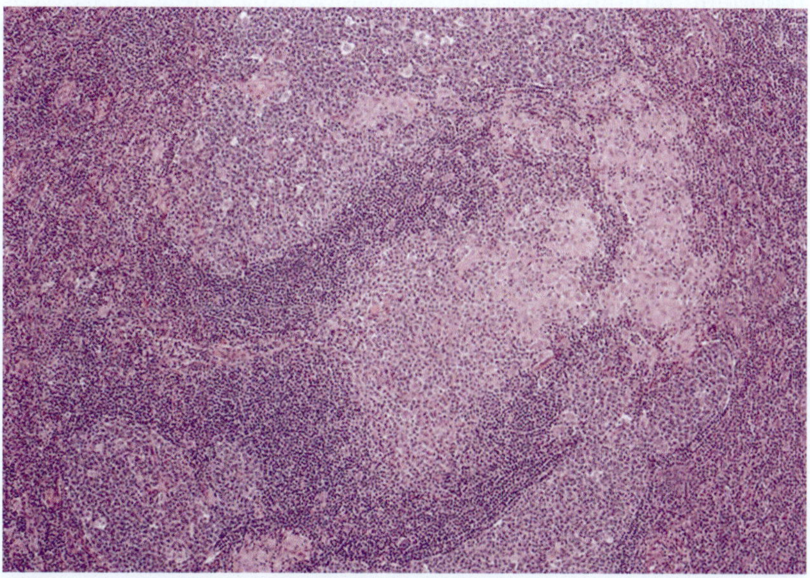

FIGURE 3.31 **Toxoplasma lymphadenitis.** The classic histologic "triad" including follicular hyperplasia, single and clustered epithelioid histiocytes impinging on the germinal centers, and collections of monocytoid B cells.

Moreover, it is important to have all elements in the triad, as many other conditions should be considered if only two morphologic criteria are present.

HISTIOCYTIC NECROTIZING LYMPHADENITIS (KIKUCHI-FUJIMOTO DISEASE)

KFD is a reactive condition of unknown etiology. It is more common in young women, although it can occur at any age. KFD was first described in Asia and appears to be more common in people of Asian ancestry. Patients typically present with cervical lymphadenopathy, although other sites (eg, axillary lymph nodes) can be involved. A subset of patients present with systemic symptoms resembling a viral illness (eg, fever, myalgias, sore throat), weight loss, and night sweats), and a minority may have skin rash. KFD is a self-limited illness in most cases, and patients require only symptomatic therapy.

Histologically, the lymph node will show areas of preserved architecture (usually with FH) with abrupt transition to pale, irregular areas composed of a mixture of cells including histiocytes (many C-shaped, "crescentic"), plasmacytoid dendritic cells, small lymphocytes, and immunoblasts. This infiltrate is associated with variable amounts of necrosis (Figure 3.32). Necrotic areas do not contain neutrophils, which is an important morphologic clue.[34] Histologically, three phases can be seen in the affected lymph nodes (with frequent morphologic overlap),

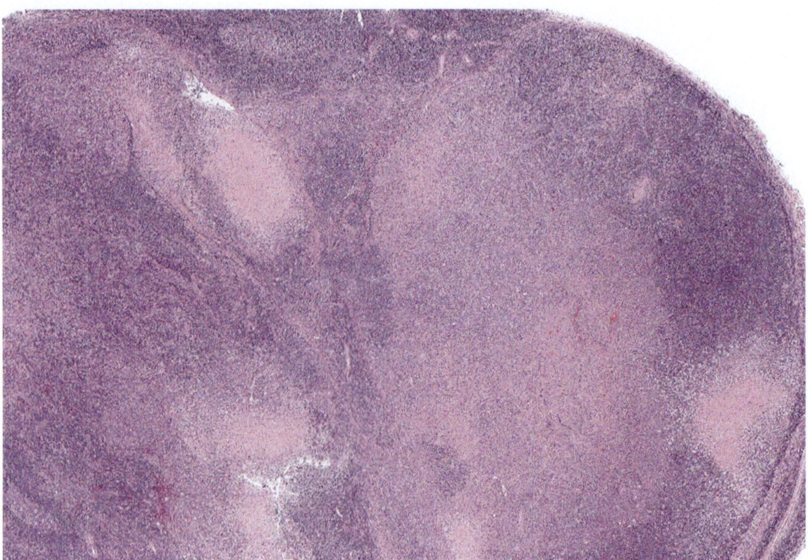

FIGURE 3.32 **Kikuchi-Fujimoto disease.** Lymph node with follicular hyperplasia and partially effaced architecture and abrupt transition to necrotic areas.

representing the disease progression. In the earliest phase (proliferative), histiocytes, admixed with other cells, will predominate, with minimal or no necrosis. Single apoptotic cells are usually seen. As the disease progresses to the necrotizing phase (the phase most commonly seen on biopsy), there will be abundant necrotic debris (Figure 3.33). In the xanthomatous phase, foamy/lipid-laden histiocytes are present to mop up the debris. This diagnosis can be difficult on small biopsies, as the abrupt transition from normal lymph node to the necrosis may not be sampled. These characteristic morphologic features are best appreciated on low-power magnification.

Some ancillary studies may be of assistance in difficult cases, although rarely are they necessary. The histiocytes will be positive for the usual histiocytic markers such as CD4, CD68, and lysozyme, and they are also positive for myeloperoxidase, an interesting aberrancy (Figure 3.34). In a small biopsy, where necrosis/karyorrhectic debris are not obvious, one should be careful not to confuse these histiocytes with myeloid blasts. CD8-positive cytotoxic T cells predominate over CD4-positive ones, which is another pitfall in a limited biopsy, as the infiltrate could be mistaken for T-cell lymphoma. Clusters of plasmacytoid dendritic cells, usually found at the periphery of the necrotic areas, may be highlighted with CD123 (Figure 3.35). CD20 will be negative in the necrosis, and this helps exclude a necrotic B-cell lymphoma. In summary, KFD is a disease that is diagnosed in most cases on H&E-stained sections. Immunohistochemical studies can be of great help in challenging cases, but they may also lead to confusion and misdiagnosis on a small biopsy. Importantly, the morphologic and

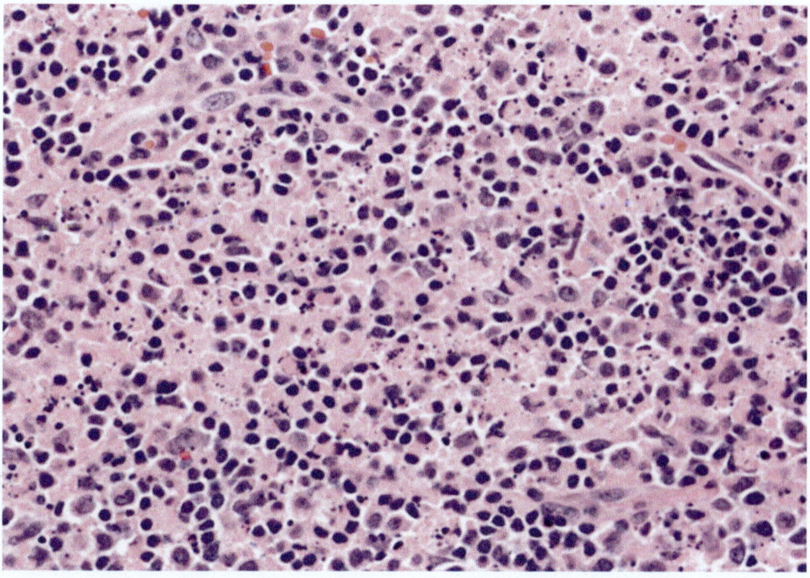

FIGURE 3.33 **Kikuchi-Fujimoto disease.** Area of necrosis with karyorrhexis without neutrophils.

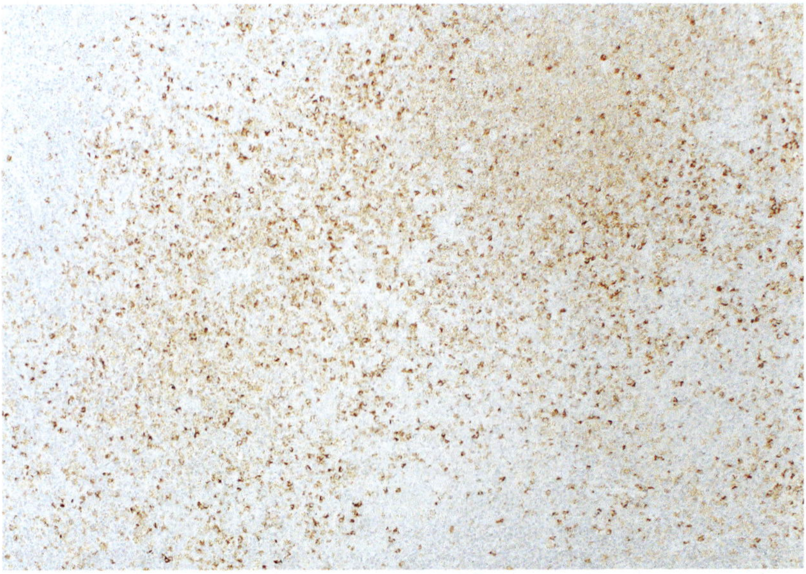

FIGURE 3.34 Histiocytes in Kikuchi-Fujimoto disease are positive for myeloperoxidase in an area of necrosis.

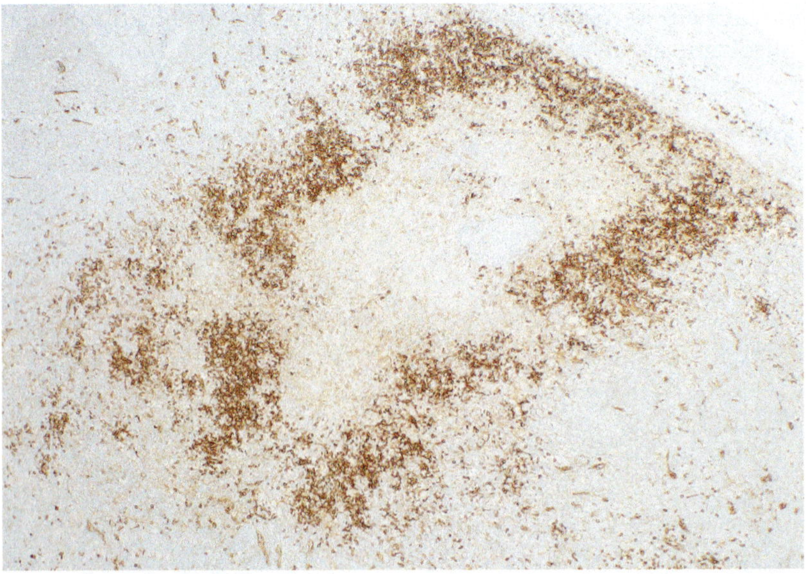

FIGURE 3.35 Collections of plasmacytoid dendritic cells positive for CD123 in Kikuchi-Fujimoto disease.

immunohistochemical features in KFD can be identical to those of SLE. The only feature that is rarely seen in SLE, but is not seen in KFD, is hematoxylin bodies (see SLE section). SLE may also have increased plasma cells compared with KFD. As they cannot be indistinguishable, it is important to give a differential diagnosis of KFD vs SLE so that the patient can be evaluated for an autoimmune disease.[35-38]

SARCOIDOSIS LYMPHADENOPATHY

Sarcoidosis is a disease of unknown etiology characterized by granulomatous inflammation in various organs. The disease can occur in young adulthood to late middle age in both men and women, although men tend to present at an earlier age. It is more common in African American patients than in Caucasians. Clinically, sarcoidosis can involve any organ in the body; however, lungs and mediastinal/hilar lymph nodes are the most frequently involved. Skin and other lymph node groups are also common sites of involvement. Significant laboratory findings include hypercalcemia, hypercalciuria, elevated angiotensin-converting enzyme and hypergammaglobulinemia.[12]

Histologically, sarcoidosis is characterized by multiple well-formed, noncaseating granulomas. Lymph node involvement can be extensive with coalescing granulomas and nearly complete obliteration of lymph node architecture (Figure 3.36). The granulomas often have multinucleated giant cells (Figure 3.37). Several types of inclusion bodies including

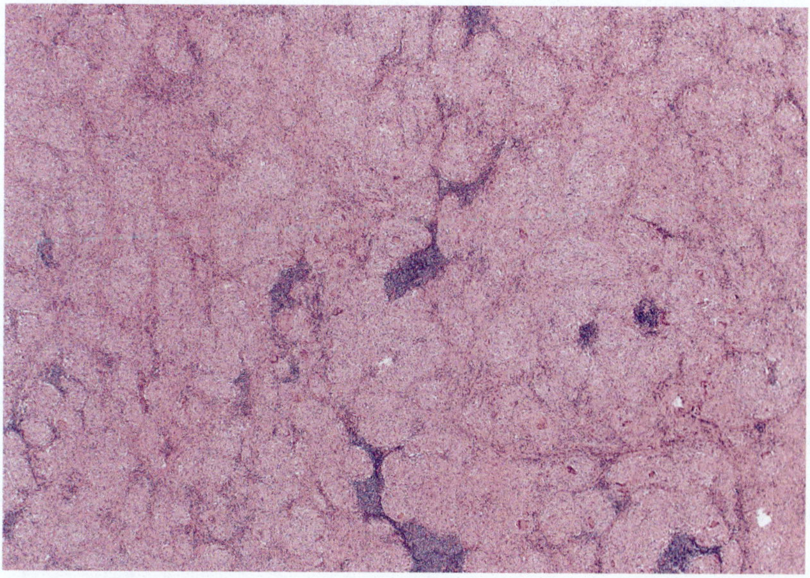

FIGURE 3.36 **Sarcoidosis.** Numerous small granulomas without necrosis obscuring the lymph node architecture.

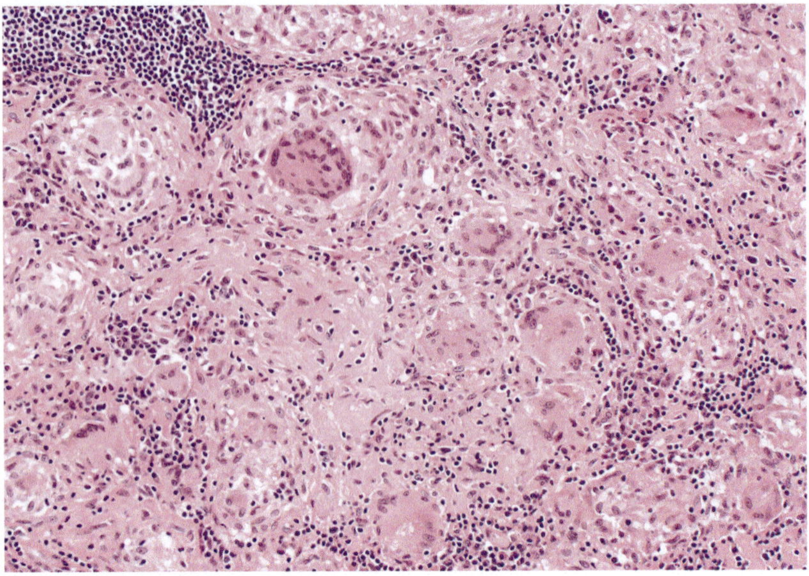

FIGURE 3.37 **Sarcoidosis.** Granulomas with hyalinization and giant cells.

asteroid, Hamazaki-Wesenberg, and Schaumann can also be seen.[12] Small areas of fibrinoid necrosis may be present, but there are typically no large areas of necrosis. In older lesions, hyalinization may be seen, which can lead to confusion with necrotizing granulomas.

The differential diagnosis of sarcoidosis includes mycobacterial and fungal infections, although these typically show necrosis/caseation. As infection must always be considered, sarcoidosis is considered a diagnosis of exclusion. Special stains for fungi and acid-fast bacilli should be routinely performed to exclude infection, although these are not as sensitive as universal PCR, which could be performed if infection is still suspected clinically. The differential diagnosis of sarcoidosis also includes a foreign-body giant cell reaction, which can be assessed with polarization of the tissue. It is also important to recognize that hilar lymph nodes often have prominent sinus histiocytosis with anthracotic pigment admixed, and therefore, it is important not to misdiagnose these normal findings as sarcoidosis or infection. Furthermore, small epithelioid granulomas can be associated with both Hodgkin and non-Hodgkin lymphomas. It is therefore important to carefully examine the biopsy to make sure that the granulomas do not disguise underlying lymphoma.

AUTOIMMUNE LYMPHADENOPATHY

Patients with autoimmune diseases frequently have lymphadenopathy, and many autoimmune conditions carry an increased risk of lymphoma. Although the large majority of enlarged lymph nodes in these individuals are benign, lymph node biopsies are performed to evaluate for a lymphoproliferative disorder. Knowledge of clinical and medication history is paramount for adequate assessment of these lymph nodes specimens.

Rheumatoid Arthritis

Rheumatoid arthritis (RA) is an autoimmune disease that typically develops in young to middle-aged adults and is more frequent in women. Clinically, RA typically affects joints, but lymphadenopathy is seen in over half of the patients during the course of the disease. The most commonly enlarged lymph nodes are the ones draining affected joints, including axillary, cervical, inguinal, and epitrochlear.[12] The finding of lymphadenopathy in the setting of RA may be concerning, since these patients have an increased incidence of lymphoma compared with the general population. Contributing to increased lymphoma risk are medications (eg, methotrexate and TNF inhibitors) that are used to treat RA. These so-called iatrogenic lymphoproliferative disorders that arise in people who take immunosuppressive medications are discussed in Chapter 8.

Morphologic findings in benign lymph nodes of patients with RA include FH and prominent interfollicular plasmacytosis. Other histologic findings include increased vascularity in the paracortex, foci of necrosis, and epithelioid granulomas.[39]

Immunohistochemistry or in situ hybridization can be used to demonstrate that the plasma cells are polyclonal. Interfollicular plasmacytosis is a nonspecific finding and can be seen in patients with other autoimmune diseases, lymph nodes draining malignancy, or in the plasma cell and multicentric variants of Castleman Disease (CD).

Systemic Lupus Erythematosus

SLE is a multisystem autoimmune disease with a marked female predominance and an age of onset in the second to fifth decade. The disease is frequently associated with lymphadenopathy, either localized (typically in cervical and axillary lymph nodes) or generalized.

The morphologic findings in the acute form of the disease may be nearly identical to those of KFD (histiocytic necrotizing lymphadenitis). Necrotic areas can be extensive and are surrounded by inflammatory cells (Figure 3.38). Necrotic foci contain cellular debris but no neutrophils. Hematoxylin bodies, darkly staining extracellular clumps of necrotic material, are seen in a small number of cases but are very helpful since they can distinguish lupus from KFD. Azzopardi effect around blood vessels (ie, deposits of degenerated nuclear material that stains with hematoxylin) may also be seen in SLE (Figure 3.39). In cases resembling KFD, a differential diagnosis should include both entities. Clinical and laboratory correlation is needed for definitive diagnosis. In chronic forms of SLE, the findings in lymph nodes are less specific and may resemble other autoimmune diseases such as RA or CD. FH is typically present with increased

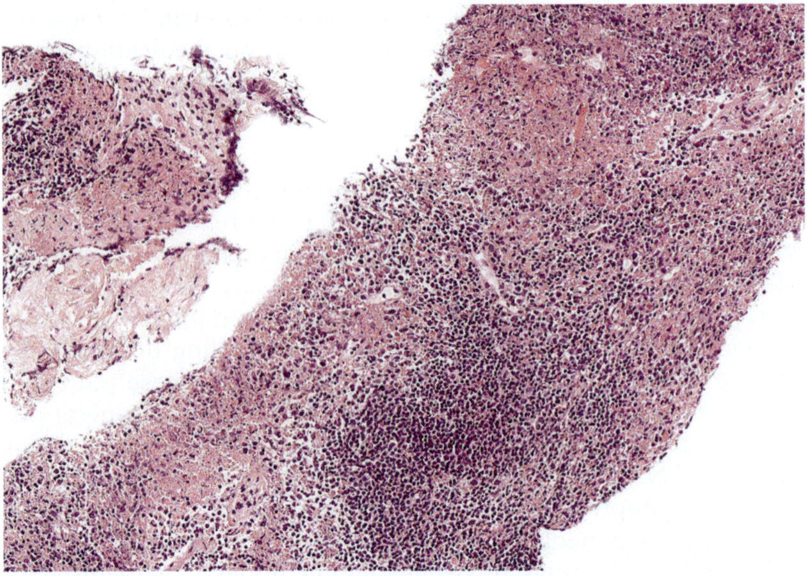

FIGURE 3.38 **Systemic lupus erythematosus lymphadenitis.** Lymph node with areas of necrosis and increased plasma cells.

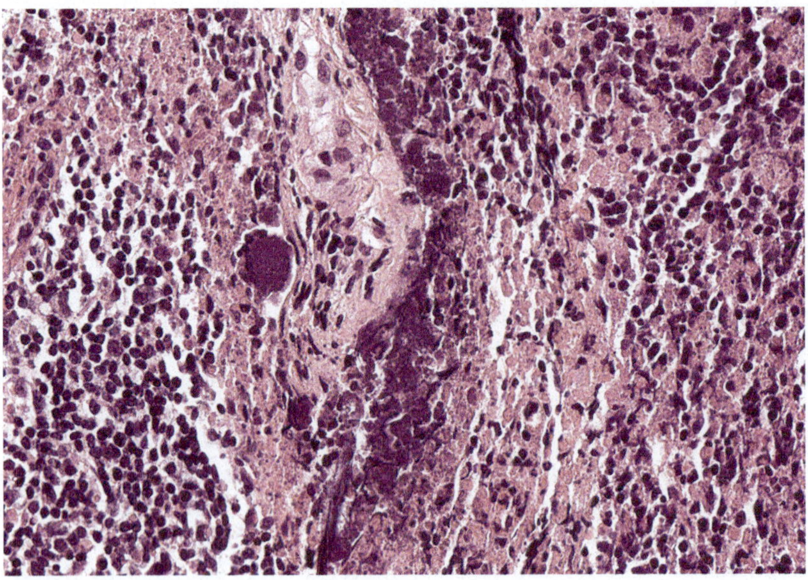

FIGURE 3.39 **Hematoxylin body adjacent to Azzopardi effect in SLE lymphadenitis.**

interfollicular plasma cells. Other nonspecific reactive patterns can sometimes be seen including immunoblastic proliferations and paracortical expansions. Core biopsies could be difficult to diagnose unless an area with an abrupt transition to necrosis is seen. If no viable tissue is present, a larger biopsy should be requested.[38,40,41] Confirmation is clinical and requires correlation with laboratory tests including antinuclear antibody (ANA), anti-double stranded DNA, and anti-Smith antibodies.

CASTLEMAN DISEASE

CD is a benign lymphoproliferative disease that involves lymph nodes and has two morphologic types including the hyaline vascular and the plasma cell variant. In some cases, both features may be prominent, and a mixed variant can be diagnosed. There are two clinical types of CD, unicentric and multicentric, which may show either morphologic pattern or be mixed. Unicentric CD presents as a localized mass, and excision of the mass typically results in resolution of symptoms. Multicentric CD is a systemic disease that presents with multiple signs and symptoms including diffuse lymphadenopathy, hepatosplenomegaly, rash, effusions, and B symptoms (ie, fever, weight loss and night sweats). Patients usually have laboratory abnormalities including cytopenias, polyclonal hypergammaglobulinemia, and elevated interleukin-6 (IL-6). Two types of multicentric CD exist, human herpesvirus 8 (HHV8)-positive and HHV8-negative (idiopathic), the positive one being the more common type. Most patients with HHV8-positive multicentric CD are HIV positive, but some are HIV negative and might have other types of immunosuppression or live in HHV8 endemic areas, such as the Mediterranean basin.[42]

Hyaline vascular CD typically presents as a single mass in young to middle-aged patients. Mediastinum is a common site of disease, but other lymph nodes can also be involved. The morphologic features include lymph node architecture distorted by a paracortical expansion with numerous high endothelial venules (Figure 3.40). The lymphoid follicles are increased and have small (regressively transformed) germinal centers, are depleted of small lymphocytes, and are frequently hyalinized. Characteristically, two or more germinal centers (so-called twinning) are present, which is a very helpful morphologic feature that is not seen frequently in other entities (Figure 3.41). Hyalinized vessels may radially penetrate the germinal centers creating a "lollipop" appearance (Figure 3.42). On low-power magnification, the increased interfollicular vascularity conveys an eosinophilic appearance between the small germinal centers. Interfollicular areas show a mixed inflammatory infiltrate, and focal clusters of plasmacytoid dendritic cells can be seen in some cases. The lymph node capsule is frequently thickened with fibrotic bands in the lymph node parenchyma. Hyaline vascular CD can be a difficult diagnosis to make on small biopsies. In stroma-rich cases, core biopsies may lead to a misdiagnosis of IgG4-related

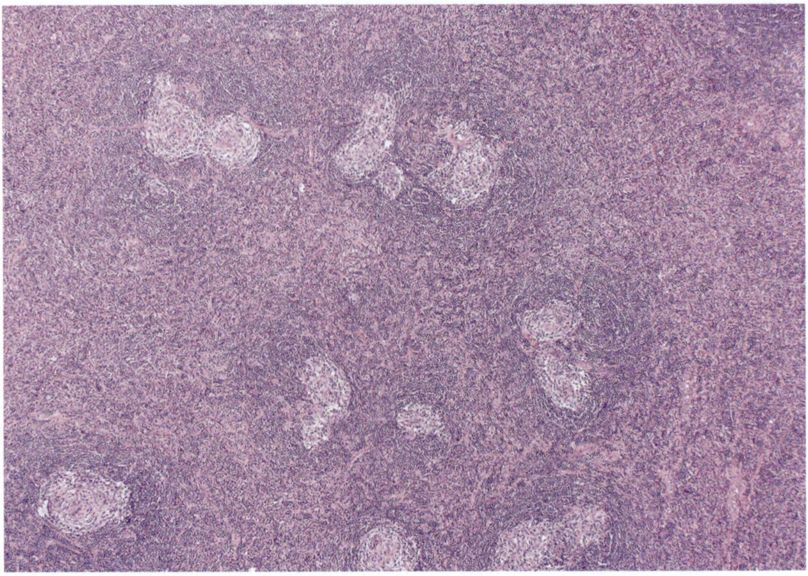

FIGURE 3.40 **Hyaline vascular Castleman disease.** Lymph node with regressively transformed germinal centers and increased interfollicular vessels.

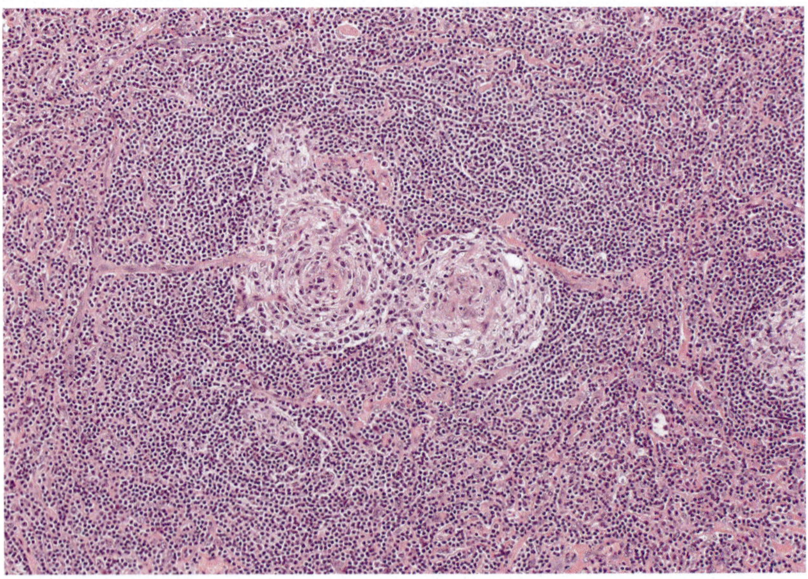

FIGURE 3.41 **Hyaline vascular Castleman disease.** Multiple germinal centers within a follicle (so-called twinning).

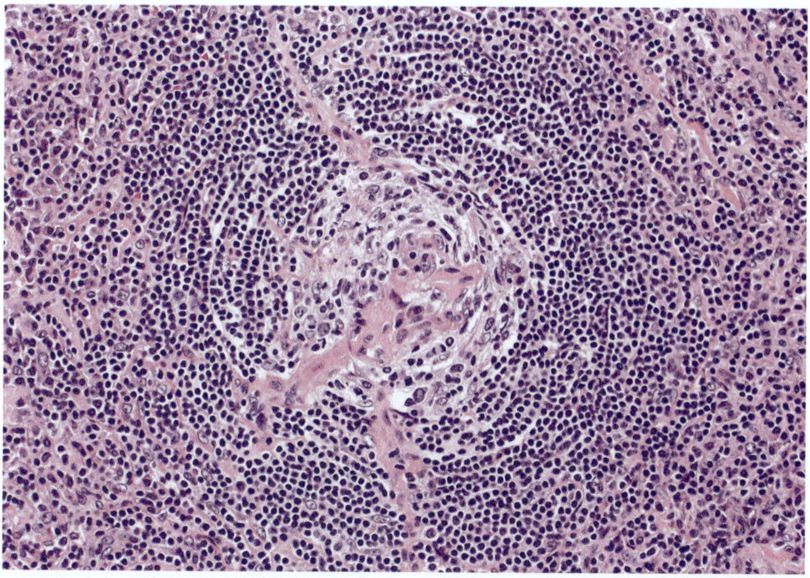

FIGURE 3.42 **Hyaline vascular Castleman disease.** Follicle with "onion skinning" of the mantle zone cells and a hyalinized vessel radially penetrating the germinal center.

lymphadenopathy or an inflammatory pseudotumor. A larger biopsy or complete excision (which is also curative) may be necessary for diagnosis.[43]

The morphologic findings in lymph nodes with the plasma cell variant include expanded paracortex and medulla by sheets of plasma cells in an interfollicular pattern (Figure 3.43). The germinal centers are usually more normal-appearing, or can be small/regressed, as in the hyaline vascular type, a feature commonly seen in multicentric CD (Figure 3.44). The interfollicular areas may also contain increased vascularity. In HHV8-positive multicentric CD, larger cells with plasmablastic or immunoblastic morphology that are HHV8 positive are typically seen in the mantle zones or germinal centers (Figure 3.45). These HHV8-positive cells show IgM staining (Figure 3.46) and lambda light chain restriction (ie, they are polyclonal by molecular studies but lambda-restricted/monotypic). Of note, the interfollicular plasma cells are polytypic when stained for kappa and lambda light chains. The differential diagnosis in these cases includes HIV lymphadenitis in the later chronic stages of disease and some lymphomas including angioimmunoblastic T-cell lymphoma. Cases that are HHV8-negative are more difficult to diagnose, as the histologic findings are less specific and the differential diagnosis is relatively broad. As there are many clinical criteria for diagnosis, a descriptive diagnosis is often required, and final diagnosis usually rests on the clinical team. The diagnostic criteria are summarized in Table 3.2, but the diagnosis requires exclusion of other mimics.[44] Differential diagnostic considerations include other autoimmune

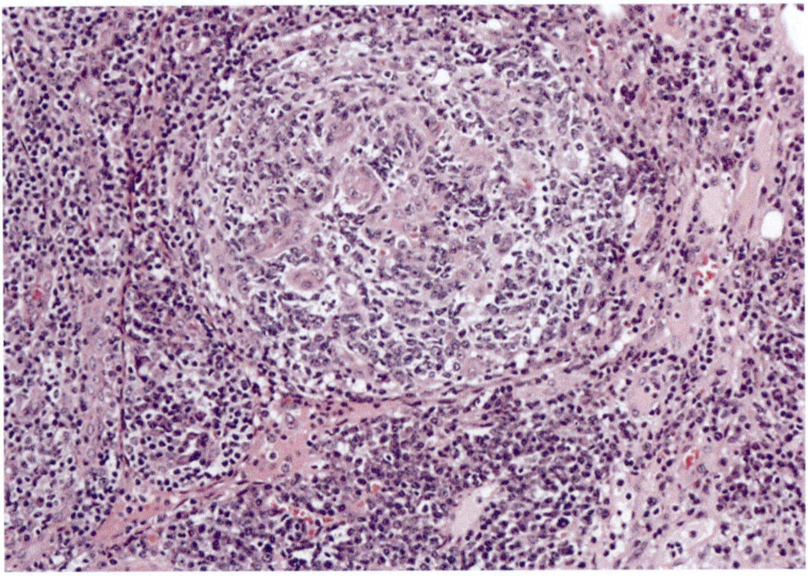

FIGURE 3.43 Plasma cell variant of Castleman disease showing sheets of plasma cells in interfollicular area.

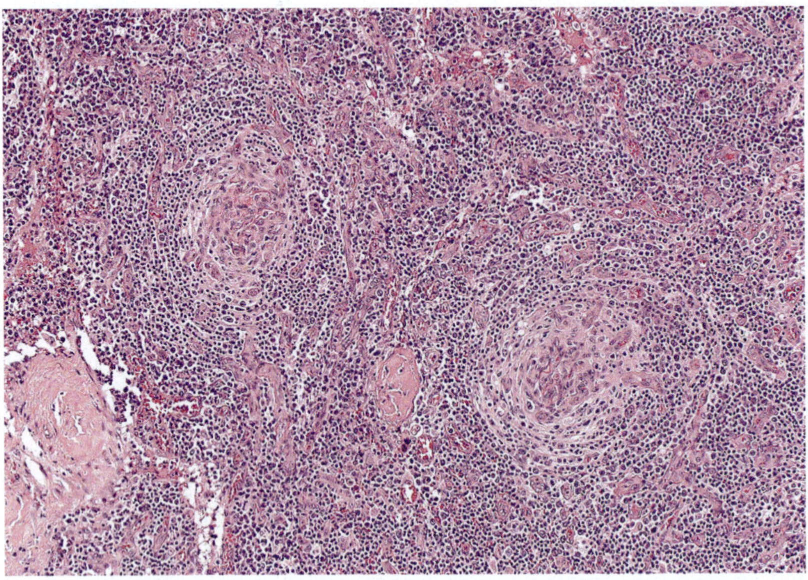

FIGURE 3.44 Multicentric Castleman disease showing regressed germinal centers and increased vascularity in the paracortex.

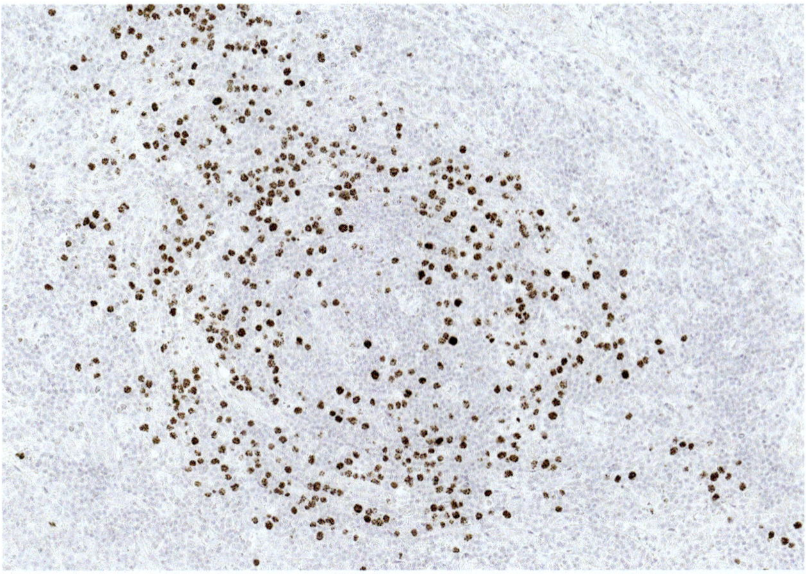

FIGURE 3.45 HHV8 immunohistochemical stain demonstrating positive cells (plasmablasts) in an HIV-positive patient with multicentric Castleman disease.

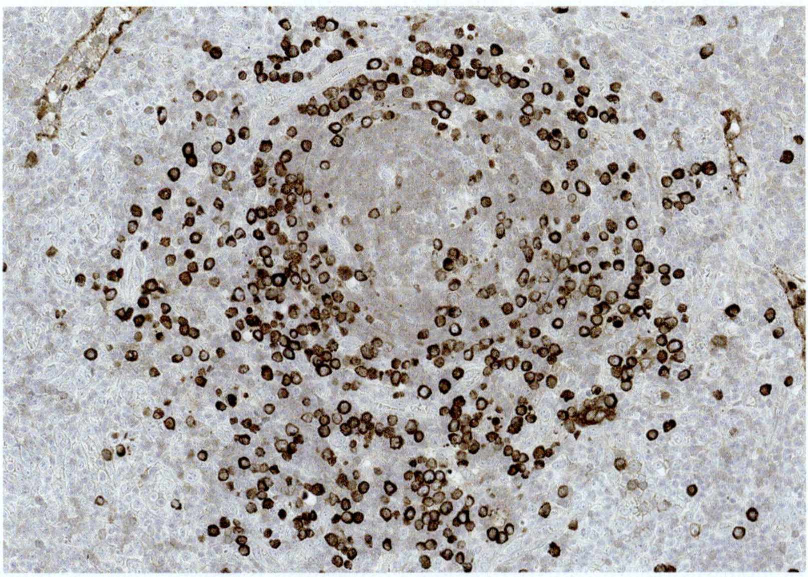

FIGURE 3.46 **IgM immunohistochemical stain showing positive plasmablasts in multicentric Castleman disease.** Plasmablasts are predominantly distributed in mantle zones.

TABLE 3.2 **Diagnostic Criteria for HHV8-negative Multicentric Castleman Disease**[44]

Criteria
Major
Histopathologic features 1. Atrophic/regressed germinal centers 2. Follicular dendritic cell prominence 3. Vascularity 4. Polytypic plasmacytosis 5. Hyperplastic germinal centers
Lymphadenopathy
Minor
Elevated C-reactive protein (CRP) or erythrocyte sedimentation rate (ESR)
Anemia
Thrombocytopenia/thrombocytosis
Hypoalbuminemia
Renal dysfunction

diseases and lymph nodes draining malignancy. IgG4-related disease is also a diagnostic consideration in patients with these findings.

DERMATOPATHIC LYMPHADENOPATHY

Dermatopathic lymphadenopathy (DL) is typically seen in regional lymph nodes draining a skin rash.[45] It can be seen in patients with reactive skin conditions as well as patients with mycosis fungoides/Sezary syndrome or angioimmunoblastic T-cell lymphoma. It may occur in lymph nodes above or below the diaphragm. If lymph nodes are not enlarged or the findings are not well-developed, dermatopathic change is the preferred term. Most of these patients have no clinical history of skin disease. Dermatopathic change is a relatively common incidental finding in lymph nodes biopsied or excised for other conditions (eg, cancer staging).

Lymph node architecture is preserved, and there is a paracortical expansion with nodular pale/mottled areas under the capsule, best appreciated on low-power magnification (Figure 3.47). These areas are composed of histiocytes, Langerhans cells, interdigitating dendritic cells, and occasional scattered histiocytes containing pigment, usually melanin or less commonly hemosiderin (Figure 3.48).[46,47] This condition should not be confused with Langerhans cell histiocytosis, which is characterized by larger clusters of Langerhans cells filling lymph node sinuses. Immunohistochemical studies are not usually warranted in routine cases

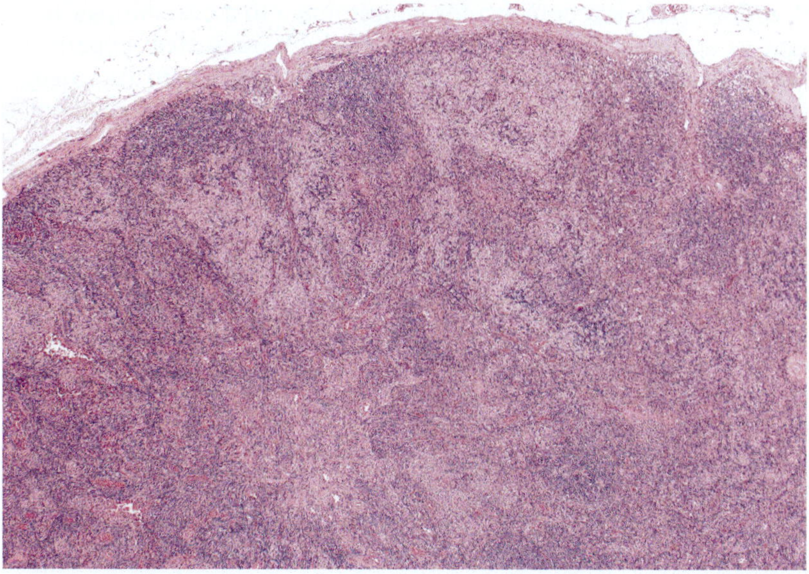

FIGURE 3.47 **Dermatopathic lymphadenopathy.** Lymph node in a patient with skin rash showing paracortical expansion with "nodules" containing numerous pale cells corresponding to histiocytes, Langerhans cells, and interdigitating dendritic cells.

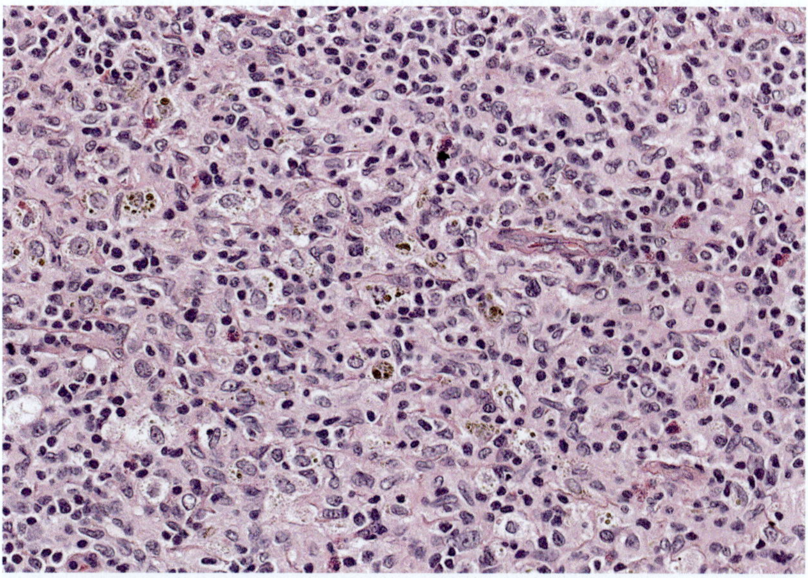

FIGURE 3.48 **Dermatopathic lymphadenopathy.** Mixed inflammatory infiltrate with numerous histiocytes showing brown pigment.

of DL unless there is a concern for lymphoma. On a core biopsy, it may be difficult to appreciate the architecture of the paracortical expansion, but a mixture of cells with abundant eosinophilic cytoplasm (ie, histiocytes, Langerhans cells, and interdigitating dendritic cells) and pigment-laden macrophages can be easily seen.

KIMURA LYMPHADENOPATHY

Kimura lymphadenopathy is a rare condition of unknown etiology that involves subcutaneous tissues and regional lymph nodes, most commonly in the head and neck region. Posterior auricular lymph nodes are typically involved. The disease is most commonly reported in Asian countries, but it has been described around the world with a male predominance. Nearly all patients present with eosinophilia and increased levels of IgE.

The morphologic findings include FH with occasional follicle lysis by infiltrating eosinophils and increased vessels in germinal centers.[48] There are interfollicular sheets of eosinophils as well as eosinophilic microabscesses (Figures 3.49 and 3.50). Thin-walled capillaries are often prominent in the paracortex. Warthin-Finkeldey type giant cells may be seen (Figure 3.51).

The diagnosis is typically suspected based on clinicopathologic findings. This condition should be distinguished from angiolymphoid hyperplasia with eosinophilia (also known as epithelioid hemangioma), which is localized to the skin and should not involve lymph nodes unless they

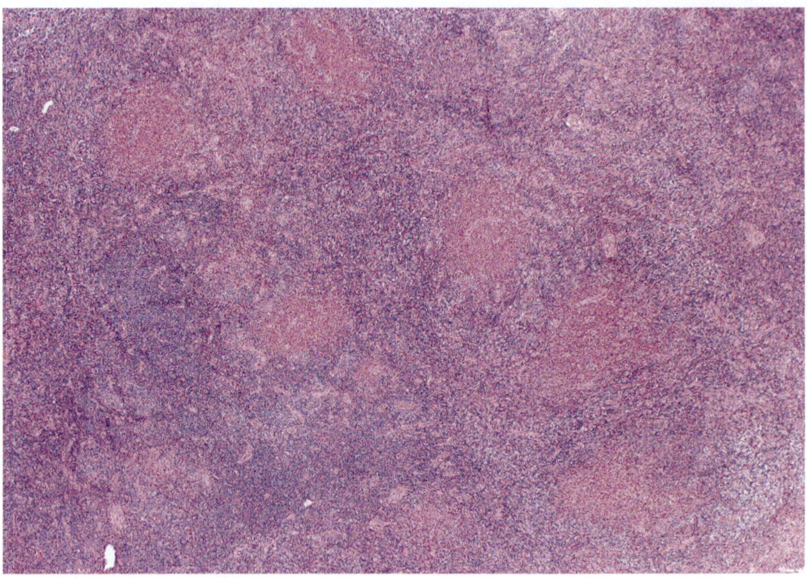

FIGURE 3.49 **Kimura disease.** Low magnification of a lymph node with eosinophilic microabscesses.

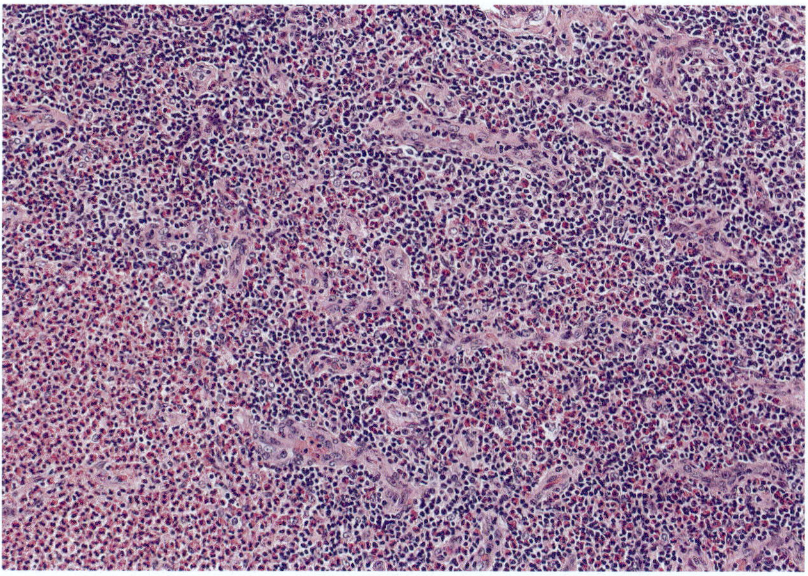

FIGURE 3.50 **Kimura disease.** Thin-walled vessels and sheets of eosinophils.

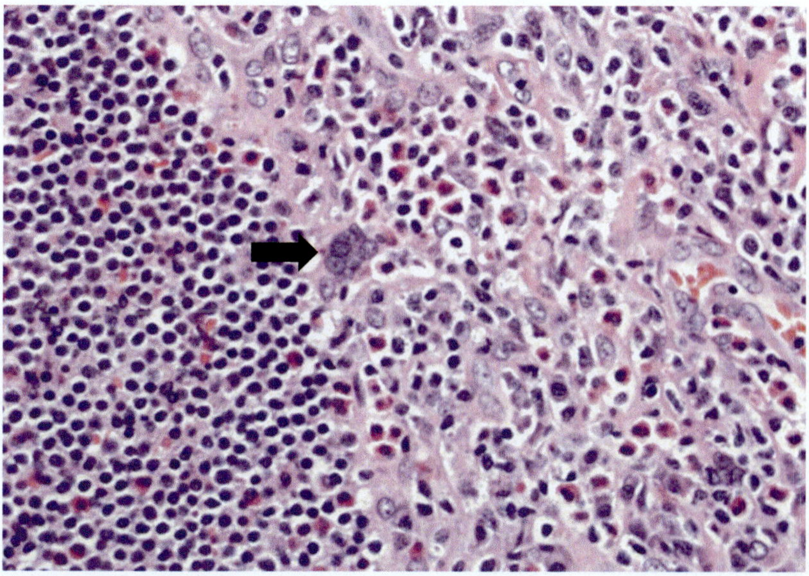

FIGURE 3.51 Warthin-Finkeldey-type giant cell (arrow) in Kimura disease with admixed eosinophils and thin-walled vessels. These cells can also be seen in measles and HIV infection.

are adjacent to the lesion. It also must be distinguished from other more common causes of eosinophilia in lymph nodes including drug/hypersensitivity reactions or parasitic infections and IgG4-related disease.[49-51]

IgG4-RELATED LYMPHADENOPATHY

IgG4-related disease (IgG4-RD) has become a more widely recognized entity in recent years and is associated with systemic sclerosis in a number of different organs and a variable clinical presentation. While the findings in some organs are quite characteristic (eg, autoimmune pancreatitis), the findings in lymph nodes are less specific and require clinical correlation. Any lymph node can be involved, and lymphadenopathy can be one of the first presenting symptoms, or it can be detected during diagnostic workup of these patients.

Enlarged lymph nodes in patients with IgG4-RD can have a variety of morphologic appearances that overlap with other reactive conditions, and there are five histologic types recognized. These are type I, multicentric Castleman-like; type II, FH; type III, PCH with plasmacytosis; type IV, FFH and PTGC; and type V, inflammatory pseudotumor-like. Only type V (the least common pattern) is specific for IgG4-related disease.[52,53]

Since FH with PTGC is relatively unusual in adults, this finding often prompts immunohistochemistry for IgG and IgG4. Moreover, increased plasma cells in germinal centers is an unusual finding that should make one consider this diagnosis. Regardless of the pattern, the diagnosis should be considered when IgG4-positive plasma cells represent ≥40% of the IgG-positive cells and the number of IgG4-positive plasma cells is >100 per high power field (Figure 3.52A and B). The distribution of plasma cells may be patchy.[8] However, an increase in IgG4-positive cells is nonspecific and not diagnostic of IgG4-related disease in isolation, and the lymph node biopsy should not be used as the sole criteria for IgG4-RD. Clinical, laboratory, and radiologic correlation is needed for definitive diagnosis of this entity.

The differential diagnosis includes a number of benign entities that result in one of the lymph node patterns seen in IgG4-related lymphadenopathy. Other differential diagnostic considerations include lymphomas that can have increased IgG4-positive plasma cells, such as marginal zone lymphoma, other B-cell lymphomas with plasmacytic differentiation, or plasmacytoma (rare in lymph nodes).[54] On a core biopsy this can be a difficult diagnosis, but one to consider in cases that show preserved architecture with plasmacytosis in the reactive follicles or paracortical areas in the appropriate clinical setting.

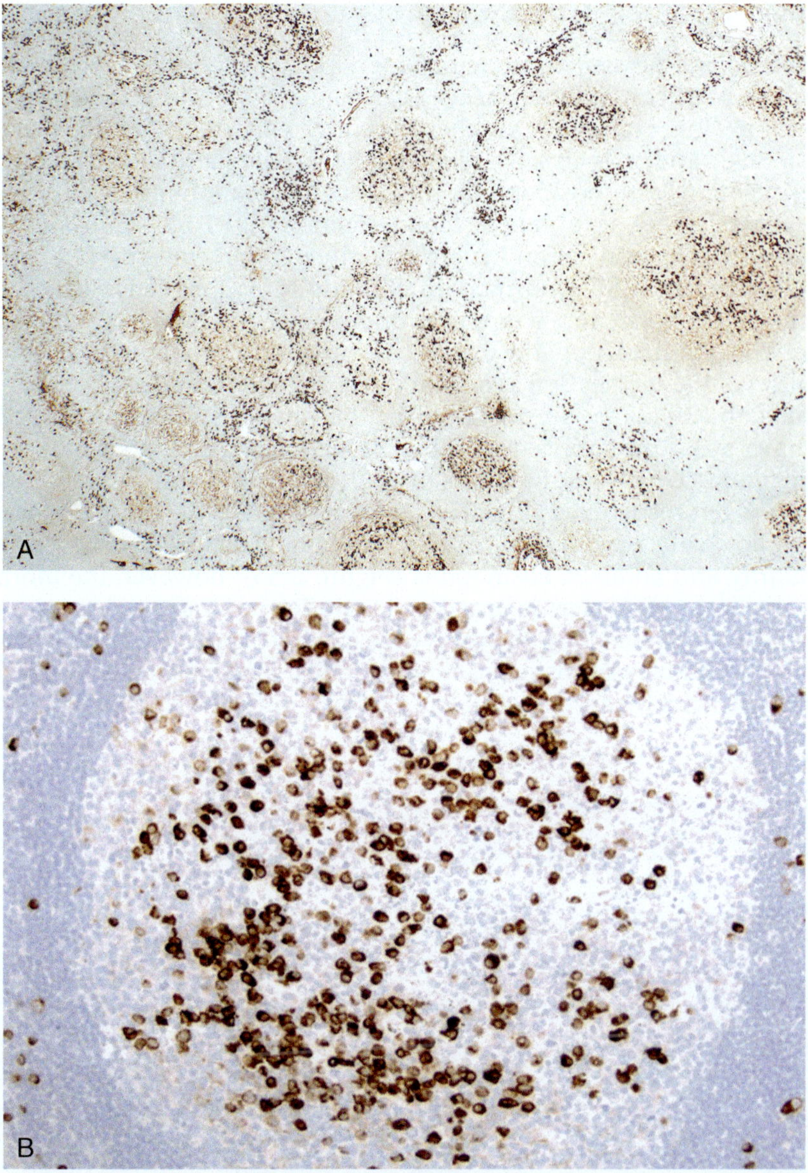

FIGURE 3.52 **IgG4-related disease.** IgG4 immunohistochemical stain showing increased but variable numbers of IgG4-positive plasma cells in the germinal centers (A). IgG4-positive plasma cells are greater than 100 per high power field (B).

DRUG-INDUCED LYMPHADENOPATHY

Many medications can cause lymphadenopathy, the well-recognized culprits being anticonvulsants such as carbamazepine, phenytoin, and phenobarbital, for example. Lymphadenopathy can be either localized or widespread, and it is usually seen is association with so-called DRESS (drug reaction with eosinophilia and systemic symptoms) syndrome. In some cases, there is a genetic component to DRESS syndrome, with increased risk of medication hypersensitivity in family members of patients who also had DRESS syndrome. In addition to lymphadenopathy, a concomitant rash, systemic symptoms, and/or peripheral eosinophilia may occur. The lymphadenopathy tends to occur several weeks to months after initiation of the medication and should resolve with cessation. It may recur if similar medications are restarted in the future. Patients with DRESS can have quite pronounced lymphadenopathy with metabolically active lymph nodes which are biopsied to rule out lymphoma. In some cases, DRESS is not recognized clinically, and lymphoma is the primary concern. Morphologically, a prominent paracortical expansion is seen with increased vascularity and admixed eosinophils (Figure 3.53); however, the morphologic spectrum of changes is broad and includes pronounced immunoblastic proliferations that may be positive for CD30 (Figures 3.54 and 3.55).[55,56] Increased numbers of histiocytes, neutrophils, and plasma cells may also be present, which can make diagnosis more difficult. Moreover, patients

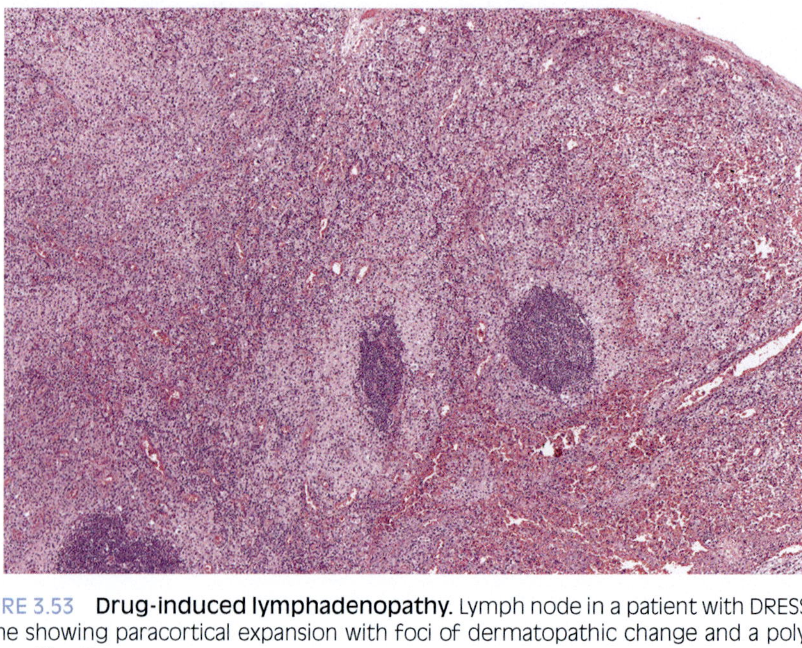

FIGURE 3.53 **Drug-induced lymphadenopathy.** Lymph node in a patient with DRESS syndrome showing paracortical expansion with foci of dermatopathic change and a polymorphic proliferation.

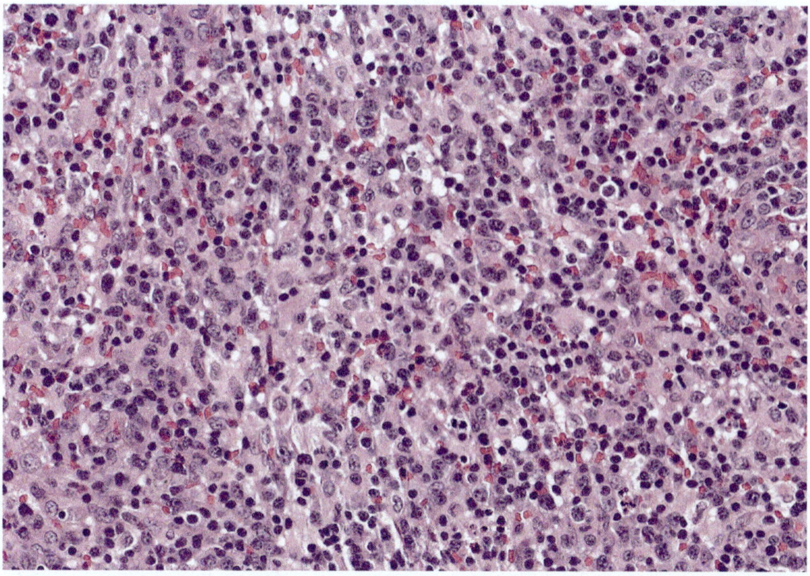

FIGURE 3.54 Increased immunoblasts, eosinophils, and plasma cells in the lymph node with drug-induced lymphadenopathy, an infiltrate that may mimic lymphoma.

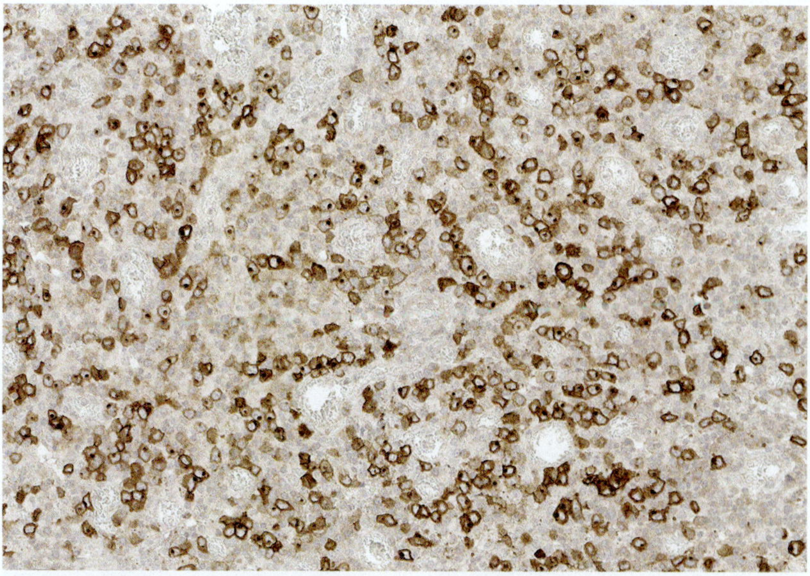

FIGURE 3.55 Numerous immunoblasts are highlighted by CD30 in drug-induced lymphadenopathy.

with rash can also have pronounced dermatopathic change in the lymph node, which further confounds morphologic assessment. One of the most commonly entertained differential diagnoses is angioimmunoblastic T-cell lymphoma. Diagnosis of drug-induced lymphadenopathy is very difficult on a core biopsy in the majority of cases. Excisional biopsy is the optimal specimen in these cases since the architecture can be carefully evaluated and correlated with immunohistochemical stains.

VASCULAR TRANSFORMATION OF SINUSES

Vascular transformation of sinuses is a finding that occurs when the sinuses become lined with endothelial cells forming vascular channels (Figures 3.56 and 3.57).[57,58] It is more common in abdominal lymph nodes but may occur at any location. It is often an incidental finding discovered during abdominal surgery for other conditions. The etiology is unknown, but it may be due to venous obstruction. The morphologic findings include a proliferation of endothelial cells that may be seen in association with sclerosis. Vascular transformation of sinuses is frequently difficult to appreciate on a small biopsy, and the differential diagnosis would include vascular neoplasms or tumors such as Kaposi sarcoma or hemangioma. If the endothelial cells are plump it could also resemble bacillary angiomatosis.

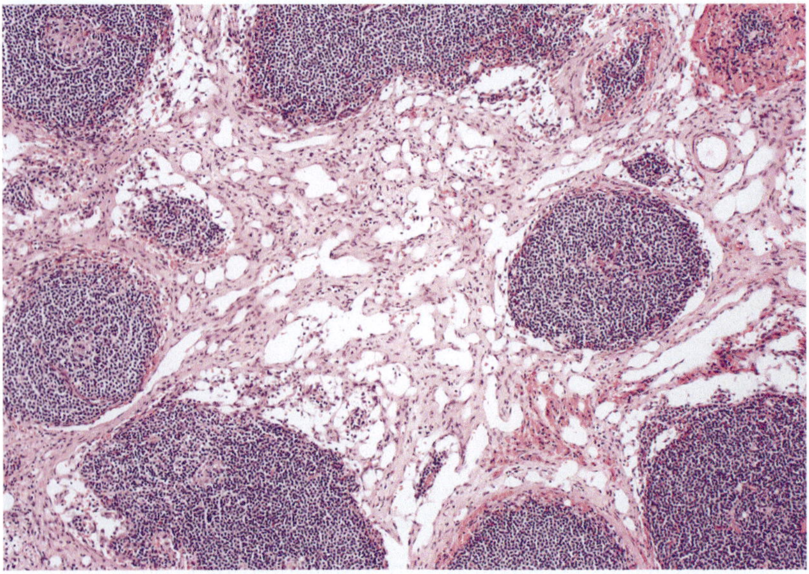

FIGURE 3.56 **Vascular transformation of sinuses.** A proliferation of thin-walled vessel in a lymph node sinus.

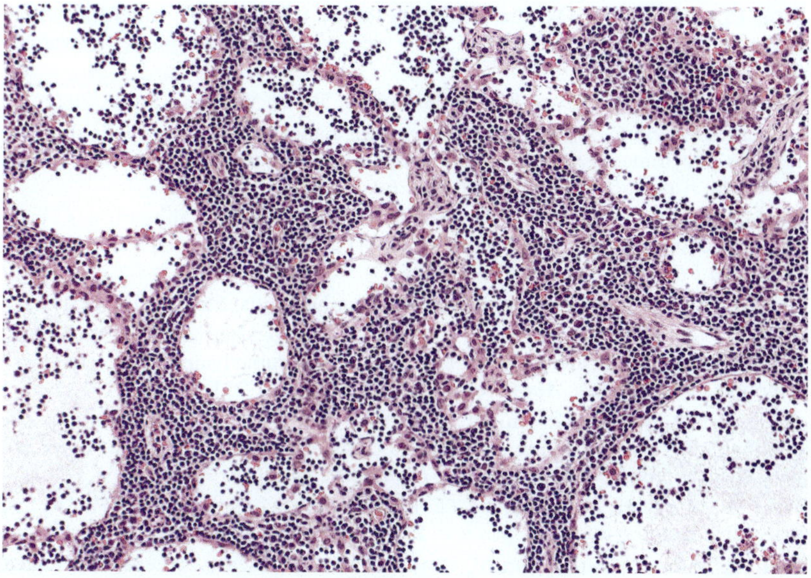

FIGURE 3.57 Another type of appearance that can be seen in vascular transformation of sinuses with plump endothelial cells.

REFERENCES

1. Kussick SJ, Kalnoski M, Braziel RM, Wood BL. Prominent clonal B-cell populations identified by flow cytometry in histologically reactive lymphoid proliferations. *Am J Clin Pathol*. 2004;121(4):464-472.
2. Weiss LM, O'Malley D. Benign lymphadenopathies. *Mod Pathol*. 2013;26(suppl 1): S88-S96.
3. Chang CC, Osipov V, Wheaton S, Tripp S, Perkins SL. Follicular hyperplasia, follicular lysis, and progressive transformation of germinal centers. A sequential spectrum of morphologic evolution in lymphoid hyperplasia. *Am J Clin Pathol*. 2003;120(3):322-326.
4. Egan C, Jaffe ES. Non-neoplastic histiocytic and dendritic cell disorders in lymph nodes. *Semin Diagn Pathol*. 2018;35(1):20-33.
5. Hartmann S, Winkelmann R, Metcalf RA, et al. Immunoarchitectural patterns of progressive transformation of germinal centers with and without nodular lymphocyte-predominant Hodgkin lymphoma. *Hum Pathol*. 2015;46(11):1655-1661.
6. Nguyen PL, Ferry JA, Harris NL. Progressive transformation of germinal centers and nodular lymphocyte predominance Hodgkin's disease: a comparative immunohistochemical study. *Am J Surg Pathol*. 1999;23(1):27-33.
7. Shaikh F, Ngan BY, Alexander S, Grant R. Progressive transformation of germinal centers in children and adolescents: an intriguing cause of lymphadenopathy. *Pediatr Blood Cancer*. 2013;60(1):26-30.
8. Grimm KE, Barry TS, Chizhevsky V, et al. Histopathological findings in 29 lymph node biopsies with increased IgG4 plasma cells. *Mod Pathol*. 2012;25(3):480-491.
9. Dunmire SK, Verghese PS, Balfour HH Jr. Primary Epstein-Barr virus infection. *J Clin Virol*. 2018;102:84-92.
10. Louissaint A Jr, Ferry JA, Soupir CP, Hasserjian RP, Harris NL, Zukerberg LR. Infectious mononucleosis mimicking lymphoma: distinguishing morphological and immunophenotypic features. *Mod Pathol*. 2012;25(8):1149-1159.

11. Lum EL, Schaenman JM, DeNicola M, Reddy UG, Shen JI, Pullarkat ST. A case report of CMV lymphadenitis in an adult kidney transplant recipient. *Transplant Proc.* 2015;47(1):141-145.
12. Medeiros L. *Ioachim's Lymph Node Pathology*. 5th ed. Wolters Kluwer; 2021.
13. Joubert M, Morin C, Moreau A, Heymann MF, Laboisse C, Gaillard F. Histopathologic features of cytomegalovirus lymphadenitis in the "immunocompetent" patient. Report of 7 cases. *Ann Pathol.* 1996;16(4):254-260.
14. Rushin JM, Riordan GP, Heaton RB, Sharpe RW, Cotelingam JD, Jaffe ES. Cytomegalovirus-infected cells express Leu-M1 antigen. A potential source of diagnostic error. *Am J Pathol.* 1990;136(5):989-995.
15. Villa D, Skinnider B. Herpes simplex virus lymphadenitis. *Blood.* 2014;123(1):12.
16. Joseph L, Scott MA, Schichman SA, Zent CS. Localized herpes simplex lymphadenitis mimicking large-cell (Richter's) transformation of chronic lymphocytic leukemia/small lymphocytic lymphoma. *Am J Hematol.* 2001;68(4):287-291.
17. Hodgson YA, Jones SG, Knight H, Sovani V, Fox CP. Herpes simplex necrotic lymphadenitis masquerading as Richter's transformation in treatment-naive patients with chronic lymphocytic leukemia. *J Hematol.* 2019;8(2):79-82.
18. Wear DJ, Margileth AM, Hadfield TL, Fischer GW, Schlagel CJ, King FM. Cat scratch disease: a bacterial infection. *Science.* 1983;221(4618):1403-1405.
19. Kudo E, Sakaki A, Sumitomo M, et al. Cat scratch disease. An epidemiological and ultrastructural study of lymphadenitis caused by Warthin-Starry positive bacteria. *Virchows Arch A Pathol Anat Histopathol.* 1988;412(6):563-572.
20. Miller-Catchpole R, Variakojis D, Vardiman JW, Loew JM, Carter J. Cat scratch disease. Identification of bacteria in seven cases of lymphadenitis. *Am J Surg Pathol.* 1986;10(4):276-281.
21. Petersen K, Earhart KC, Wallace MR. Bacillary angiomatosis in a patient with chronic lymphocytic leukemia. *Infection.* 2008;36(5):480-484.
22. Schmidt R, Carson PJ, Jansen RJ. Resurgence of syphilis in the United States: an assessment of contributing factors. *Infect Dis (Auckl).* 2019;12:1178633719883282.
23. Liu Z, Zhang C, Kakudo K, et al. Diagnostic pitfalls in pathological diagnosis of infectious disease: patients with syphilitic lymphadenitis often present with inconspicuous history of infection. *Pathol Int.* 2016;66(3):142-147.
24. Farhi DC, Wells SJ, Siegel RJ. Syphilitic lymphadenopathy. Histology and human immunodeficiency virus status. *Am J Clin Pathol.* 1999;112(3):330-334.
25. Duffield AS, Borowitz MJ. Syphilitic lymphadenitis with abscess formation involving cervical lymph nodes. *Blood.* 2018;131(6):707.
26. Porter JD, McAdam KP. The re-emergence of tuberculosis. *Annu Rev Public Health.* 1994;15:303-323.
27. Ramanathan VD, Jawahar MS, Paramasivan CN, et al. A histological spectrum of host responses in tuberculous lymphadenitis. *Indian J Med Res.* 1999;109:212-220.
28. Evans MJ, Smith NM, Thornton CM, Youngson GG, Gray ES. Atypical mycobacterial lymphadenitis in childhood – a clinicopathological study of 17 cases. *J Clin Pathol.* 1998;51(12):925-927.
29. Jarzembowski JA, Young MB. Nontuberculous mycobacterial infections. *Arch Pathol Lab Med.* 2008;132(8):1333-1341.
30. van de Vosse E, van Wengen A, van der Meide WF, Visser LG, van Dissel JT. A 38-year-old woman with necrotising cervical lymphadenitis due to Histoplasma capsulatum. *Infection.* 2017;45(6):917-920.
31. Gurney JW, Conces DJ. Pulmonary histoplasmosis. *Radiology.* 1996;199(2):297-306.
32. Gupta N, Arora SK, Rajwanshi A, Nijhawan R, Srinivasan R. Histoplasmosis: cytodiagnosis and review of literature with special emphasis on differential diagnosis on cytomorphology. *Cytopathology.* 2010;21(4):240-244.

33. Lin MH, Kuo TT. Specificity of the histopathological triad for the diagnosis of toxoplasmic lymphadenitis: polymerase chain reaction study. *Pathol Int.* 2001;51(8):619-623.
34. Dorfman RF. Histiocytic necrotizing lymphadenitis of Kikuchi and Fujimoto. *Arch Pathol Lab Med.* 1987;111(11):1026-1029.
35. Dorfman RF, Berry GJ. Kikuchi's histiocytic necrotizing lymphadenitis: an analysis of 108 cases with emphasis on differential diagnosis. *Semin Diagn Pathol.* 1988;5(4):329-345.
36. Onciu M, Medeiros LJ. Kikuchi-Fujimoto lymphadenitis. *Adv Anat Pathol.* 2003;10(4):204-211.
37. Perry AM, Choi SM. Kikuchi-Fujimoto disease: a review. *Arch Pathol Lab Med.* 2018;142(11):1341-1346.
38. Dumas G, Prendki V, Haroche J, et al. Kikuchi-Fujimoto disease: retrospective study of 91 cases and review of the literature. *Medicine (Baltimore).* 2014;93(24):372-382.
39. Benaglio F, Vitolo B, Scarabelli M, et al. The draining lymph node in rheumatoid arthritis: current concepts and research perspectives. *Biomed Res Int.* 2015;2015:420251.
40. Eisner MD, Amory J, Mullaney B, Tierney L Jr, Browner WS. Necrotizing lymphadenitis associated with systemic lupus erythematosus. *Semin Arthritis Rheum.* 1996;26(1):477-482.
41. Kojima M, Nakamura S, Morishita Y, et al. Reactive follicular hyperplasia in the lymph node lesions from systemic lupus erythematosus patients: a clinicopathological and immunohistological study of 21 cases. *Pathol Int.* 2000;50(4):304-312.
42. Dispenzieri A, Fajgenbaum DC. Overview of Castleman disease. *Blood.* 2020;135(16):1353-1364.
43. Wang W, Medeiros LJ. Castleman disease. *Surg Pathol Clin.* 2019;12(3):849-863.
44. Fajgenbaum DC, Uldrick TS, Bagg A, et al. International, evidence-based consensus diagnostic criteria for HHV-8-negative/idiopathic multicentric Castleman disease. *Blood.* 2017;129(12):1646-1657.
45. Cooper RA, Dawson PJ, Rambo ON. Dermatopathic lymphadenopathy a clinicopathologic analysis of lymph node biopsy over a fifteen-year period. *Calif Med.* 1967;106(3):170-175.
46. Garces S, Yin CC, Miranda RN, et al. Clinical, histopathologic, and immunoarchitectural features of dermatopathic lymphadenopathy: an update. *Mod Pathol.* 2020;33(6):1104-1121.
47. Gould E, Porto R, Albores-Saavedra J, Ibe MJ. Dermatopathic lymphadenitis. The spectrum and significance of its morphologic features. *Arch Pathol Lab Med.* 1988;112(11):1145-1150.
48. Jaffe ES, Arber DA, Campo E, Harris NL, Quintanilla-Martinez L. *Hematopathology.* 2nd ed. Elsevier; 2017.
49. Abuel-Haija M, Hurford MT. Kimura disease. *Arch Pathol Lab Med.* 2007;131(4):650-651.
50. Chen H, Thompson LD, Aguilera NS, Abbondanzo SL. Kimura disease: a clinicopathologic study of 21 cases. *Am J Surg Pathol.* 2004;28(4):505-513.
51. Kuo TT, Shih LY, Chan HL. Kimura's disease. Involvement of regional lymph nodes and distinction from angiolymphoid hyperplasia with eosinophilia. *Am J Surg Pathol.* 1988;12(11):843-854.
52. Wallace ZS, Naden RP, Chari S, et al. The 2019 American College of Rheumatology/European League Against Rheumatism classification criteria for IgG4-related disease. *Ann Rheum Dis.* 2020;79(1):77-87.
53. Wick MR, O'Malley DP. Lymphadenopathy associated with IgG4-related disease: diagnosis & differential diagnosis. *Semin Diagn Pathol.* 2018;35(1):61-66.
54. Bledsoe JR, Wallace ZS, Deshpande V, et al. Atypical IgG4+ plasmacytic proliferations and lymphomas: characterization of 11 cases. *Am J Clin Pathol.* 2017;148(3):215-235.

55. Abbondazo SL, Irey NS, Frizzera G. Dilantin-associated lymphadenopathy. Spectrum of histopathologic patterns. *Am J Surg Pathol.* 1995;19(6):675-686.
56. Chen HC, Wang RC, Tsai HP, Medeiros LJ, Chang KC. Morphologic spectrum of lymphadenopathy in drug reaction with eosinophilia and systemic symptoms syndrome. *Arch Pathol Lab Med.* 2022;146(9):1084-1093.
57. Chan JK, Warnke RA, Dorfman R. Vascular transformation of sinuses in lymph nodes. A study of its morphological spectrum and distinction from Kaposi's sarcoma. *Am J Surg Pathol.* 1991;15(8):732-743.
58. Ghosh P, Saha K, Ghosh AK. Vascular transformation of bilateral cervical lymph node sinuses: a rare entity masquerading as tumor recurrence. *J Maxillofac Oral Surg.* 2015;14(suppl 1):397-400.

4

PRECURSOR LYMPHOID NEOPLASMS, MYELOID SARCOMA, AND BLASTIC PLASMACYTOID DENDRITIC CELL NEOPLASM

ANAMARIJA M. PERRY

Precursor/immature hematopoietic neoplasms can involve lymph nodes and extranodal tissues, and in rare cases the initial diagnosis is made on a lymph node biopsy. This chapter covers four of the most frequently encountered acute leukemias seen in the lymph node, including B- and T-lymphoblastic leukemia/lymphoma (ALL/LBL), myeloid sarcoma, and blastic plasmacytoid dendritic cell neoplasm (BPDCN). Especially in a small biopsy, all of the precursor neoplasms discussed in this chapter can look very similar on hematoxylin and eosin (H&E)-stained sections and typically show sheets of cells with features of blasts, including round to variably irregular/convoluted nuclei, fine/dusty chromatin, and variably prominent nucleoli. Some morphologic features and/or clinical presentation can suggest a certain entity, but definitive diagnosis requires comprehensive immunophenotypic and genetic studies. Flow cytometry can be particularly useful in this setting. If fresh tissue is available and a diagnosis of acute leukemia in tissue is suspected, conventional cytogenetic studies can be useful. Molecular and/or fluorescence in situ hybridization studies, either on fresh or paraffin-embedded tissue can also be applied if needed. A lymph node biopsy does not supplant the need for a bone marrow aspirate and biopsy; however, if the bone marrow is not involved, complete genetic and immunophenotypic workup may be necessary on a paraffin block. For a newly diagnosed blastic neoplasm in tissue, the immunohistochemistry workup should include myeloid markers (myeloperoxidase (MPO), lysozyme, and CD117), B-cell markers (CD19, CD20, and PAX5), T-cell marker CD3, markers of immature cells (CD34 and TdT), and CD43, a general hematopoietic marker that will often stain blasts of myeloid and T-cell lineage. CD45 may be considered if nonhematolymphoid small round blue cell tumors are in the differential diagnosis. If BPDCN is a consideration, CD4, CD56, CD123, CD303, and

TCL1 should be performed, as well as the lineage markers above. Finally, some mature lymphoid neoplasms can have blastoid cytology such as high-grade B-cell lymphoma and blastoid variant of mantle cell lymphoma, which are addressed in more detail in Chapter 5. The phenotypes of different precursor neoplasms discussed in this chapter are summarized in Table 4.1.

B-LYMPHOBLASTIC LEUKEMIA/LYMPHOMA

B-lymphoblastic leukemia/lymphoma (B-ALL/LBL) is a neoplasm of lymphoid progenitors committed to B-cell lineage (B lymphoblasts). Similar to the 2017 World Health Organization (WHO) Classification, the 2022 International Consensus Classification (ICC) recognizes two broad categories, B-ALL/LBL with recurrent genetic abnormalities and B-ALL/LBL, not otherwise specified.[1,2] B-ALL comprises 80% of all acute leukemias in childhood and 20% of acute leukemias in adulthood. Children under 6 years of age are most affected. The patients usually present with extensive bone marrow involvement resulting in cytopenia(s) and a variable number of circulating blasts in peripheral blood. In the clinical and pathology practice, the distinction between B-ALL and B-LBL is arbitrary and defined as follows. If the blasts in the bone marrow and/or peripheral blood comprise ≥25% of cells, diagnosis of B-ALL is made. However, if the disease is primarily in lymph nodes or extranodal sites, without or with minimal blood and bone marrow involvement, the term B-LBL is used. B-lymphoblastic lymphoma comprises only 10% of all lymphoblastic lymphomas. The most common sites of involvement are skin, lymph nodes, and bone, but other extranodal sites can be involved. The majority of patients who present with B-LBL are children under 18 years of age.[1,3-6] Children have significantly higher cure rates than adults.[7,8] B-ALL/LBL is an aggressive disease that requires intensive chemotherapy protocols, as well as other therapeutic modalities in some cases.

Morphology

Lymph nodes are typically diffusely involved by sheets of blasts with frequent perinodal extension. In some cases, the infiltrate is paracortical with sparing of B-cell follicles. Occasionally, tingible body macrophages are seen, imparting a “starry sky” appearance. On H&E sections, lymphoblasts are usually small to medium sized with round to irregular nuclei, fine/dusty chromatin, inconspicuous to variably prominent nucleoli, and scant cytoplasm (Figures 4.1 and 4.2). Of note, B- and T-LBL are indistinguishable based on morphology alone. Lymphoblast morphology is best appreciated in bone marrow aspirate and peripheral blood smears, but touch preparations stained with a Wright-Giemsa or similar stain can be useful for cytologic evaluation. In most cases lymphoblasts have scant cytoplasm, fine chromatin, and inconspicuous nucleoli, while in some cases they are larger with more abundant cytoplasm and prominent nucleolus (Figure 4.3). Azurophilic cytoplasmic granules and vacuoles can be seen in some cases, as well as lymphoblasts with cytoplasmic pseudopods (“hand-mirror” cells) (Figure 4.4).[1,9]

TABLE 4.1 Phenotypic Findings in Precursor Neoplasms

	Most Commonly Expressed and/or Characteristic Markers	Other Pertinent/Helpful Markers	Markers That May be Expressed in Some Cases
B-lymphoblastic leukemia/lymphoma	CD19 CD22 (cytoplasmic and surface) CD24 cCD79a PAX5	CD10 CD20 CD34 CD45 (usually dim) CD99 TdT	Myeloid markers CD13 CD15 CD33 T-cell markers CD2 CD7
T-lymphoblastic leukemia/lymphoma	CD2 cCD3 CD4 CD5 CD7 CD8 CD43	CD1a CD10 CD34 CD45 CD99 TdT	Myeloid markers CD13 CD15 CD33 CD117 B-cell markers CD79a
Myeloid sarcoma	CD13 CD33 CD68 CD117 Lysozyme MPO	CD4 CD34 CD43 CD45 CD56 CD99 TdT	B-cell markers CD19 PAX5 T-cell markers CD2 CD5 CD7
Blastic plasmacytoid dendritic cell neoplasm	CD4 CD56 CD123 CD303 (BDCA-2) TCL-1	CD7 CD33 CD45 CD68 CD99 TdT	Myeloid markers CD13 CD117 B-cell markers CD79a T-cell markers CD2 cCD3 CD5

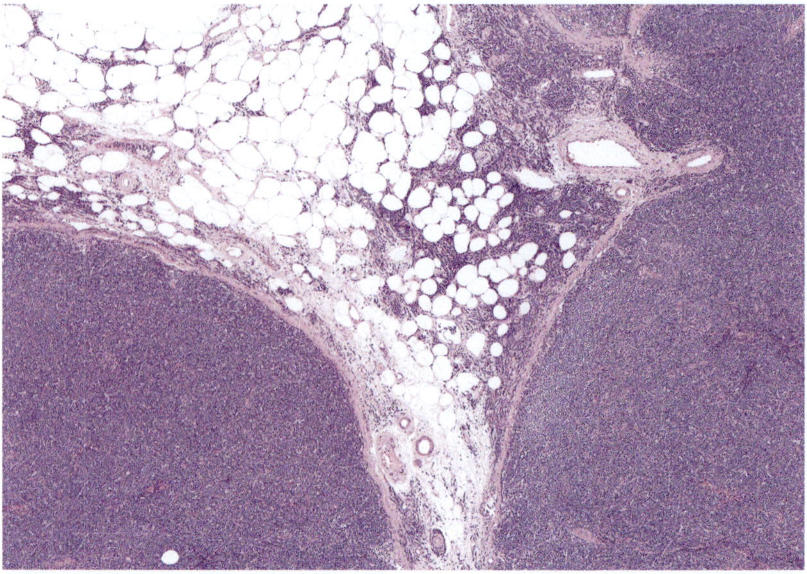

FIGURE 4.1 **B-lymphoblastic lymphoma.** Lymphoblasts are diffusely effacing lymph node architecture and extending into perinodal adipose tissue.

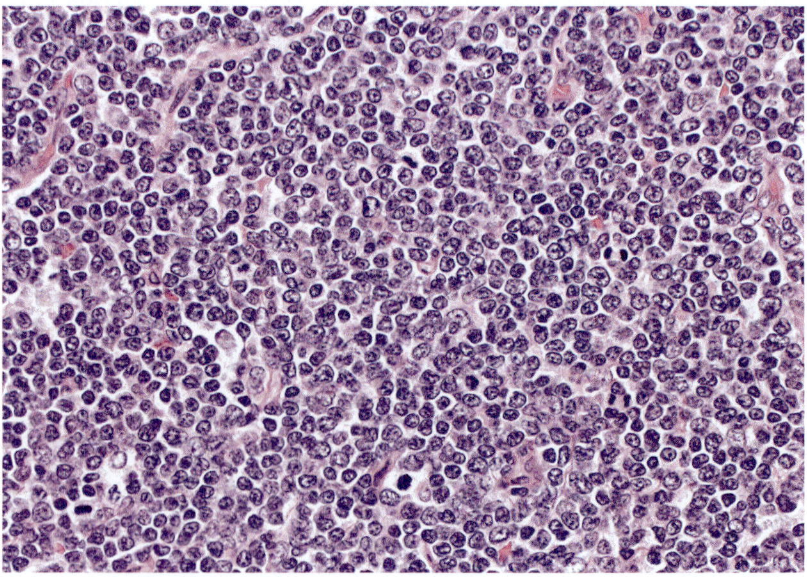

FIGURE 4.2 **B-lymphoblastic lymphoma.** Lymphoblasts are medium sized with fine chromatin and variably prominent nucleoli.

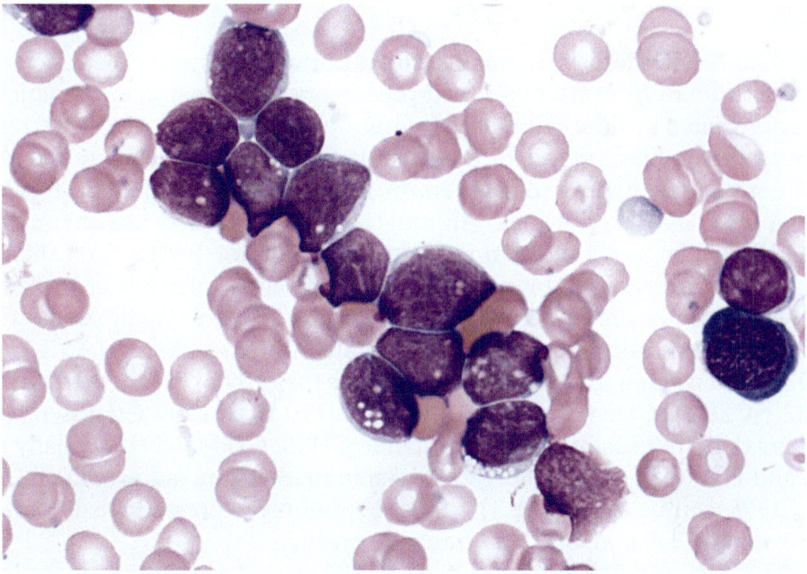

FIGURE 4.3 **B-lymphoblastic lymphoma.** Bone marrow aspirate smear with lymphoblasts showing high nuclear to cytoplasmic ratio, inconspicuous nucleoli, and vacuolated cytoplasm.

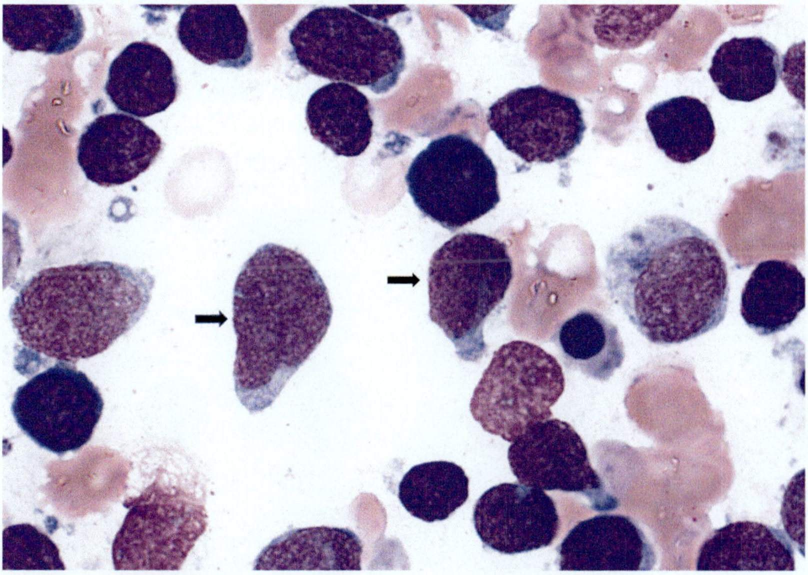

FIGURE 4.4 **B-lymphoblastic lymphoma.** Lymphoblasts with cytoplasmic pseudopods (arrows), so-called "hand-mirror" cells.

Phenotype

Leukemic B lymphoblasts virtually always show phenotypic aberrancies that distinguish them from normal B-cell precursors (ie, hematogones), which are best appreciated by flow cytometry. Immunophenotype of B-ALL/LBL reflects different maturational stages of B cells in the bone marrow (Figure 4.5).[10] The most consistently expressed markers in B-ALL/LBL are CD19, cytoplasmic CD79a (cCD79a), and cCD22. Although all listed markers are characteristic of B-cell lineage, none of them is by itself specific for B-ALL, and diagnosis typically requires a combination of markers or high intensity of expression, another characteristic best evaluated by flow cytometry. Weak partial CD19 and cCD22 expression can be present in acute myeloid leukemia (AML), while cCD79a can be seen in T-ALL and AML. The majority of cases express surface CD22 (sCD22), CD24, and PAX5, while CD20 is variably expressed. Other markers that are usually expressed include CD10, CD34, CD45 (usually dim), TdT, and HLA-DR (Figure 4.6A-C). Myeloid markers, including CD13, CD15, and CD33, can be expressed. The most commonly expressed T-cell marker is CD43, while CD2 and CD7 can rarely be positive.[1,3,11,12]

The differential diagnosis of B-ALL/LBL includes other precursor hematopoietic neoplasms, which have to be excluded by comprehensive immunophenotyping. High-grade B-cell lymphoma with TdT expression is an aggressive B-cell neoplasm that can pose significant diagnostic challenge and has to be distinguished from B-LBL. The approach to high-grade B-cell lymphoma is discussed in more detail in Chapter 5. Lastly, it is important to keep in mind that scattered benign TdT-positive cells can be "normally" seen in virtually all pediatric lymph nodes and >70% of lymph nodes in adults biopsied for other neoplasms (Figure 4.7). These cells are usually found in interfollicular areas, scattered singly or in small clusters, and are positive for CD34, CD10, CD79a, and occasionally CD7, consistent with hematogones.[13,14]

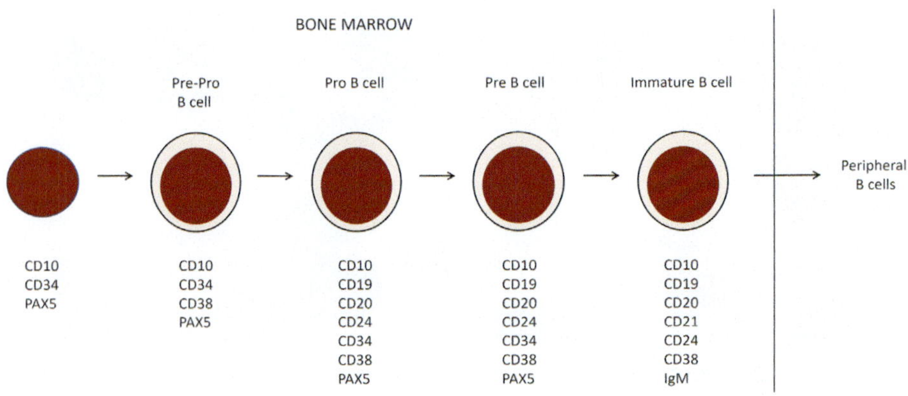

FIGURE 4.5 Maturational stages of B cell in the bone marrow and the antigens expressed during different stages.

Genetics

The complex and rapidly expanding genetic landscape of B-ALL/LBL is beyond the scope of this text and will be only briefly discussed. Genetic abnormalities carry prognostic significance and are routinely used for risk stratification. By conventional cytogenetic analysis, abnormalities are

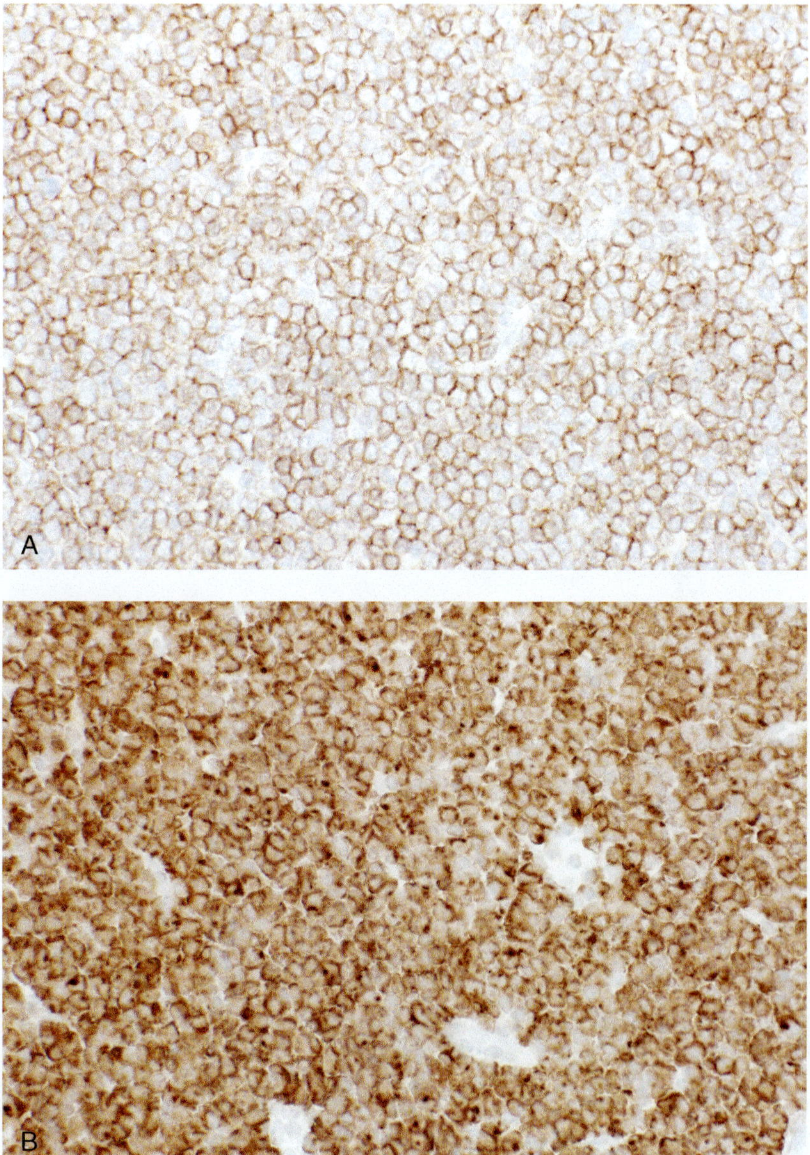

FIGURE 4.6 (*Continued*)

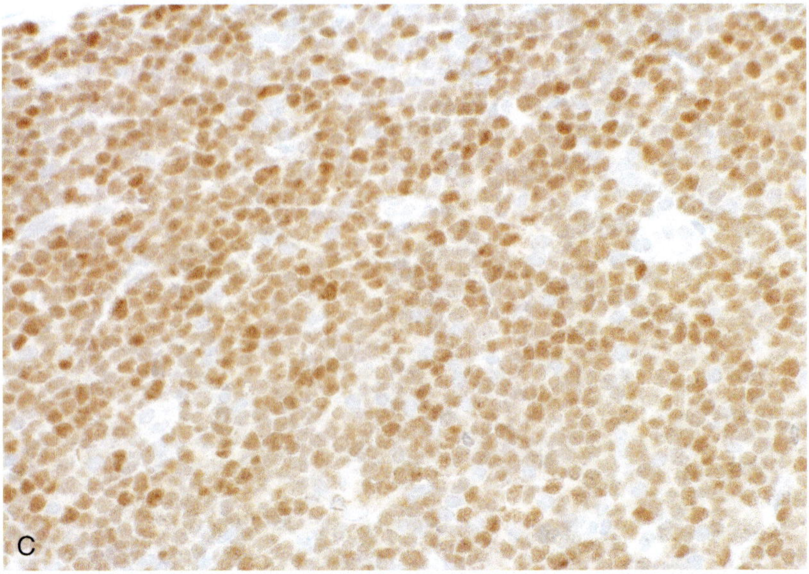

FIGURE 4.6 **Immunohistochemical staining of B-lymphoblastic lymphoma.** The lymphoblasts stain weakly for CD19 (A) and strongly for CD10 (B) and TdT (C).

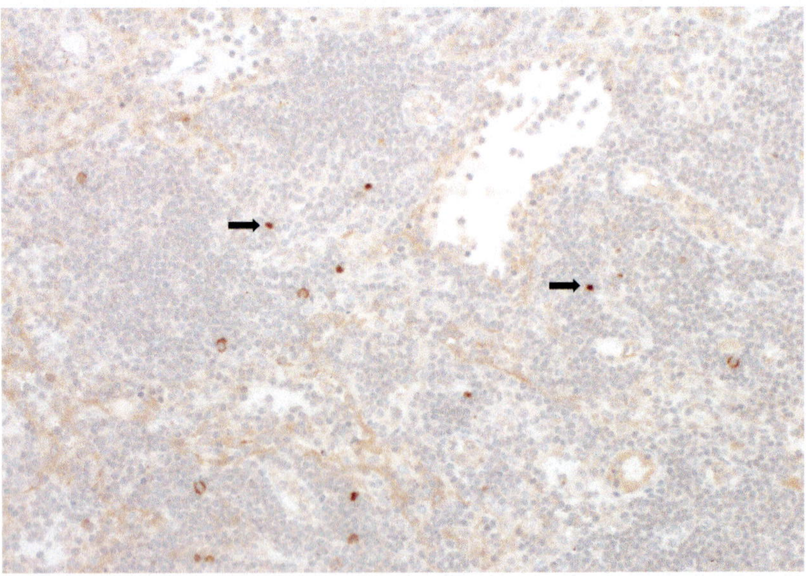

FIGURE 4.7 **Scattered benign TdT-positive cell (arrows) in a reactive lymph node from a child.**

found in 60% to 70% of cases. For a complete list of B-ALL/LBL entities that are defined by recurrent genetic abnormality, please refer to the 2022 ICC of myeloid neoplasms and acute leukemia.[15] Currently, there are >20 subtypes of B-ALL, with variable prevalence in different age groups that have distinct gene expression profiles. Major types of genetic alterations that occur in B-ALL include chromosomal aneuploidy (ie, hyper- or hypodiploidy), rearrangements that deregulate different oncogenes or result in chimeric transcription factors, and point mutations.[8,16-18] Clonal immunoglobulin heavy chain (IGH) rearrangement can be detected in virtually all cases of B-ALL/LBL, while a subset has immunoglobulin kappa (IGK) and immunoglobulin lambda (IGL) light chain rearrangements. In over half of cases, clonal T-cell receptor (TCR) gene rearrangements can be demonstrated.

T-LYMPHOBLASTIC LEUKEMIA/LYMPHOMA

T-lymphoblastic leukemia/lymphoma (T-ALL/LBL) is a neoplasm of lymphoid progenitor cells (lymphoblasts) committed to T-cell lineage. The disease involves bone marrow, peripheral blood, as well as thymus, lymph nodes, and a variety of extranodal sites including testis and central nervous system. Similar to B-ALL/LBL, if the blasts in the bone marrow and/or peripheral blood comprise ≥25% of cells, diagnosis of T-ALL is made, while cases with primarily thymic, nodal, or other extranodal involvement are termed T-LBL. T-LBL typically occurs in adolescents and young adults and is more common in males; however, it can occur over a broad age range including infants and the elderly. While T-ALL comprises only 15% of childhood lymphoblastic leukemias, T-LBL accounts for nearly 90% of all lymphoblastic lymphomas. Both pediatric and adult patients frequently present with a clinical picture of "lymphoma" often with advanced stage (III or IV) of disease. Thymus and lymph nodes above the diaphragm are the most common sites of involvement. Adolescent and young adult patients typically present with an anterior mediastinal mass, associated with pleural and pericardial effusions.[1,6,19,20] Complications such as airway compression, superior vena cava syndrome, and cardiac tamponade can occur. T-ALL/LBL is an aggressive disease that requires intensive chemotherapy regimens. Children have an overall better prognosis than adult patients.[6,21]

Morphology

Lymph node architecture is usually diffusely replaced by sheets of blasts with frequent involvement of capsule and perinodal fibroadipose tissue (Figure 4.8). In cases of partial involvement paracortical infiltration is frequently seen. Some cases show "pseudofollicular" pattern with strands of fibrous tissue taking on a nodular appearance. Blasts vary in size and can have round or irregular (convoluted) nuclei with scant cytoplasm. Chromatin is fine/dusty, and nucleoli are usually inconspicuous (Figures 4.9 and 4.10). In our experience, some cases have blasts that morphologically resemble mature lymphocytes and can be difficult to recognize on H&E-stained sections, especially if the section is thick or the lymph node is partially involved (Figure 4.11).[1]

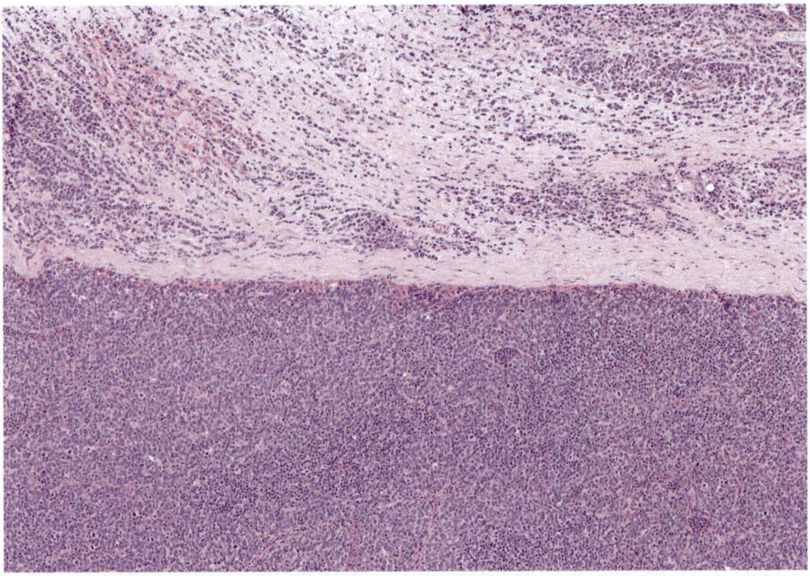

FIGURE 4.8 **T-lymphoblastic lymphoma.** Lymph node is diffusely effaced by sheets of blasts, and infiltrate also involves thickened lymph node capsule. Lymphoblasts are invading the capsule in a linear pattern.

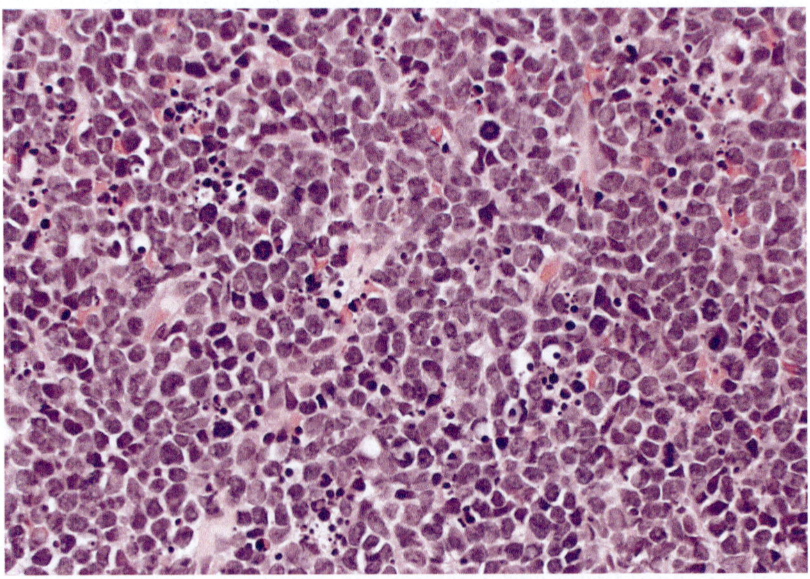

FIGURE 4.9 **T-lymphoblastic lymphoma shows a diffuse infiltrate of medium-sized lymphoblasts with irregular nuclei, fine chromatin, and inconspicuous nucleoli.**

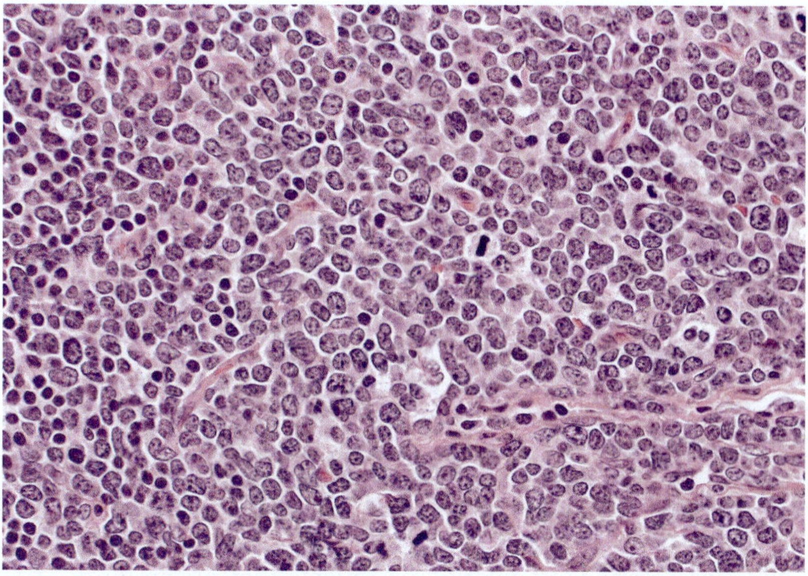

FIGURE 4.10 **T-lymphoblastic lymphoma.** In this case, lymphoblasts show more variability in size, the chromatin is open, and small nucleoli can be appreciated.

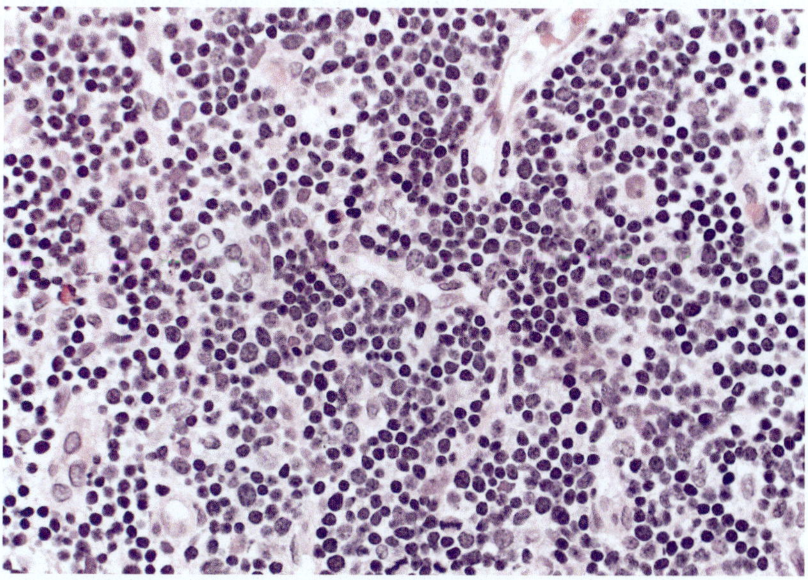

FIGURE 4.11 **T-lymphoblastic lymphoma.** Lymphoblasts are small with round nuclei and are reminiscent of small lymphocytes, which can pose diagnostic challenge.

Phenotype

Immunophenotype of T-ALL/LBL varies and reflects different maturational stages of T cells in bone marrow and thymus (Figure 4.12).[22] The cytoplasmic CD3 (cCD3) is the most reliable (lineage specific) marker that indicates T-lineage commitment. Surface CD3 (sCD3) appears later in the maturation. The most commonly expressed markers in T-ALL/LBL include CD2, cCD3, CD5, CD7, and CD43. Most cases have a phenotype of a late cortical thymocyte with expression of both CD4 and CD8, as well as CD1a. TdT is expressed in 90% of cases (Figure 4.13A and B). Other markers that are variably expressed include CD10, CD34 (small subset), CD99, as well as CD45 and CD52 (both expressed in >95% of cases). Myeloid markers can be expressed as well, the most common being CD33. Others include CD13, CD15, and rarely CD117. T-ALL can express CD79a, but the other B-cell markers are usually negative. Approximately one-third of cases will express a TCR, most commonly alpha/beta and rarely gamma/delta.[1,3,11,23,24]

Early T-cell precursor (ETP)-ALL is a recognized subgroup of T-ALL in WHO classification. Its phenotype reflects that of the more primitive early T-cell precursors, which recently migrated from bone marrow to thymus and retained some multilineage potency. These cases are positive for cCD3 and CD7 and are usually negative or weakly subset positive for CD5, a useful feature to identify them. In addition, one or more markers of myeloid or stem cell lineage, including CD34, CD117, CD11b, CD13, CD33, CD65, and HLA-DR, should be present. The presence of the more mature thymocyte markers, including CD8 and CD1a, excludes the diagnosis of ETP-ALL.[1,25,26]

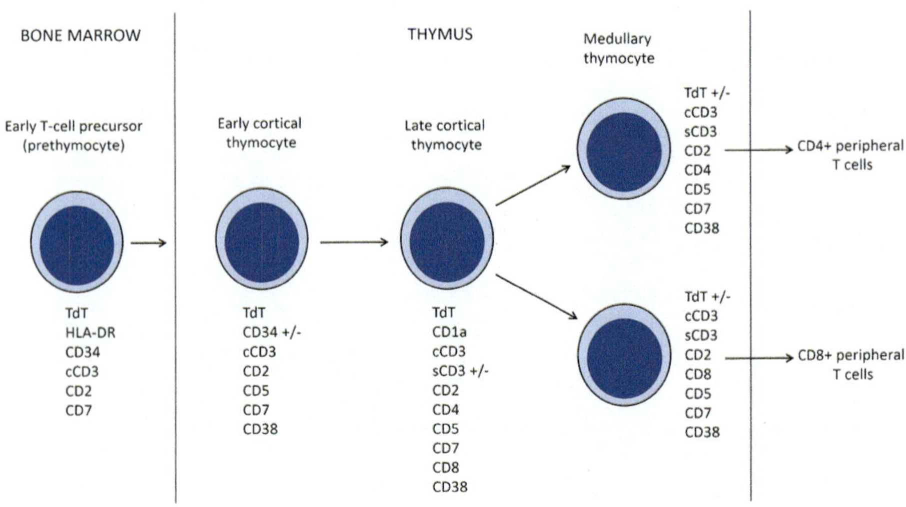

FIGURE 4.12 Maturational stages of T cell in the bone marrow and thymus, and the antigens expressed during different stages.

In addition to other precursor hematopoietic neoplasms, the differential diagnosis of T-ALL/LBL includes nonneoplastic thymic tissue, lymphocyte-rich thymoma, and indolent T-cell lymphoblastic proliferation. Biopsy of ectopic or hyperplastic thymus can pose a diagnostic challenge and can be confused with T-LBL. Benign thymic tissue will show intact

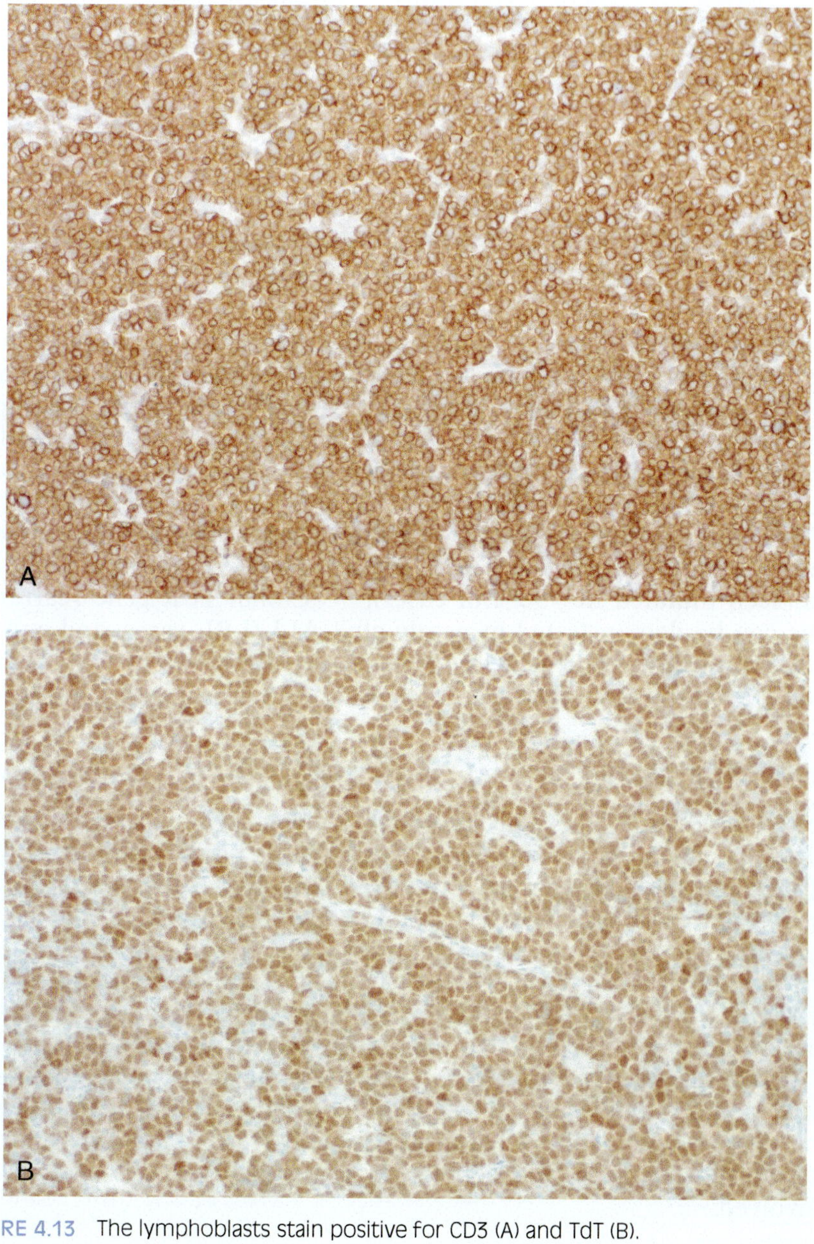

FIGURE 4.13 The lymphoblasts stain positive for CD3 (A) and TdT (B).

architecture with well-delineated cortex and medulla, and small bland lymphocytes with round nuclei and indistinct nucleoli. Flow cytometry can be very helpful in identifying these cases as it will demonstrate a full spectrum of normal thymic maturational pattern with the presence of single-positive CD4 or CD8 and double-positive CD4 and CD8 T cells. Furthermore, cytokeratin stain with highlight thymic epithelium, which is usually absent in T-ALL/LBL. Rarely, one can encounter indolent T-cell lymphoblastic proliferation, a nonclonal expansion of TdT-positive T cells within lymph nodes. This occurs often in association with other pathologic conditions, including Castleman disease, follicular dendritic sarcoma, carcinoma, and some autoimmune conditions. The distribution can be nodal or nonnodal. In the lymph nodes, these proliferations manifest as confluent groups of TdT-positive T cells that usually do not efface lymph node architecture. However, they can be very challenging on a core/limited biopsy and larger biopsy is frequently needed for definitive distinction from T-LBL.[27]

Genetics

By conventional cytogenetic analysis, abnormalities are found in >50% of cases. Recurrent translocations include TRA/D, TRB, and TRG loci as well as 11q23 locus (*KMT2A*) with different partners.[1,28] Gene expression profiling studies identified mutually exclusive subgroups of T-ALL with characteristic transcriptional profile with ectopic expression of one specific transcription factor (including TAL1, TXL1, TXL3, HOXA 9/10, LMO2, and NKX 2-1), as a consequence of chromosomal abnormality. The most commonly mutated genes in T-ALL include *NOTCH1* and *CDKN2A/2B* (each seen mutated in >50% of cases).[29-31] Clonal TCR gene rearrangements can be demonstrated in nearly all T-ALL/LBL cases, and approximately 20% have IGH gene rearrangement. All cases of T-ALL carry multiple genomic abnormalities.

MYELOID SARCOMA

Myeloid sarcoma (MS) is a proliferation of myeloid blasts in an extramedullary site that forms a tumor mass and disrupts tissue architecture. It is diagnostically equivalent to acute myeloid leukemia (AML), regardless of blast count in peripheral blood and bone marrow. Most cases of MS occur synchronous or metachronous (preceding or in the setting of relapse) to AML. Some cases represent the blast phase of myelodysplastic (MDS), myeloproliferative (MPN), or MDS/MPN neoplasms. Very rarely (<1% of cases), MS occurs as an isolated neoplasm, but a subset of those patients will develop AML. Of all patients with AML, up to 10% have evidence of MS. Median age of diagnosis is in the 7th decade with slight male predominance. Most common sites of involvement are skin, soft tissue, breast, gastrointestinal tract, lymph nodes, and spleen, but virtually any site can be involved.[1,32-37]

Morphology

Lymph nodes involved by MS can be partially involved by an interfollicular expansion of blasts or can be diffusely effaced. Cellular morphology of the infiltrate varies, and many cases show myelomonocytic or purely monocytic differentiation. Of note, patients with monocytic AML have a higher frequency of extramedullary involvement. Blasts vary in size from small to large with typically high nuclear to cytoplasmic ratio, variably irregular nuclei, fine chromatin, and inconspicuous to prominent nucleoli. Some cases show evidence of granulocytic maturation including scattered eosinophilic precursors. In some cases, erythroid precursors and/or megakaryocytes can be seen. Mitotic figures, apoptosis, and areas of necrosis are frequently seen (Figures 4.14-4.16). In cases that show monocytic differentiation blasts and/or promonocytes are large with irregular/convoluted nuclei and abundant cytoplasm (Figure 4.17).[3,33,36]

Phenotype

Phenotyping of myeloid sarcoma is best done by flow cytometry. In a patient with a history of AML or other myeloid neoplasm, MS is in the differential diagnosis of any new "mass," particularly in the skin, soft tissue, or gastrointestinal tract, as well as in cases of lymphadenopathy.

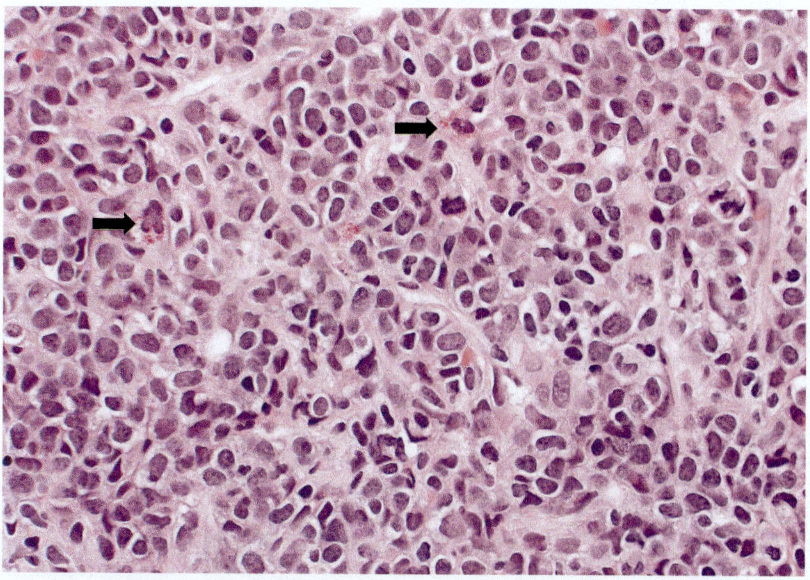

FIGURE 4.14 **Myeloid sarcoma.** Sheets of medium-sized blasts with slightly irregular nuclei, fine chromatin, and inconspicuous nucleoli. Rare scattered eosinophilic precursors are seen, a helpful diagnostic clue (arrows).

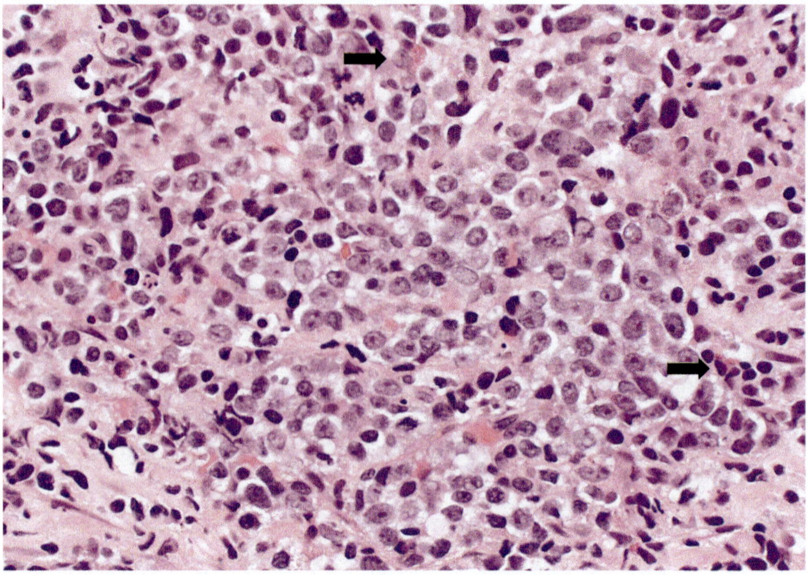

FIGURE 4.15 **Myeloid sarcoma.** In this case, myeloid blasts are reminiscent of immunoblasts, which can raise the differential diagnosis of diffuse large B-cell lymphoma. Subtle scattered eosinophilic precursors are seen (arrows).

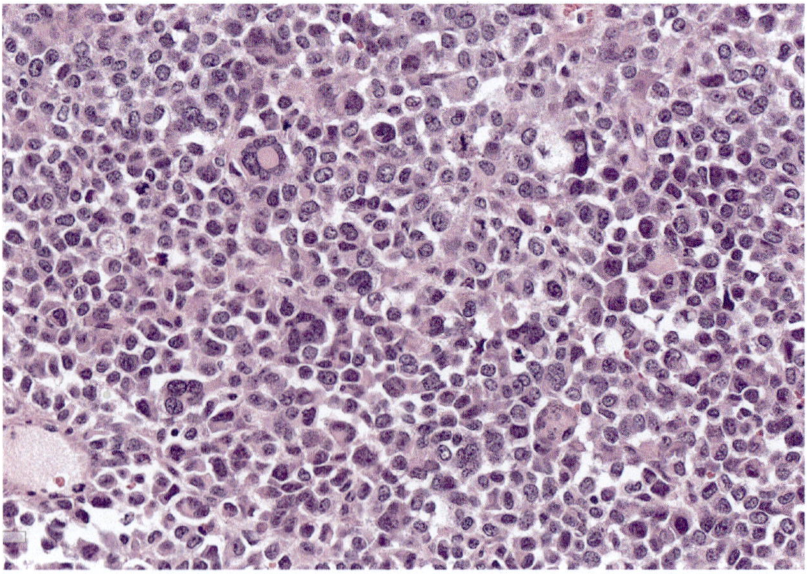

FIGURE 4.16 **Myeloid sarcoma.** This case shows granulocytic maturation and scattered dysplastic megakaryocytes.

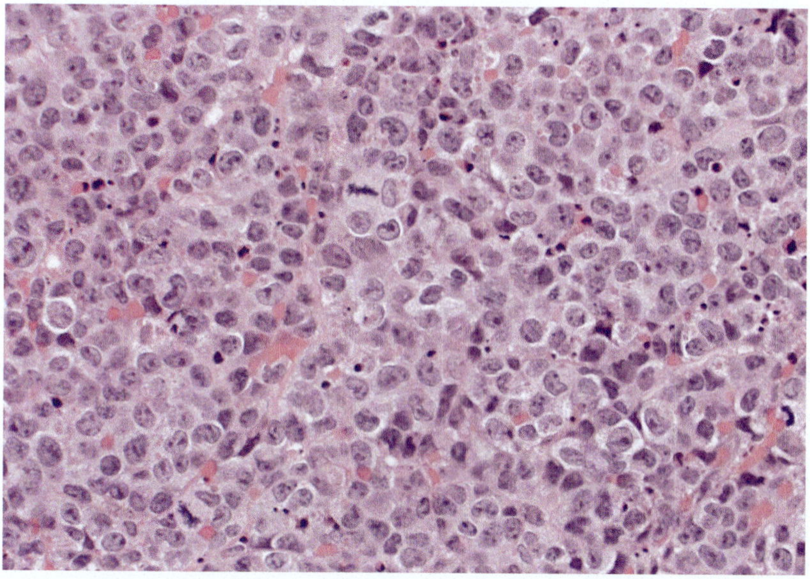

FIGURE 4.17 **Myeloid sarcoma with monoblastic differentiation.** Sheets of monoblasts and promonocytes with round to irregular/folded nuclei, fine chromatin, small nucleoli, and abundant cytoplasm.

The most commonly expressed markers in MS are CD13, CD33, CD68, CD117, lysozyme, and MPO (Figure 4.18A and B). MPO will be partially expressed in tumors with myelomonocytic differentiation and negative in purely monoblastic cases. Other commonly expressed markers include CD4, CD43, and CD45. CD34, CD56, CD99, and TdT are variably expressed but can be helpful in diagnosis. Cases of monoblastic MS will be positive for lysozyme, CD4, CD11c, CD14, CD68, and CD163 and usually negative for CD34 and MPO. B-cell markers, including CD19 and PAX5, can be positive in some cases and are associated with AML with t(8;21)(q22;q22). T-cell markers, such as CD2, CD5, and CD7 can be occasionally seen.[33,36,38]

Diagnosis of MS is frequently challenging, especially on a small biopsy in a patient with no previous history of AML or myeloid neoplasm. Morphologically, MS can look very similar to large B- and T-cell lymphomas, as well as more mature histiocytic neoplasms. The presence of immature myeloid cells, and especially scattered eosinophilic myelocytes, should immediately raise the differential diagnosis of MS. Other precursor neoplasm mentioned in this chapter should be ruled out by comprehensive immunophenotyping.

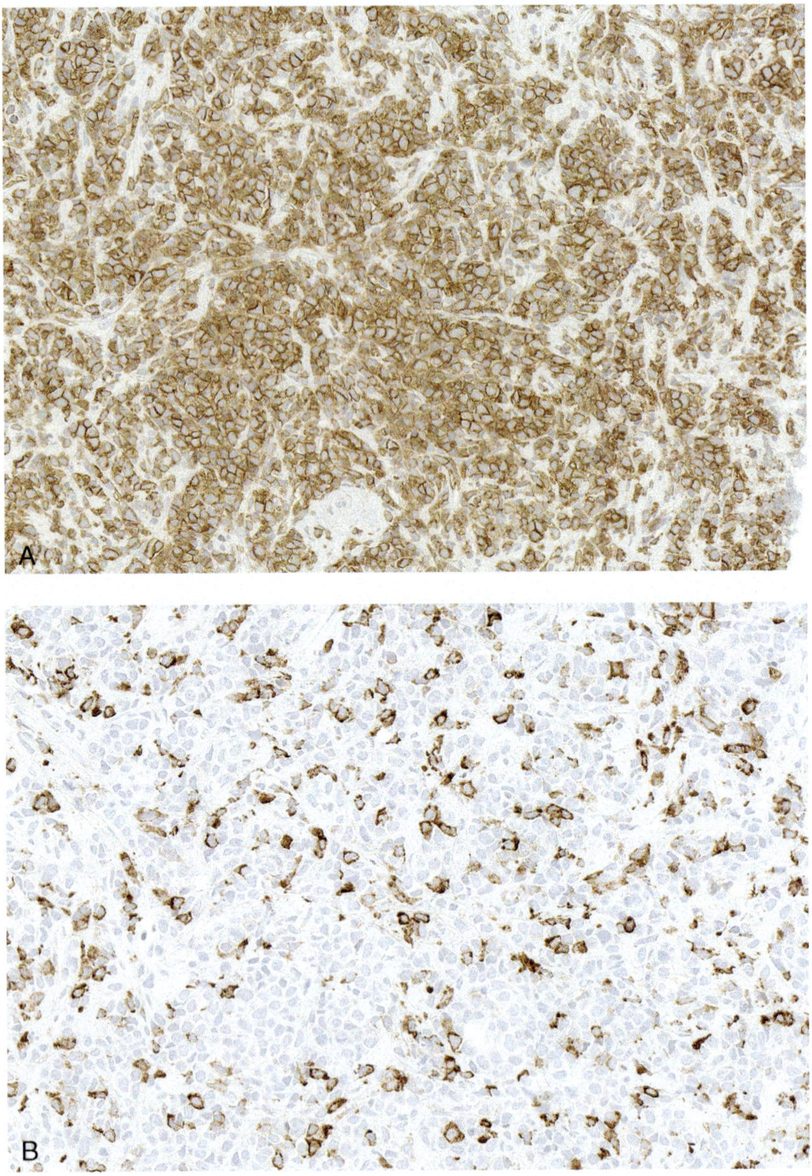

FIGURE 4.18 Myeloid blasts are diffusely positive for CD117 (A) and partially positive for myeloperoxidase (B).

Genetics

Genetic landscape of myeloid sarcoma is vast and parallels the one of AML. It is worth mentioning that cases of AML with t(8;21)(q22;q22.1); *RUNX1-RUNX1T1*, AML with inv(16)(p13.1q22); *CBFB-MYH11*, and AML with t(9;11)(p21.3;q23.3); *KMT2A-MLL3* have a higher frequency of MS.[1,39,40]

BLASTIC PLASMACYTOID DENDRITIC CELL NEOPLASM

Blastic plasmacytoid dendritic cell neoplasm (BPDCN) is a rare and aggressive disease that arises from the precursors of plasmacytoid dendritic cells (PDCs). The median age of patients is 60 years, but it occurs over a broad age range and has a bimodal pattern of occurrence with higher incidence in younger people (<20 years) and in people >60 years of age. Males are more frequently affected than females.[1,41-43] Clinically, the most commonly involved sites are skin (the most common site), bone marrow, and peripheral blood, as well as lymph nodes. A number of patients present with isolated skin lesions, which typically quickly disseminate into other sites if left untreated. Involvement of bone marrow is associated with cytopenia(s), frequently with circulating blasts. BPDCN can involve other sites, including the central nervous system.[1,44-46] Treatment involves a multimodal approach including chemotherapy and stem cell transplantation, as well as targeted therapy with CD123-directed cytotoxin (tagraxofusp). Reported median survival is relatively poor, ranging from 12 to 16 months, with children having somewhat better outcomes. Introduction of tagraxofusp into therapy led to improved clinical responses.[41,42,44,45,47]

Morphology

Biopsies of an enlarged lymph node or skin lesion are often initial specimens where diagnosis of BPDCN is made. The neoplastic cells usually replace the lymph node architecture, but some cases can show interfollicular involvement with sparing of B-cell follicles. The neoplastic cells are usually small blasts with irregular nuclei, fine chromatin, and variably prominent nucleoli. Apoptotic bodies and mitoses, as well as tingible body macrophages are frequently observed (Figures 4.19 and 4.20). Skin involvement is characterized by diffuse infiltrates in the dermis and subcutaneous fat with sparing of the epidermis (Figure 4.21A and B). The morphology of BPDCN is best appreciated in bone marrow smears where the blasts show round to elongated nuclei with finely dispersed chromatin and unipolar cytoplasmic projections with cytoplasmic microvacuoles (Figure 4.22).[1,3,46]

Phenotype

Blasts characteristically express CD4, CD56, CD123, CD303 (BDCA-2), and TCL-1, although loss of one or more markers is not uncommon. However, with the exception of CD303, these markers are not specific and can be seen in AML and other neoplasms. Diagnosis of BPDCN on a tissue biopsy should be done with extreme caution if any of the characteristic markers is negative (Figure 4.23A and B). Other commonly expressed but nonspecific markers include bright HLA-DR, CD38, CD7, CD33, CD45, and CD68 (perinuclear dot pattern). In addition, CD2,

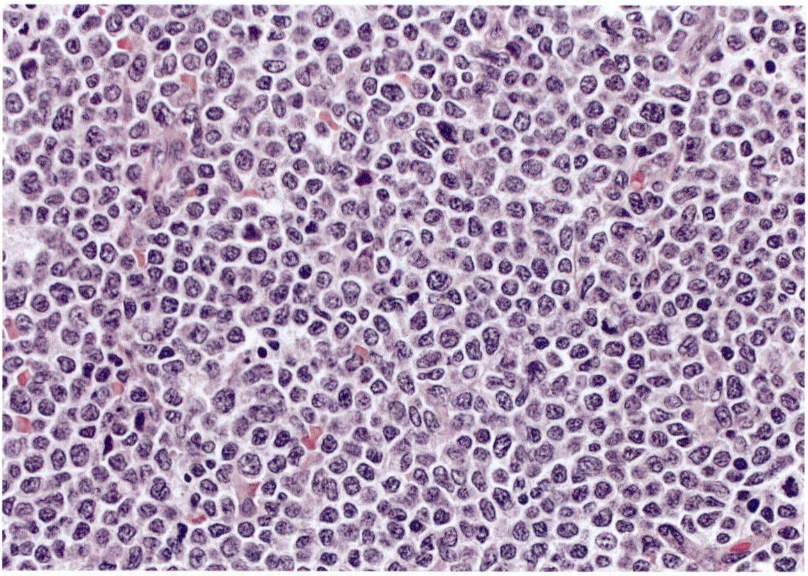

FIGURE 4.19 **Blastic plasmacytoid dendritic cell neoplasm.** Blasts show variability in size, irregular nuclei, open chromatin, and inconspicuous to small nucleoli.

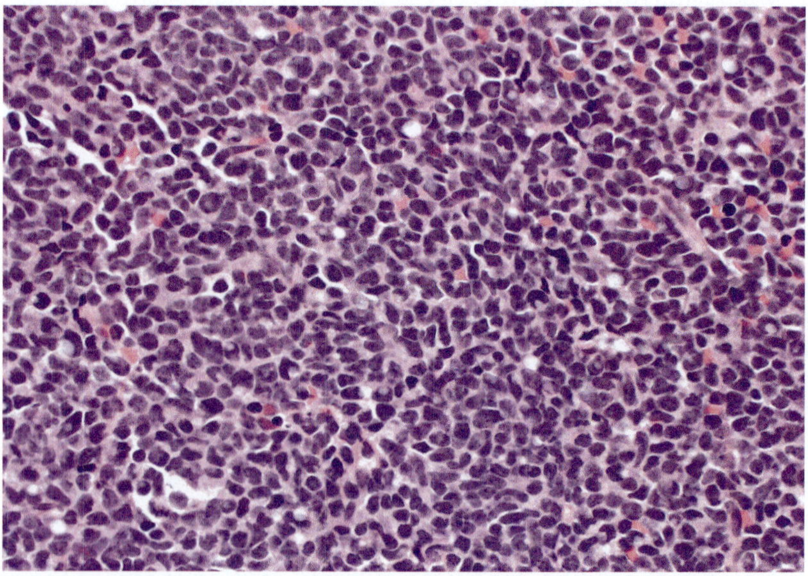

FIGURE 4.20 **Blastic plasmacytoid dendritic cell neoplasm.** In this case, blasts show irregular and frequently elongated nuclei, fine chromatin, inconspicuous nucleoli, and scant cytoplasm.

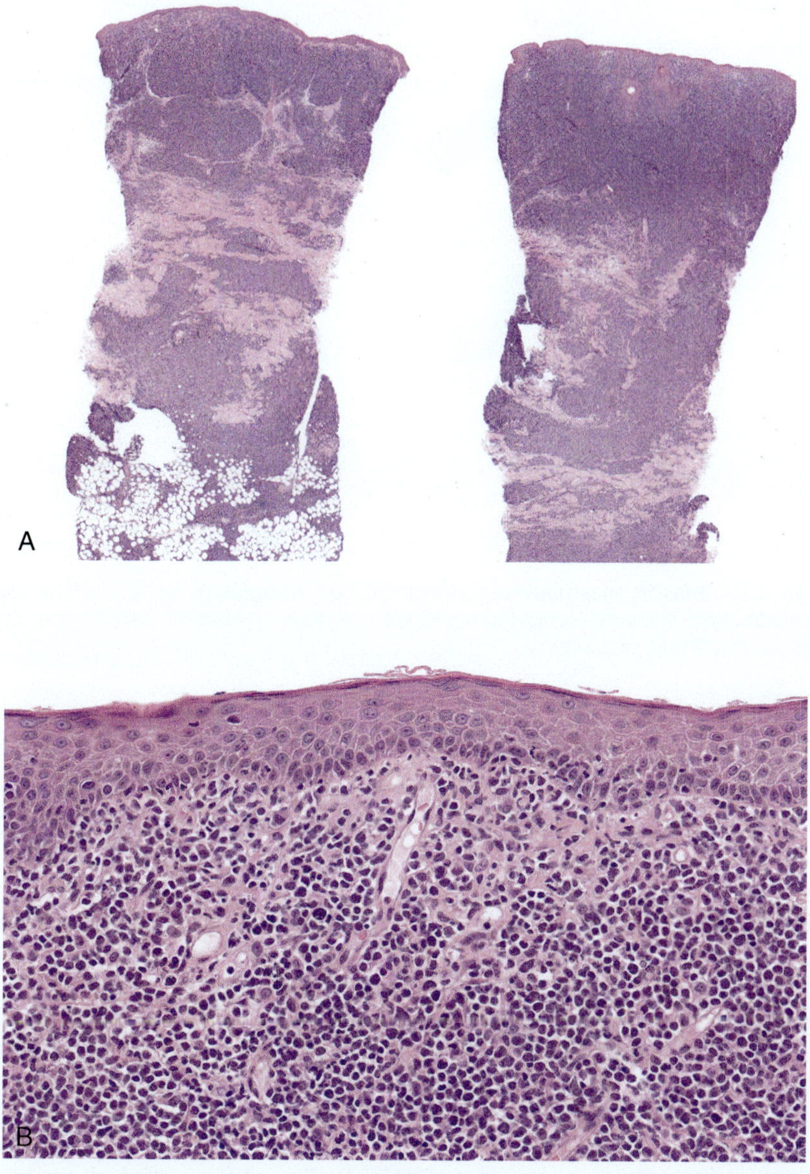

FIGURE 4.21 **Blastic plasmacytoid dendritic cell neoplasm involving the skin.** Blasts diffusely infiltrate dermis and subcutaneous fat (A), while the epidermis is spared (B).

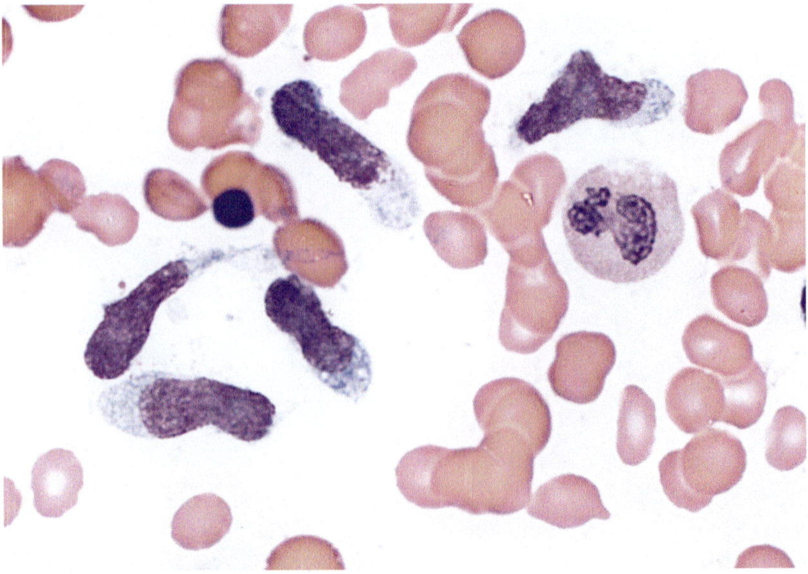

FIGURE 4.22 **Blastic plasmacytoid dendritic cell neoplasm.** Bone marrow aspirate smear with blasts showing elongated nuclei with unipolar cytoplasmic projections containing small cytoplasmic vacuoles.

CD5, CD13, CD71, CD79a, CD99, CD117, and TdT can also be positive. BPDCN should be negative for CD3, as well as CD19, CD20, CD34, lysozyme, and MPO.[1,3,46] In evaluating suspected cases of BPDCN, comprehensive flow cytometry evaluation is very useful to rule out other immature neoplasms in the differential diagnosis. Furthermore, flow cytometry is essential in evaluating for minimal residual disease after chemotherapy and for distinguishing between reactive PDCs and BPDCN. Proliferation (clusters or sheets) of benign or mature PDCs can be seen in a number of entities such as Castleman disease, Kikuchi-Fujimoto disease, and chronic myelomonocytic leukemia. In comparison with BPDCN, reactive PDCs are consistently positive for CD2, CD4, CD123, CD38, CD33, CD38 (bright), and CD303; negative for CD7; and usually negative for CD56.[48] The differential diagnosis of BPDCN primarily includes acute myeloid leukemia and acute lymphoblastic leukemia/lymphoma.

Genetics

Most cases of BPDCN have complex karyotypes, with predominance of genomic losses and with recurrent chromosomal targets being 5q, 6q, chromosome 9, 12p, 13q, and 15q.[49,50] The most commonly mutated genes are *TET2, ASXL1, NRAS, IKAROS* family, and *ZEB2*.[51,52]

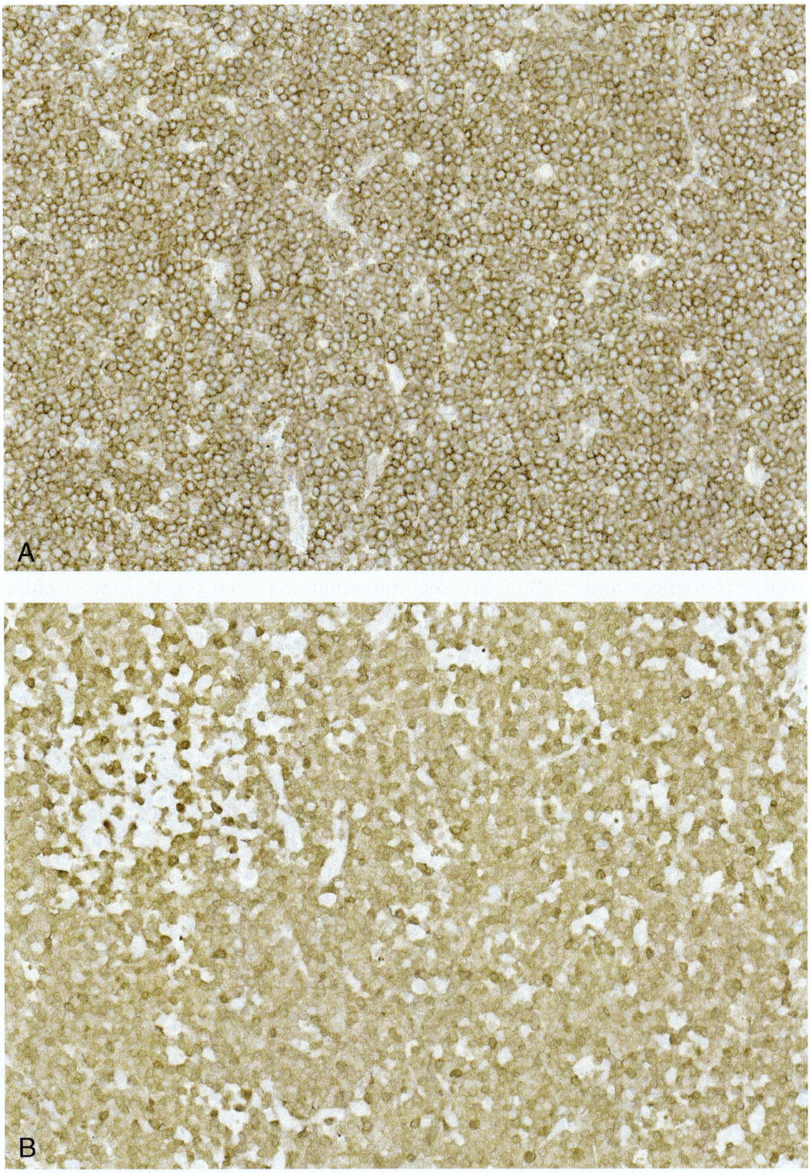

FIGURE 4.23 The neoplastic cells in blastic plasmacytoid dendritic cell neoplasm are positive for CD123 (A) and TCL-1 (B).

REFERENCES

1. Swerdlow SH, Campo E, Harris NL, et al. *WHO Classification of Tumours of Haematopoietic and Lymphoid Tissues*. IARC; 2017.
2. Arber DA, Orazi A, Hasserjian RP, et al. International Consensus Classification of Myeloid Neoplasms and Acute Leukemia: integrating morphological, clinical, and genomic data. *Blood*. 2022;140(11):1200-1228. doi:10.1182/blood.2022015850

3. Medeiros LJ. *Ioachim's Lymph Node Pathology*. 5th ed. Wolters Kluwer; 2021.
4. Lin P, Jones D, Dorfman DM, Medeiros LJ. Precursor B-cell lymphoblastic lymphoma: a predominantly extranodal tumor with low propensity for leukemic involvement. *Am J Surg Pathol.* 2000;24(11):1480-1490.
5. Maitra A, McKenna RW, Weinberg AG, Schneider NR, Kroft SH. Precursor B-cell lymphoblastic lymphoma. A study of nine cases lacking blood and bone marrow involvement and review of the literature. *Am J Clin Pathol.* 2001;115(6):868-875.
6. Burkhardt B, Hermiston ML. Lymphoblastic lymphoma in children and adolescents: review of current challenges and future opportunities. *Br J Haematol.* 2019;185(6):1158-1170.
7. Rafei H, Kantarjian HM, Jabbour EJ. Recent advances in the treatment of acute lymphoblastic leukemia. *Leuk Lymphoma.* 2019;60(11):2606-2621.
8. Inaba H, Mullighan CG. Pediatric acute lymphoblastic leukemia. *Haematologica.* 2020;105(11):2524-2539.
9. Bennett JM, Catovsky D, Daniel MT, et al. The morphological classification of acute lymphoblastic leukaemia: concordance among observers and clinical correlations. *Br J Haematol.* 1981;47(4):553-561.
10. Wilkinson MGL, Rosser EC. B cells as a therapeutic target in paediatric rheumatic disease. *Front Immunol.* 2019;10:214.
11. Oschlies I, Burkhardt B, Chassagne-Clement C, et al. Diagnosis and immunophenotype of 188 pediatric lymphoblastic lymphomas treated within a randomized prospective trial: experiences and preliminary recommendations from the European childhood lymphoma pathology panel. *Am J Surg Pathol.* 2011;35(6):836-844.
12. Thalhammer-Scherrer R, Mitterbauer G, Simonitsch I, et al. The immunophenotype of 325 adult acute leukemias: relationship to morphologic and molecular classification and proposal for a minimal screening program highly predictive for lineage discrimination. *Am J Clin Pathol.* 2002;117(3):380-389.
13. Onciu M, Lorsbach RB, Henry EC, Behm FG. Terminal deoxynucleotidyl transferase-positive lymphoid cells in reactive lymph nodes from children with malignant tumors: incidence, distribution pattern, and immunophenotype in 26 patients. *Am J Clin Pathol.* 2002;118(2):248-254.
14. Pizzi M, Brignola S, Righi S, et al. Benign TdT-positive cells in pediatric and adult lymph nodes: a potential diagnostic pitfall. *Hum Pathol.* 2018;81:131-137.
15. Campo E, Jaffe ES, Cook JR, et al. The International Consensus Classification of Mature Lymphoid Neoplasms: a report from the Clinical Advisory Committee. *Blood.* 2022;140(11):1229-1253. doi:10.1182/blood.2022015851
16. Roberts KG, Mullighan CG. The biology of B-progenitor acute lymphoblastic leukemia. *Cold Spring Harb Perspect Med.* 2020;10(7).
17. Mullighan CG, Goorha S, Radtke I, et al. Genome-wide analysis of genetic alterations in acute lymphoblastic leukaemia. *Nature.* 2007;446(7137):758-764.
18. Iacobucci I, Mullighan CG. Genetic basis of acute lymphoblastic leukemia. *J Clin Oncol.* 2017;35(9):975-983.
19. Cortelazzo S, Ponzoni M, Ferreri AJ, Hoelzer D. Lymphoblastic lymphoma. *Crit Rev Oncol Hematol.* 2011;79(3):330-343.
20. Lamvik J, Waage A, Wahl SG, Naess I, Paulsen PQ, Hammerstrom J. Adult acute lymphoblastic leukemia, Burkitt's lymphoma and lymphoblastic lymphoma in middle Norway 1985-2004. *Haematologica.* 2006;91(10):1428-1429.
21. Teachey DT, O'Connor D. How I treat newly diagnosed T-cell acute lymphoblastic leukemia and T-cell lymphoblastic lymphoma in children. *Blood.* 2020;135(3):159-166.
22. Litwack G. *Human Biochemistry*. Academic Press; 2018.
23. Jaffe ES, Arber DA, Campo E, Harris NL, Quintanilla-Martinez L. *Hematopathology*. 2nd ed. Elsevier; 2017.

24. Patel JL, Smith LM, Anderson J, et al. The immunophenotype of T-lymphoblastic lymphoma in children and adolescents: a Children's Oncology Group report. *Br J Haematol.* 2012;159(4):454-461.
25. Jain N, Lamb AV, O'Brien S, et al. Early T-cell precursor acute lymphoblastic leukemia/lymphoma (ETP-ALL/LBL) in adolescents and adults: a high-risk subtype. *Blood.* 2016;127(15):1863-1869.
26. Khogeer H, Rahman H, Jain N, et al. Early T precursor acute lymphoblastic leukaemia/lymphoma shows differential immunophenotypic characteristics including frequent CD33 expression and in vitro response to targeted CD33 therapy. *Br J Haematol.* 2019;186(4):538-548.
27. Ohgami RS, Arber DA, Zehnder JL, Natkunam Y, Warnke RA. Indolent T-lymphoblastic proliferation (iT-LBP): a review of clinical and pathologic features and distinction from malignant T-lymphoblastic lymphoma. *Adv Anat Pathol.* 2013;20(3):137-140.
28. Harrison CJ, Foroni L. Cytogenetics and molecular genetics of acute lymphoblastic leukemia. *Rev Clin Exp Hematol.* 2002;6(2):91-113, discussion 200-112.
29. Girardi T, Vicente C, Cools J, De Keersmaecker K. The genetics and molecular biology of T-ALL. *Blood.* 2017;129(9):1113-1123.
30. Liu Y, Easton J, Shao Y, et al. The genomic landscape of pediatric and young adult T-lineage acute lymphoblastic leukemia. *Nat Genet.* 2017;49(8):1211-1218.
31. Pear WS, Aster JC. T cell acute lymphoblastic leukemia/lymphoma: a human cancer commonly associated with aberrant NOTCH1 signaling. *Curr Opin Hematol.* 2004;11(6):426-433.
32. Shallis RM, Gale RP, Lazarus HM, et al. Myeloid sarcoma, chloroma, or extramedullary acute myeloid leukemia tumor: a tale of misnomers, controversy and the unresolved. *Blood Rev.* 2021;47:100773.
33. Kawamoto K, Miyoshi H, Yoshida N, Takizawa J, Sone H, Ohshima K. Clinicopathological, cytogenetic, and prognostic analysis of 131 myeloid sarcoma patients. *Am J Surg Pathol.* 2016;40(11):1473-1483.
34. Claerhout H, Van Aelst S, Melis C, et al. Clinicopathological characteristics of de novo and secondary myeloid sarcoma: a monocentric retrospective study. *Eur J Haematol.* 2018;100(6):603-612.
35. Goyal G, Bartley AC, Patnaik MM, Litzow MR, Al-Kali A, Go RS. Clinical features and outcomes of extramedullary myeloid sarcoma in the United States: analysis using a national data set. *Blood Cancer J.* 2017;7(8):e592.
36. Pileri SA, Ascani S, Cox MC, et al. Myeloid sarcoma: clinico-pathologic, phenotypic and cytogenetic analysis of 92 adult patients. *Leukemia.* 2007;21(2):340-350.
37. Movassaghian M, Brunner AM, Blonquist TM, et al. Presentation and outcomes among patients with isolated myeloid sarcoma: a Surveillance, Epidemiology, and End Results database analysis. *Leuk Lymphoma.* 2015;56(6):1698-1703.
38. Shang L, Chen X, Liu Y, et al. The immunophenotypic characteristics and flow cytometric scoring system of acute myeloid leukemia with t(8;21) (q22;q22); RUNX1-RUNX1T1. *Int J Lab Hematol.* 2019;41(1):23-31.
39. Cancer Genome Atlas Research Network; Ley TJ, Miller C, Ding L, et al. Genomic and epigenomic landscapes of adult de novo acute myeloid leukemia. *N Engl J Med.* 2013;368(22):2059-2074.
40. Khwaja A, Bjorkholm M, Gale RE, et al. Acute myeloid leukaemia. *Nat Rev Dis Prim.* 2016;2:16010.
41. Guru Murthy GS, Pemmaraju N, Atallah E. Epidemiology and survival of blastic plasmacytoid dendritic cell neoplasm. *Leuk Res.* 2018;73:21-23.
42. Jegalian AG, Buxbaum NP, Facchetti F, et al. Blastic plasmacytoid dendritic cell neoplasm in children: diagnostic features and clinical implications. *Haematologica.* 2010;95(11):1873-1879.

43. Li Y, Sun V, Sun W, Pawlowska A. Blastic plasmacytoid dendritic cell neoplasm in children. *Hematol Oncol Clin North Am.* 2020;34(3):601-612.
44. Pagano L, Valentini CG, Grammatico S, Pulsoni A. Blastic plasmacytoid dendritic cell neoplasm: diagnostic criteria and therapeutical approaches. *Br J Haematol.* 2016;174(2):188-202.
45. Laribi K, Baugier de Materre A, Sobh M, et al. Blastic plasmacytoid dendritic cell neoplasms: results of an international survey on 398 adult patients. *Blood Adv.* 2020;4(19):4838-4848.
46. Julia F, Dalle S, Duru G, et al. Blastic plasmacytoid dendritic cell neoplasms: clinico-immunohistochemical correlations in a series of 91 patients. *Am J Surg Pathol.* 2014;38(5):673-680.
47. Pemmaraju N, Lane AA, Sweet KL, et al. Tagraxofusp in blastic plasmacytoid dendritic-cell neoplasm. *N Engl J Med.* 2019;380(17):1628-1637.
48. Wang W, Khoury JD, Miranda RN, et al. Immunophenotypic characterization of reactive and neoplastic plasmacytoid dendritic cells permits establishment of a 10-color flow cytometric panel for initial workup and residual disease evaluation of blastic plasmacytoid dendritic cell neoplasm. *Haematologica.* 2021;106(4):1047-1055.
49. Sakamoto K, Takeuchi K. Cytogenetics of blastic plasmacytoid dendritic cell neoplasm: chromosomal rearrangements and DNA copy-number alterations. *Hematol Oncol Clin North Am.* 2020;34(3):523-538.
50. Leroux D, Mugneret F, Callanan M, et al. CD4(+), CD56(+) DC2 acute leukemia is characterized by recurrent clonal chromosomal changes affecting 6 major targets: a study of 21 cases by the Groupe Francais de Cytogenetique Hematologique. *Blood.* 2002;99(11):4154-4159.
51. Menezes J, Acquadro F, Wiseman M, et al. Exome sequencing reveals novel and recurrent mutations with clinical impact in blastic plasmacytoid dendritic cell neoplasm. *Leukemia.* 2014;28(4):823-829.
52. Sapienza MR, Abate F, Melle F, et al. Blastic plasmacytoid dendritic cell neoplasm: genomics mark epigenetic dysregulation as a primary therapeutic target. *Haematologica.* 2019;104(4):729-737.

5

MATURE B-CELL NEOPLASMS

DANIEL P. LARSON and REBECCA L. KING

SMALL B-CELL LYMPHOMA

The approach to small B-cell lymphomas (SBCLs) in the lymph node biopsy, whether excisional or core needle, should begin with an assessment of the underlying architecture of the lymph node on hematoxylin & eosin (H&E) stained sections. Once effacement or distortion of the architecture is identified or suspected, immunophenotyping should be performed to narrow the differential diagnosis. As with all the lymphomas in this book, the World Health Organization Classification and 2022 International Consensus Classification (ICC) provide guidelines for diagnosis and classification and should guide the pathologist's selection of ancillary studies. Although many of the SBCLs have characteristic morphologic features, for example back-to-back nodules in follicular lymphoma (FL) or monocytoid B cells in marginal zone lymphoma (MZL), there is significant overlap in the growth patterns of FL, MZL, mantle cell lymphoma (MCL), chronic lymphocytic leukemia/small lymphocytic lymphoma (CLL/SLL), and lymphoplasmacytic lymphoma (LPL). In addition, unlike in large B-cell lymphomas, these lymphomas often lack cytologic atypia diagnostic of malignancy, and thus reactive lymphoid hyperplasia and SBCL often remain in the differential diagnosis of one another. It is for this reason as well, that in the absence of a tissue biopsy, fine needle aspiration specimens should not be used to render a diagnosis of SBCL, except in extenuating circumstances.

Phenotyping can be performed using either flow cytometry (FCM) or immunohistochemistry (IHC) (Chapter 2), although in most cases at least some IHC will be necessary to integrate the morphologic features with the atypical or clonal cell population identified by FCM. In addition, FCM may find small clones in otherwise reactive-appearing lymphoid hyperplasia and should not be used in isolation to diagnose a SBCL when the morphologic features are not supportive. As such, the majority of the discussion here will focus on the use of IHC in diagnosing SBCL.

TABLE 5.1 Classic Phenotypic Findings in Common Small B-cell Lymphomas

Marker	Follicular	Mantle Cell	Marginal Zone	CLL/SLL	LPL
CD20	+	+	+	+ (dim)	+
PAX5	+	+	+	+	+
CD5	–	+	–	+	–
CD10	+	–	–	–	–
BCL6	+	–	–	–	–
BCL2	+	+	+/–	+	+/–
Cyclin D1	–	+	–	–[a]	–
LEF1	–	–	–	+	–
SOX11	–	+	–	–	–

[a]CLL/SLL can have dim cyclin D1 staining in proliferation centers which is not associated with a CCND1 rearrangement.

CLL/SLL, chronic lymphocytic leukemia/small lymphocytic lymphoma; LPL, lymphoplasmacytic lymphoma.

In the majority of cases, workup of a lymph node specimen for SBCL should include a panel to address the following entities: FL, MZL, MCL, CLL/SLL, and LPL (Table 5.1). A reliable B-cell marker (CD20) and T-cell marker (CD3) are essential in assessing immunoarchitecture and will aid in interpretation of the remaining stains. Additional B-cell markers such as CD79a and PAX5 may be useful in certain settings. For example, CD79a may be useful in the setting of a lymphoplasmacytic population, as it highlights B cells as well as plasma cells and plasmacytoid B cells that may have lost CD20. PAX5, a nuclear marker, may offer a more crisp picture of the extent of the B-cell compartment compared with CD20 (a membranous stain) especially when crush artifact is present (Figure 5.1). From there, a panel including markers useful in FL (CD10, BCL6, BCL2, CD21), CLL/SLL (CD5, CD23, LEF1), MCL (CD5, cyclin D1, SOX11), and MZL (IRTA1, MNDA, CD43) may be used. A suggested panel for the workup of SBCL is: CD3, CD20, CD10, BCL6, BCL2, cyclin D1, CD5, and CD23 with other stains added depending on the differential diagnosis or clinical circumstance. Ki-67, a marker of cell proliferation, may be useful in certain circumstances such as for prognostic purposes in MCL. An IgD stain may be useful in highlighting normal primary follicle or mantle zone cells, but also may stain some SBCLs. CD43 is sometimes used in this setting, as it may be aberrantly expressed in MZL, CLL, and MCL. CD21 can be useful as a follicular dendritic cell marker, as staining with CD23 and CD21

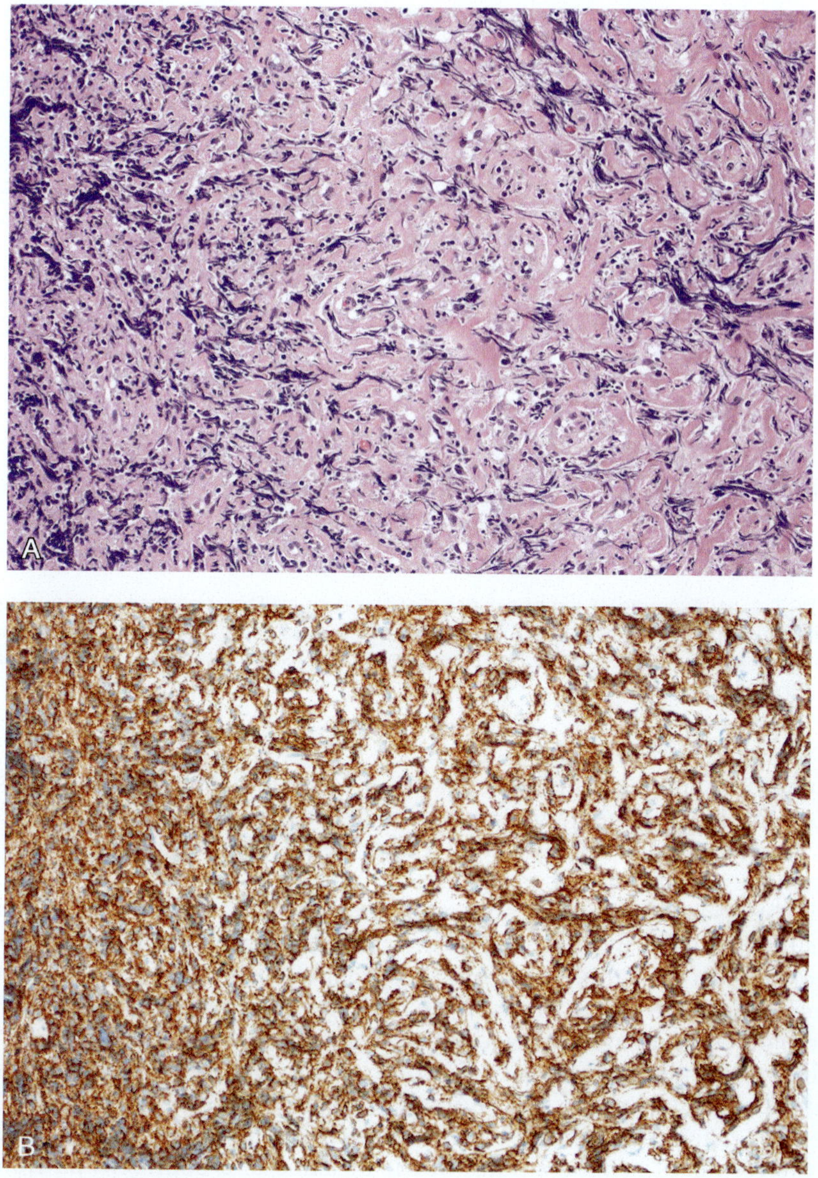

FIGURE 5.1 (*Continued*)

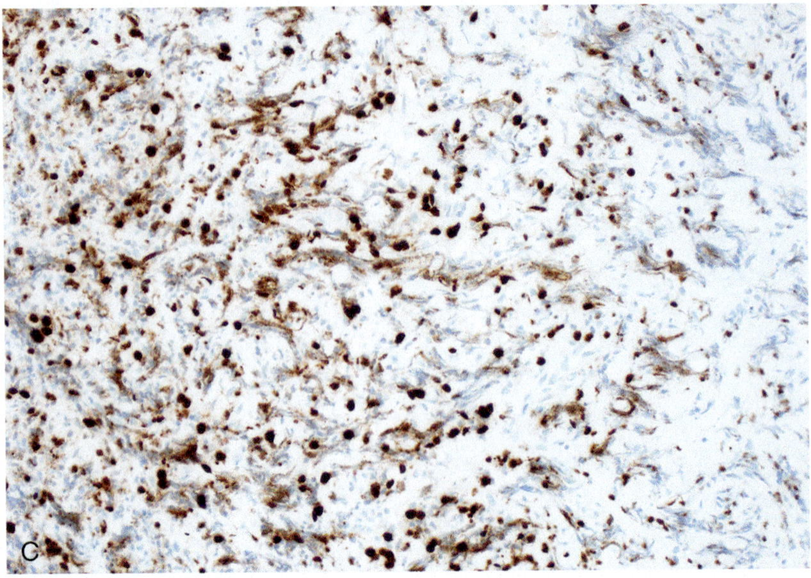

FIGURE 5.1 A, Example of lymphoid tissue with crush artifact, commonly seen in retroperitoneal lymph node biopsies. B, CD20 shows extensive staining due to antigen spreading from crushed cells. C, PAX5, a nuclear stain, more clearly shows the B-cell compartment in crushed tissue.

frequently highlight different subsets of follicular dendritic meshworks. Stains for kappa and lambda may be useful in confirming light chain restriction or localizing the light chain restricted population, although these have several caveats as discussed in Chapter 2.

The use of molecular and cytogenetic testing in the diagnosis and classification of SBCLs remains limited to a few specific indications,[1] although with the rapidly changing landscape of available next-generation sequencing (NGS) tests, this is likely to evolve over time. Currently, single-gene molecular assays, targeted fluorescence in situ hybridization (FISH) testing, and immunoglobulin gene rearrangement (IgGR) studies can be used in cases where the morphologic and phenotypic findings are insufficient to reach a diagnosis. However, caution must be used in interpreting the results of genetic studies in the absence of a confident pathologic diagnosis.

FOLLICULAR LYMPHOMA

Follicular lymphoma (FL) is the second most common lymphoma in Western countries and is likely to be encountered frequently in a general pathology practice. Median age of FL patients is 60 years with a slight female predominance.[2] FL can involve lymph nodes and extranodal sites at any location in the body. It is generally regarded as an indolent lymphoma, which is treatable, but not curable.[2] Unlike in other SBCLs, histologic grading is performed (see below).[1] Grades 1 and 2 are considered "low grade" while grade 3A is often more aggressive, although this is variable. Grade 3B, in contrast, is an aggressive disease usually requiring more intensive chemotherapy. The risk of transformation in the era of modern therapy has been estimated at 2% per year with a 5-year overall transformation rate at approximately 10%.[2,3] In that setting, diagnostic workup should proceed as directed for diffuse large B-cell lymphoma (DLBCL) (see below).

Morphology

The classic pattern of FL in a lymph node is effacement of the architecture by a nodular infiltrate representing abnormal secondary follicles, growing back-to-back, with uniform shape and size (Figure 5.2). However, in practice there is wide variability of the growth patterns that can be seen in FL, and in small biopsies the underlying pattern can be challenging to appreciate. Patterns in FL range from entirely diffuse growth (Figure 5.3), without underlying follicular dendritic cells, to serpiginous "follicles" mimicking a diffuse pattern, to large expansile follicles (Figure 5.4), and unusual variants such as the floral variant (Figure 5.5), which may mimic progressive transformation of germinal centers (PTGC). Importantly, interfollicular growth should not be interpreted as a diffuse pattern. In the retroperitoneum, core biopsies of lymph nodes involved by FL often show diffuse growth of lymphocytes in dense fibrosis, which can make diagnosis challenging unless multiple well-preserved cores are obtained (Figure 5.1). Lymph nodes also may show variability of the growth pattern within a single biopsy. When true diffuse and nodular growth is present in the biopsy, it is recommended to estimate a percentage of each in the diagnosis. This however might be only feasible or practical on an excisional biopsy.[2]

The neoplastic follicles in FL comprise a mixture of two types of B cells, centrocytes (small, angulated or cleaved cells) and centroblasts (large, round cells with often multiple small nucleoli), recapitulating the composition of normal germinal centers (Figure 5.6). In reactive germinal centers, polarization can usually be appreciated with a dark zone and light zone representing variability in the proportion of centroblasts (Figure 5.7). In FL, however, polarization is lost and can be a clue to the neoplastic nature of the infiltrate. Other morphologic clues that can help distinguish reactive from neoplastic follicles include a loss of tingible body macrophages within the germinal centers, and attenuation or complete loss of the surrounding mantle zones.

Per the ICC, grading of FL is required and is done based on counting the mean number of centroblasts per 10 consecutive 400× microscopic fields.[1,2] Grading is not equivalent to Ki-67 or other proliferation index markers, and these should not be used in lieu of morphologic grading. Grading is as follows: grade 1 if ≤5 centroblasts per 400× field, grade 2 if 6 to 15 centroblasts per 400× field, and grade 3 if >15 centroblasts per 400×

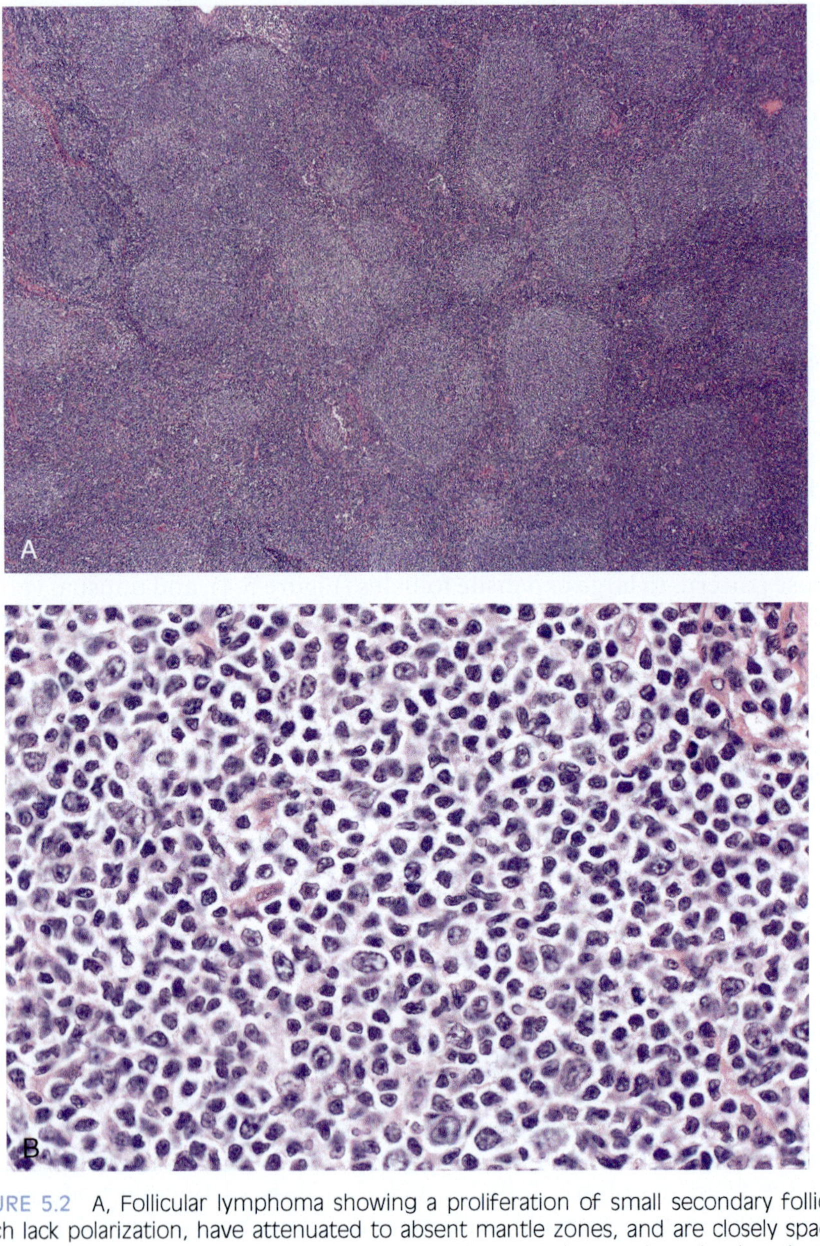

FIGURE 5.2 A, Follicular lymphoma showing a proliferation of small secondary follicles, which lack polarization, have attenuated to absent mantle zones, and are closely spaced. B, High power of follicular lymphoma, grade 1-2, shows a mixture of predominantly small cells with angulated nuclei (centrocytes) and few larger centroblasts.

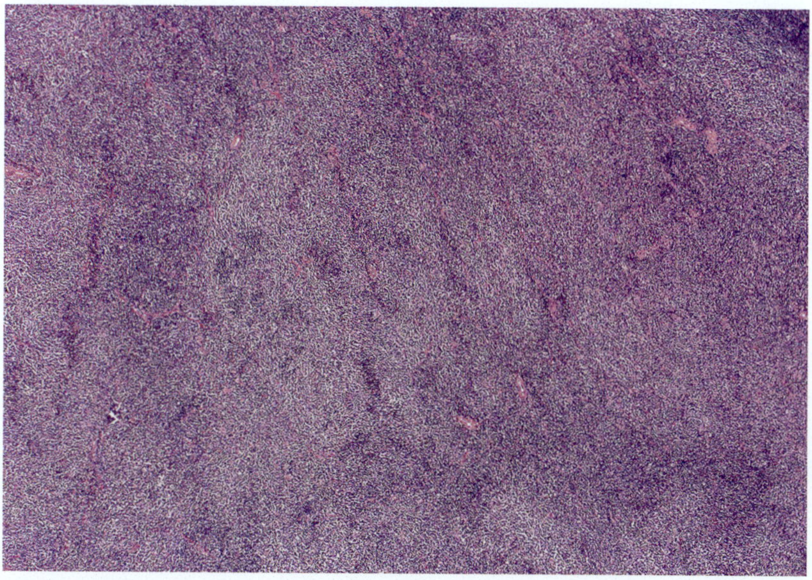

FIGURE 5.3 **Diffuse growth in follicular lymphoma.** This pattern is only acceptable in low grade (1-2).

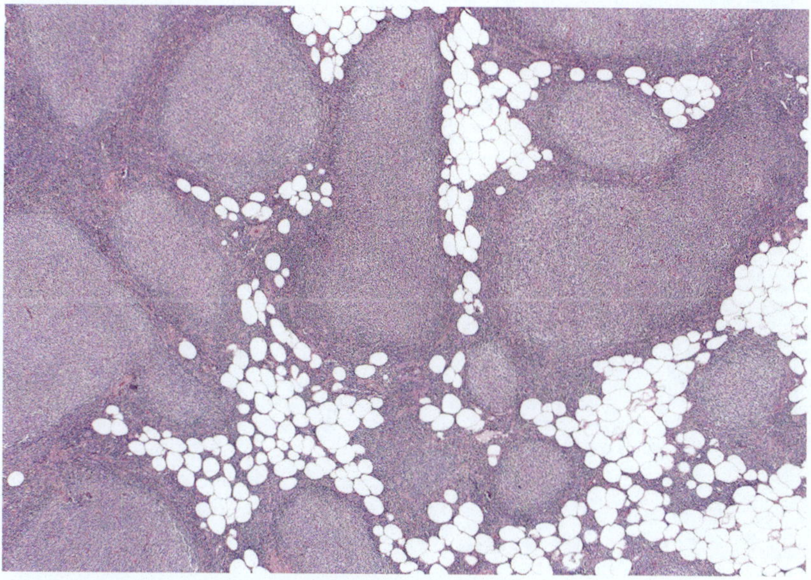

FIGURE 5.4 **Expansile follicles in follicular lymphoma.**

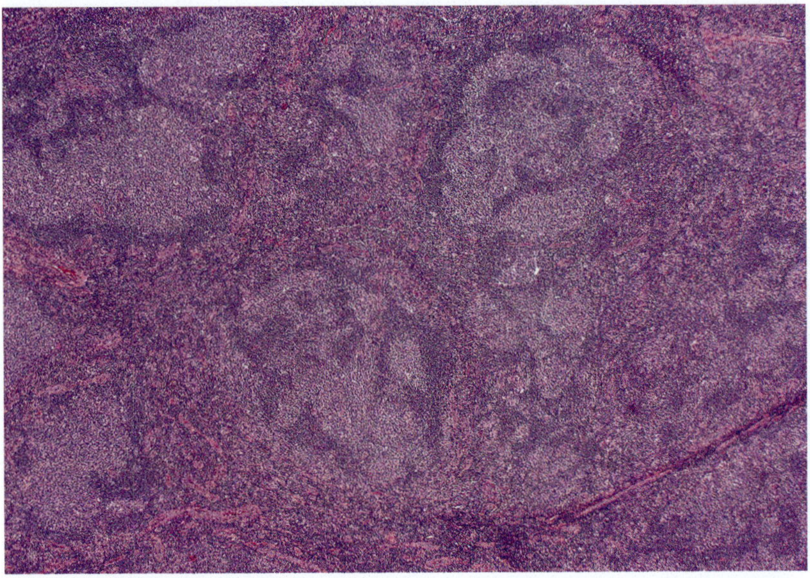

FIGURE 5.5 Follicular lymphoma with a floral growth pattern mimicking progressive transformation of germinal centers.

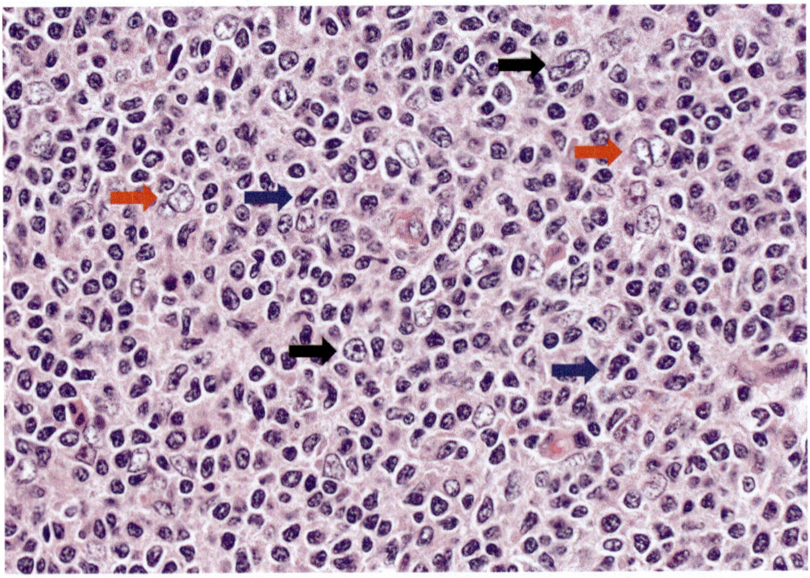

FIGURE 5.6 High-power magnification of follicular lymphoma showing centrocytes (blue arrows), centroblasts (black arrows), and follicular dendritic cells (red arrows).

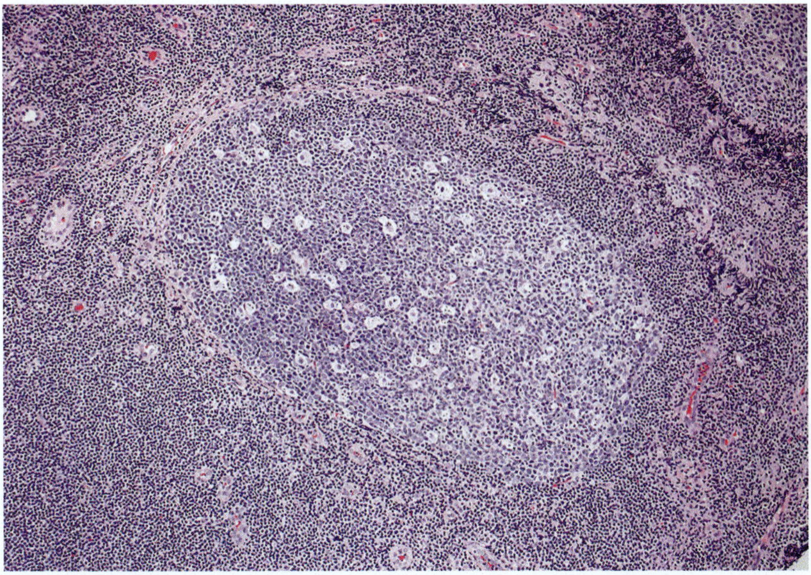

FIGURE 5.7 Reactive germinal center with retained polarization showing a dark zone (left) and light zone (right).

field. Grade 3 is subclassified as grade 3A (Figure 5.8) and 3B (Figure 5.9), with grade 3B having essentially 100% centroblasts and grade 3A being composed of a mixture of both cell types. If distinction between 3A and 3B is challenging, CD10 expression and *BCL2* rearrangement favor grade 3A.[1,4] Care must be taken not to mistake follicular dendritic cells, which have oval nuclei and may have prominent nucleoli, for centroblasts (Figure 5.6). Grades 1 and 2 are now grouped together (FL, grade 1-2) due to lack of clinical utility and reproducibility in splitting these. Importantly, only grade 1-2 cases can have a diffuse growth pattern; diffuse growth of grade 3 FL is diagnostic of DLBCL.

As with growth patterns, cytology in FL can vary and can make grading challenging, especially on small biopsies. One variant seen frequently (~10%) is FL with marginal zone differentiation, in which the FL takes on a monocytoid appearance similar to MZL (Figure 5.10).[5] Distinction from MZL with follicular colonization is essential in this setting. Overt plasmacytic differentiation in FL is rare, although it can occur and does not preclude the diagnosis.[6] Rare cases with signet-ring cell features can be seen (Figure 5.11).

Phenotype

FL expresses pan B-cell markers (CD20, CD19, PAX5, CD79a), and will typically express both germinal center markers CD10 and BCL6. However, CD10 may be absent, especially in grade 3 cases.[4] FL should be included in

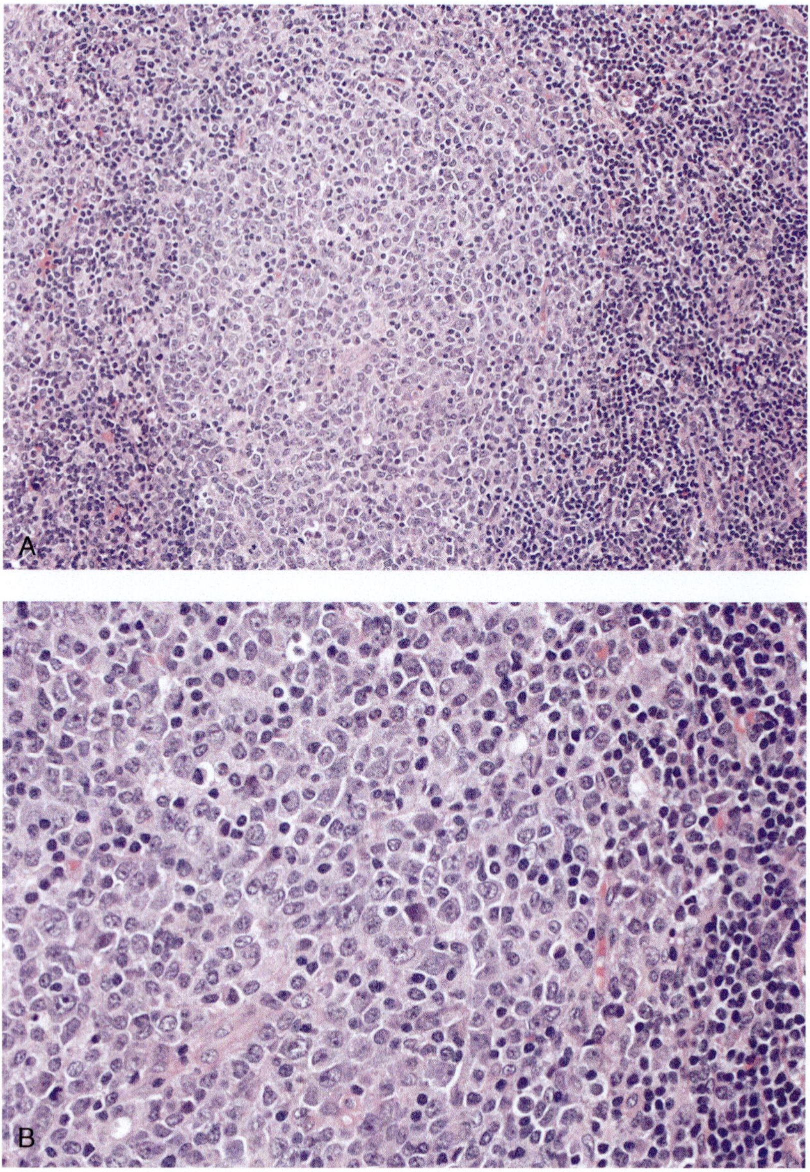

FIGURE 5.8 A and B, Follicular lymphoma grade 3A showing greater than 15 centroblasts per high power field.

the differential diagnosis of a CD10-/CD5- B-cell clone identified by FCM of a lymph node. CD10 and/or BCL6 may be positive within the neoplastic follicles but lost in the interfollicular component of the clone. Aberrant BCL2 expression is typically seen within the neoplastic germinal center B cells (GCB) and is a useful diagnostic feature (Figure 5.12). This aberrant expression of BCL2 may be helpful in differentiating follicular hyperplasia

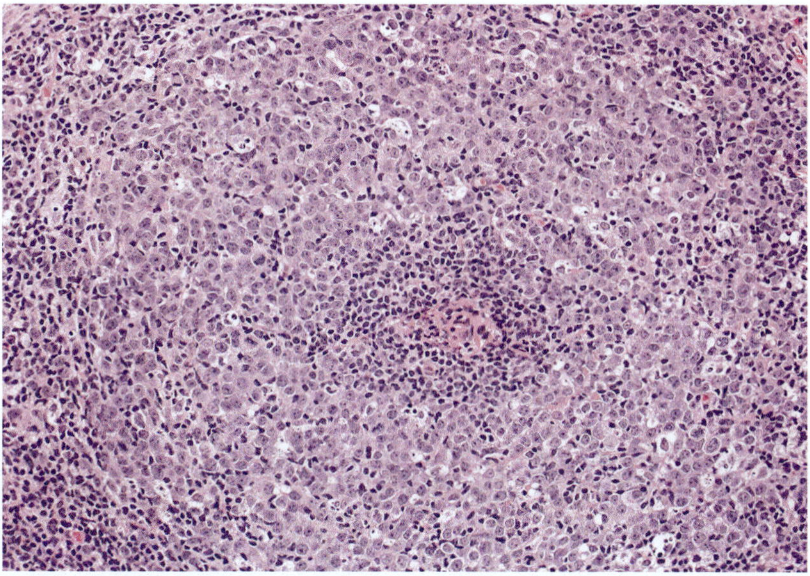

FIGURE 5.9 **Follicular lymphoma grade 3B.** The follicle (which in this example also shows an unusual targetoid pattern) is composed entirely of centroblasts.

from FL; however, expression of BCL2 does not help differentiate FL from other SBCLs as it is positive in most SBCLs. BCL2 must be interpreted in comparison to a CD3 stain, as normal T cells will express BCL2 and can be present in significant numbers within germinal centers. Additionally, BCL2 can be negative in up to 15% of low-grade FL and up to 50% of FL grade 3.[1,7] CD23 expression is common, and CD5 expression is rare, but has been reported on FL. Cyclin D1, LEF1, and SOX11 are negative. CD21 and/or CD23 should be used to identify follicular dendritic meshworks underlying the infiltrate, and can help exclude a true diffuse component.

Ki-67 is typically low (<30%) in keeping with the indolent nature of the disease. This feature also may help distinguish neoplastic germinal centers from reactive ones, since reactive germinal centers have a Ki-67 of close to 100%. Cases of FL with a low-grade histologic appearance may show a high proliferation index with Ki-67.[8] Data remain uncertain on the significance of this finding and reporting Ki-67 in cases of FL is not required.

Genetics

IgGR studies will reveal a clonal rearrangement in the majority of FL cases.[9] Of note, false negative results can occur in FL due to ongoing somatic hypermutation in GCBs.[9] As with any other lymphoma, lack of a clone by IgGR does not preclude the diagnosis.

Expression of BCL2 in GCBs in FL is mediated most frequently by the t(14;18)(q32;q21), which juxtaposes the *BCL2* gene onto the IGH promoter. This translocation is present in ~90% of grade 1-2 and fewer cases of grade

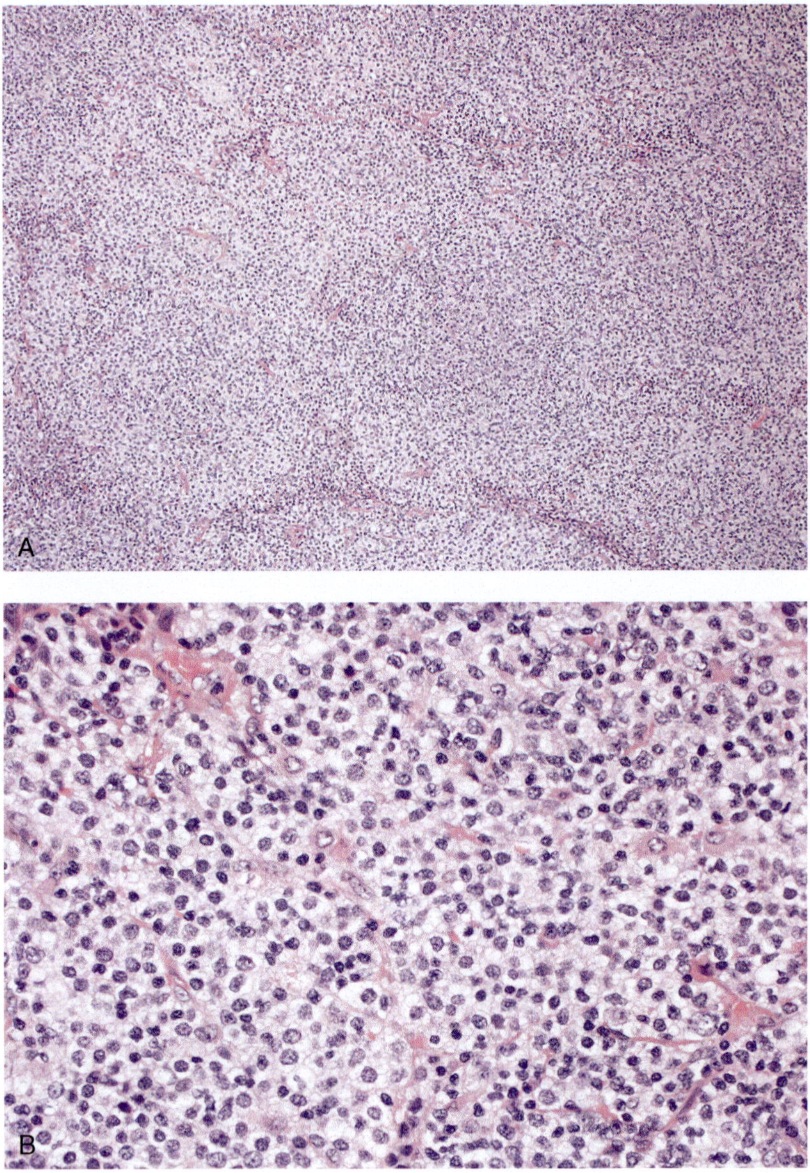

FIGURE 5.10 (*Continued*)

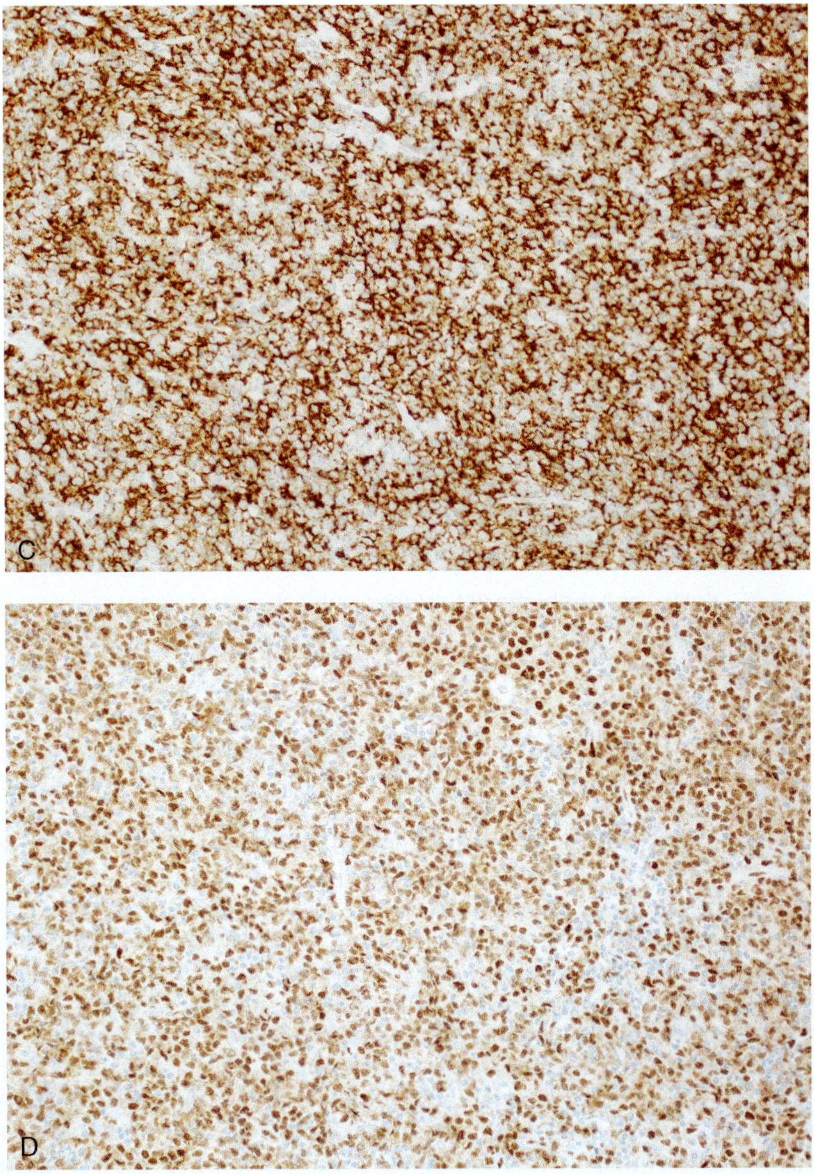

FIGURE 5.10 A and B, Follicular lymphoma with marginal zone differentiation. This case shows a monocytoid cytology with abundant pale cytoplasm. Phenotyping shows expression of CD10 (C) and BCL6 (D).

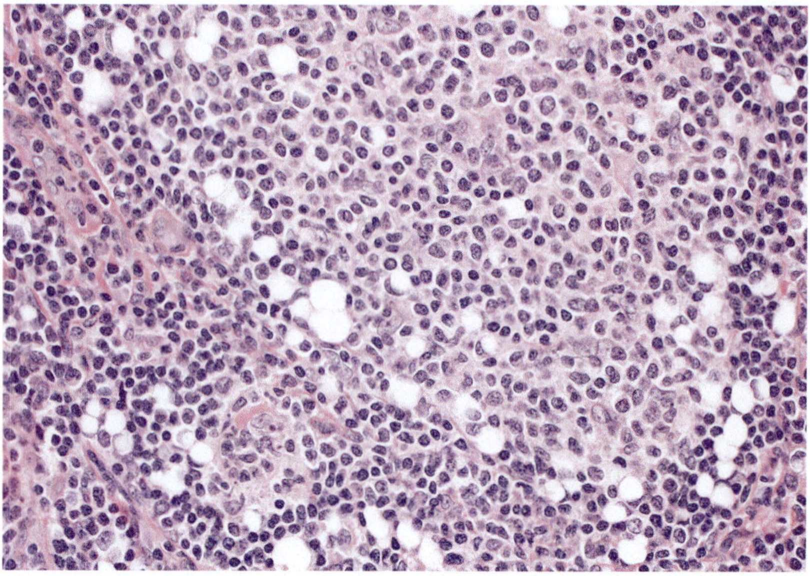

FIGURE 5.11 Follicular lymphoma with signet-ring cell morphology.

3 FL.[4] A subset of cases may have *BCL6* (3q27) rearrangements (~15%), with or without IGH::*BCL2*.[10,11] Rearrangements of *BCL6* and *BCL2* can be identified by interphase FISH testing on paraffin-embedded tissue sections.

FISH testing for *BCL2* may aid distinguishing a FL with marginal zone differentiation from a MZL, as *IGH-BCL2* rearrangements would support a diagnosis of FL in this context. *BCL6* FISH should be used with caution here, as MZL can harbor *BCL6* rearrangements.[10-12] FISH may also be useful on small biopsies where high numbers of T cells preclude accurate interpretation of BCL2 IHC on the B cells. Importantly, neither *BCL2* nor *BCL6* rearrangements are specific for FL, and neither should be used to render a diagnosis of FL in the absence of morphologic findings. Most cases of FL do not require the use of FISH for diagnosis.

One provisional variant of FL in the 2022 ICC classification is entitled t(14;18)-negative CD23+ follicle center cell lymphoma.[1] These typically present as large masses in inguinal lymph nodes and with low-stage disease. They frequently, but not always, have a diffuse growth pattern. They have distinct genetic features including lack of *BCL2* rearrangements, presence of deletion at 1p36, and *STAT6* mutations.[13] In the appropriate setting, the 1p36 deletion can be identified by FISH and *STAT6* mutations by NGS. However, 1p36 deletion is not specific for this type of FL and is seen commonly in standard *BCL2*-rearranged FL.[13] In general, 1p36 FISH is not necessary for diagnosis of diffuse FL.

MYC rearrangement, typically considered a marker of high-grade BCLs, has been found incidentally in <5% of otherwise typical FL.[14] The significance of this finding is still uncertain,[14] and FL with *MYC* and *BCL2*

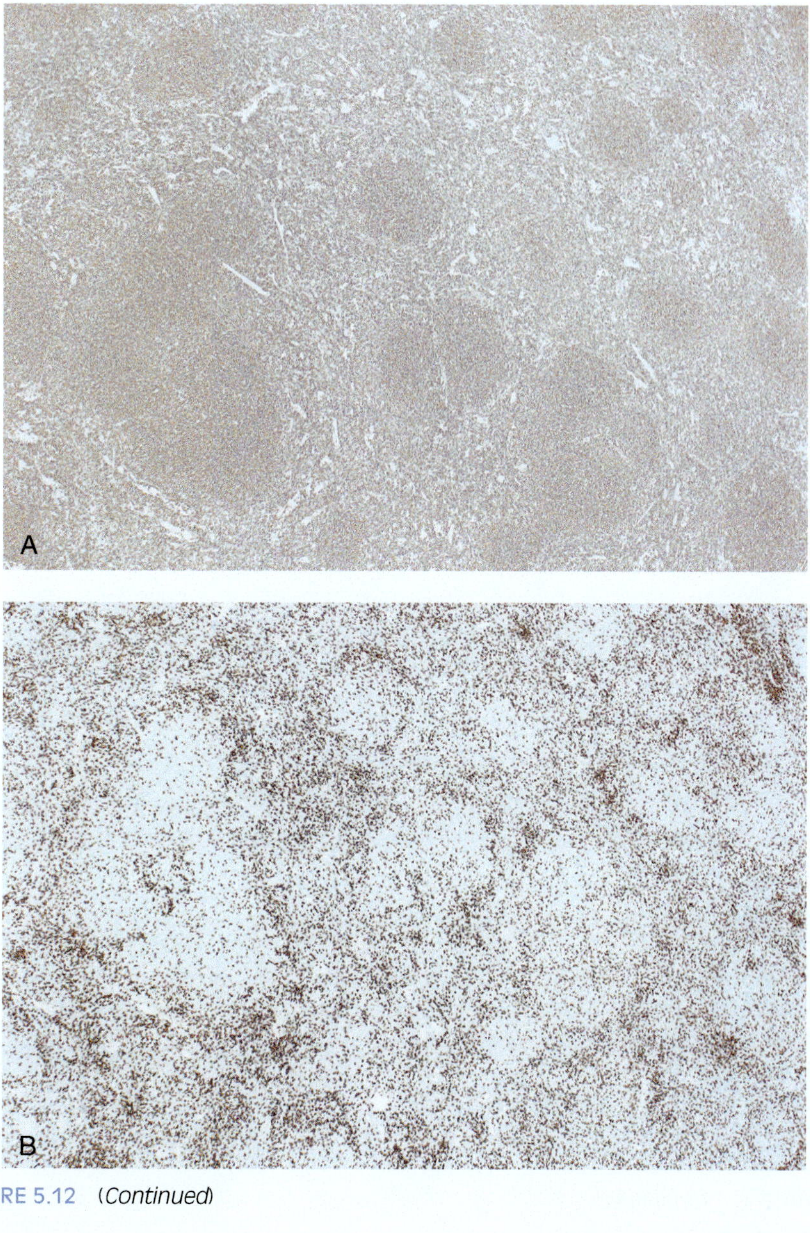

FIGURE 5.12 (*Continued*)

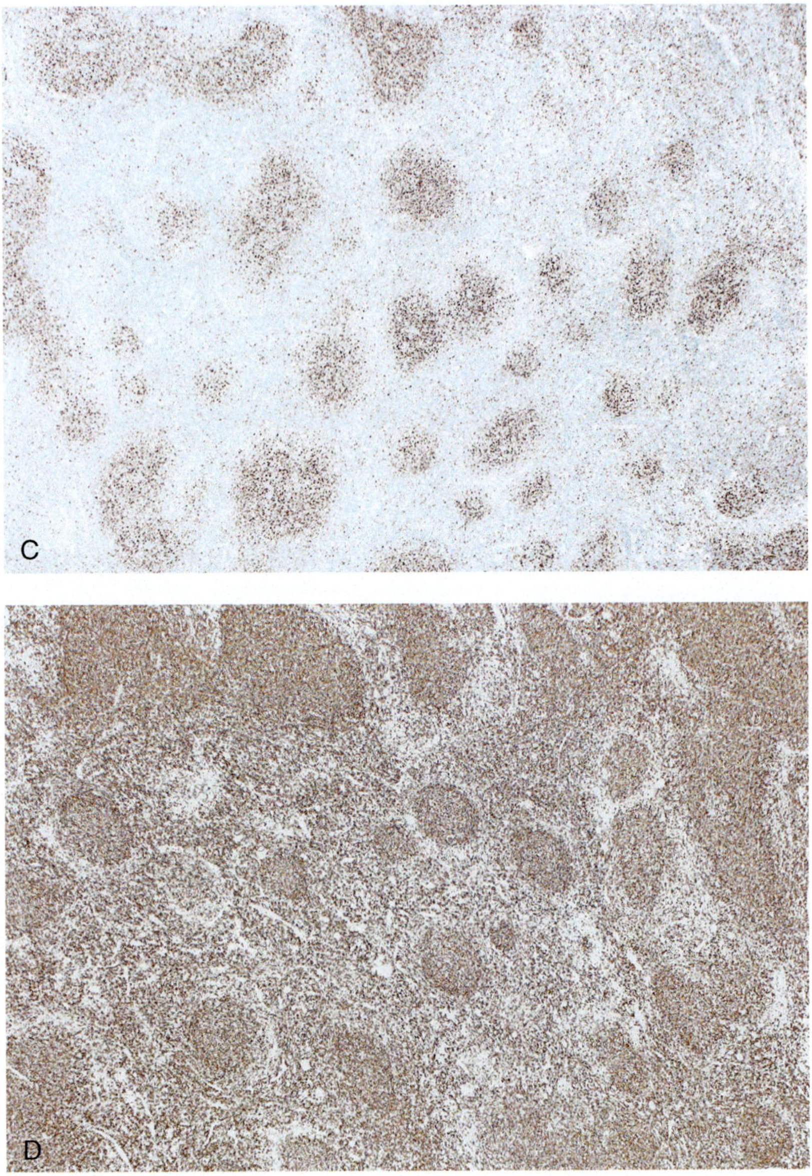

FIGURE 5.12 *(Continued)*

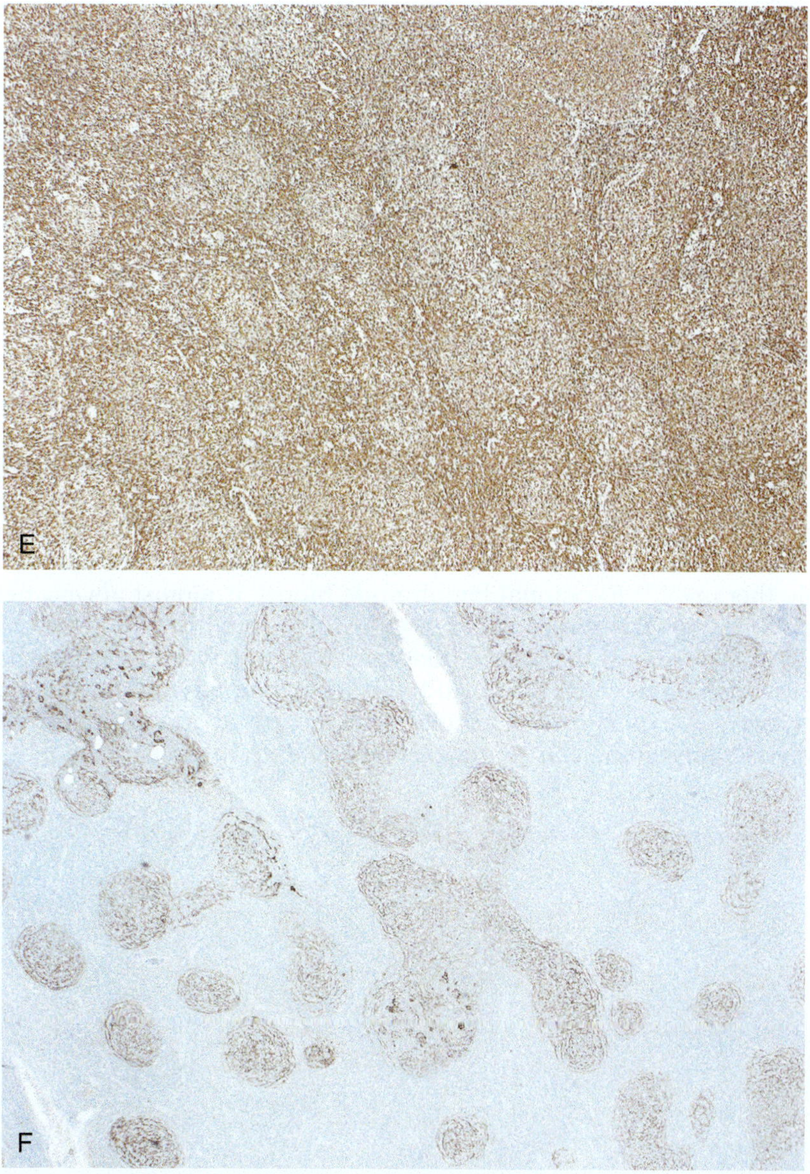

FIGURE 5.12 **Immunohistochemical staining pattern in follicular lymphoma**. A, CD20 stains B cells effacing the architecture with a nodular pattern. B, CD3 shows interfollicular T cells. C, BCL6 stains germinal centers but is downregulated in the interfollicular component of the tumor. D, CD10 stain the germinal center B cells, which extend beyond the follicles into the interfollicular space. E, BCL2 shows aberrant staining within CD10/BCL6 positive cells. F, CD21 shows underlying follicular dendritic meshworks within the neoplastic nodules.

and/or *BCL6* rearrangement should not be considered within the high-grade BCL category.[1] *MYC* FISH is not recommended in the standard workup of FL.

Numerous recurrent mutations have been identified in FL through NGS studies, although testing for these is limited to settings in which targeted therapy may be a consideration and is generally not performed at diagnosis in routine clinical practice. The most well-established example is *EZH2*, which is mutated in 25% of FL and for which EZH2 inhibitors may be considered for therapy.[15]

PEDIATRIC-TYPE FL

Pediatric-type FL (PT-FL) is a distinct clinicopathologic entity.[1] It is a nodal FL with a predilection for localized disease in the head/neck area that often, but not always, presents in children.[16-18] As such, with the appropriate clinicopathologic features, this entity may be considered even in adult patients. Distinction from standard FL is critical, as these lesions typically are localized and have excellent prognosis, sometimes even without systemic therapy.[16-18] Excisional lymph node biopsy is almost always needed when this diagnosis is a consideration.

Architecture of the lymph node in PT-FL is effaced by expansile follicles, which often resemble florid follicular hyperplasia more than typical FL (Figure 5.13). A rim of normal architecture at the periphery of the involved lymph node can sometimes be a clue to the neoplastic nature of

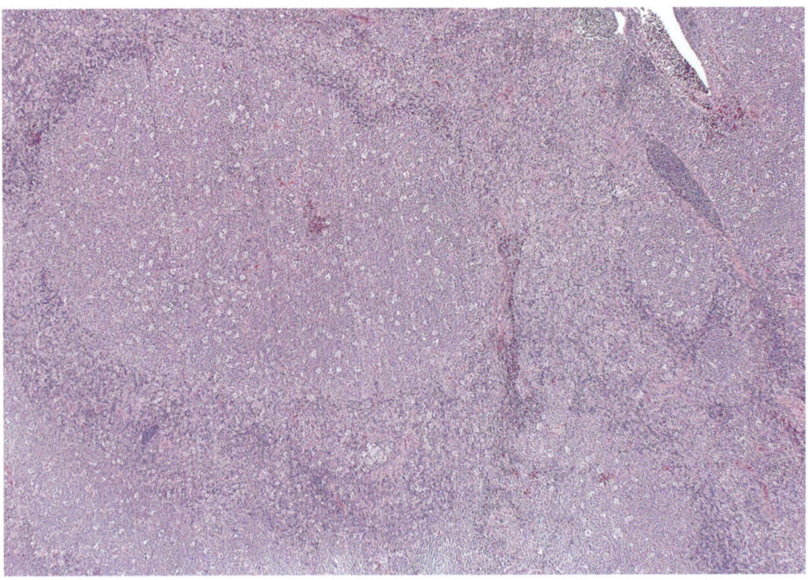

FIGURE 5.13 Pediatric-type follicular lymphoma showing expansile follicles with abundant tingible body macrophages mimicking reactive follicular hyperplasia.

the proliferation. The follicles often have a prominent tingible body macrophage population, again imparting an appearance similar to reactive follicles. They are composed of a monomorphous cell population, which does not quite have the features of either centrocytes or centroblasts. The cells instead are medium in size with a blastoid appearance and inconspicuous nucleoli (Figure 5.14). Mantle zones are often lost or attenuated. Grading is not performed here, as these have an overall indolent behavior in spite of their aggressive cytologic appearance.[16-18]

By IHC (Figure 5.14) most cases express both CD10 and BCL6 and are negative for BCL2. If BCL2 expression is seen, it is typically weak and variable, as by definition these cases must lack the IGH::*BCL2* rearrangement. Ki-67 staining is useful here, as these cases should have a Ki-67 >30% (although in most cases it is quite high [80%-100%]).[16] MUM1 staining is typically negative, and these cases are negative for rearrangements of the *IRF4* gene, distinguishing this entity from "large B-cell lymphoma with *IRF4* rearrangement" (discussed below).

Proof of light chain restriction and/or clonality by IgGR is often necessary to establish this diagnosis and distinguish PT-FL from florid follicular hyperplasia. FISH studies should be performed to exclude rearrangements of *BCL2*, *BCL6*, and *IRF4* prior to rendering this diagnosis. Recent genetic studies suggest possible relationship to pediatric-type MZL; however these remain separate entities in the 2022 ICC.

IN SITU FOLLICULAR NEOPLASIA

In situ follicular neoplasia (ISFN), formerly termed "follicular lymphoma in situ" is defined as having GCBs with the phenotype, cytology, and often genetic features of FL, but which are restricted exclusively to intact, nonexpanded germinal centers.[1,19] These germinal centers should be present in an otherwise reactive lymph node, and there should be no evidence of follicular expansion or presence of the clonal population outside of the germinal center (Figures 5.15 and 5.16). This finding is usually incidental, and the risk of overt FL is low.[20] However, a subset of patients may have subsequent or concurrent FL.[20] ISFN must also be distinguished from partial involvement of a lymph node by overt FL in which there is architectural distortion or involvement outside the germinal center.

NODAL MARGINAL ZONE LYMPHOMA

Nodal marginal zone lymphoma (NMZL) is rare (<2% of all lymphoid neoplasms) compared to FL but can present in a similar age group (median age 60 years) and with similar features as FL.[2,21] As the name implies, patients typically have lymphadenopathy, although bone marrow and peripheral blood involvement can occur making distinction from the other types of MZL (splenic MZL and extranodal MZL of mucosa-associated

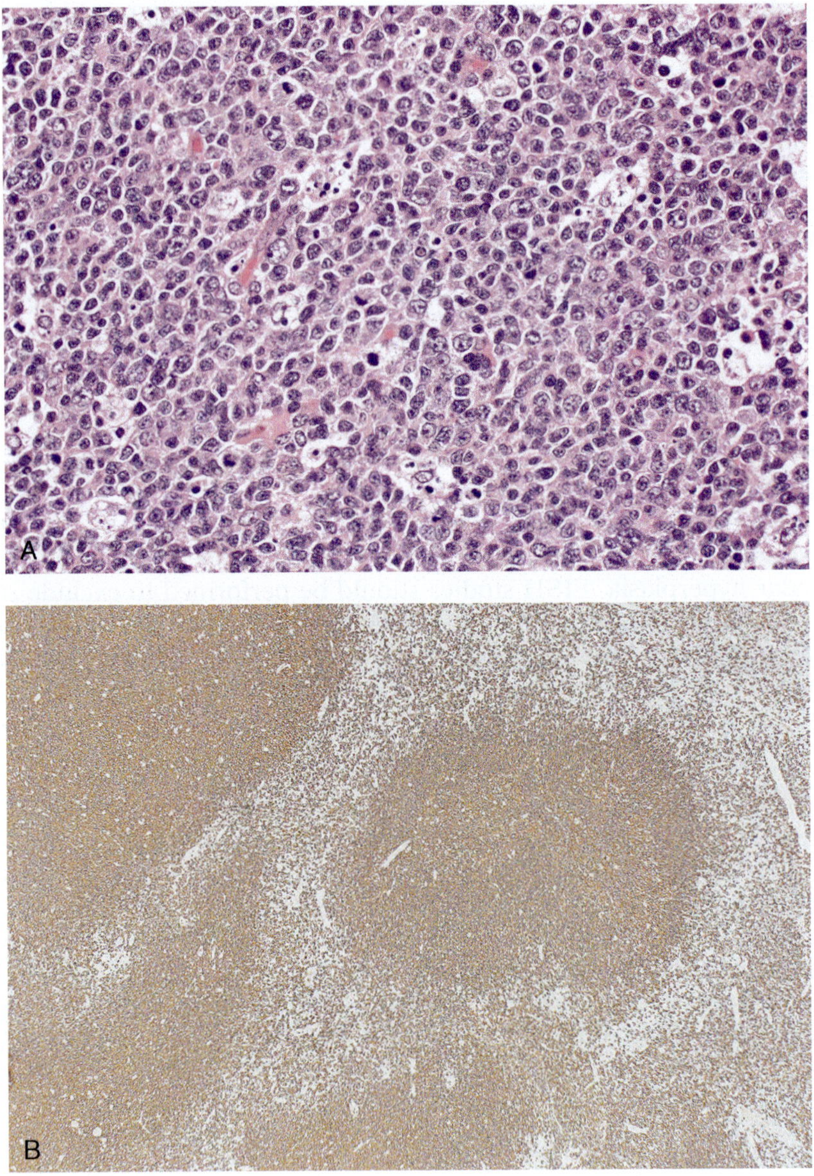

FIGURE 5.14 (*Continued*)

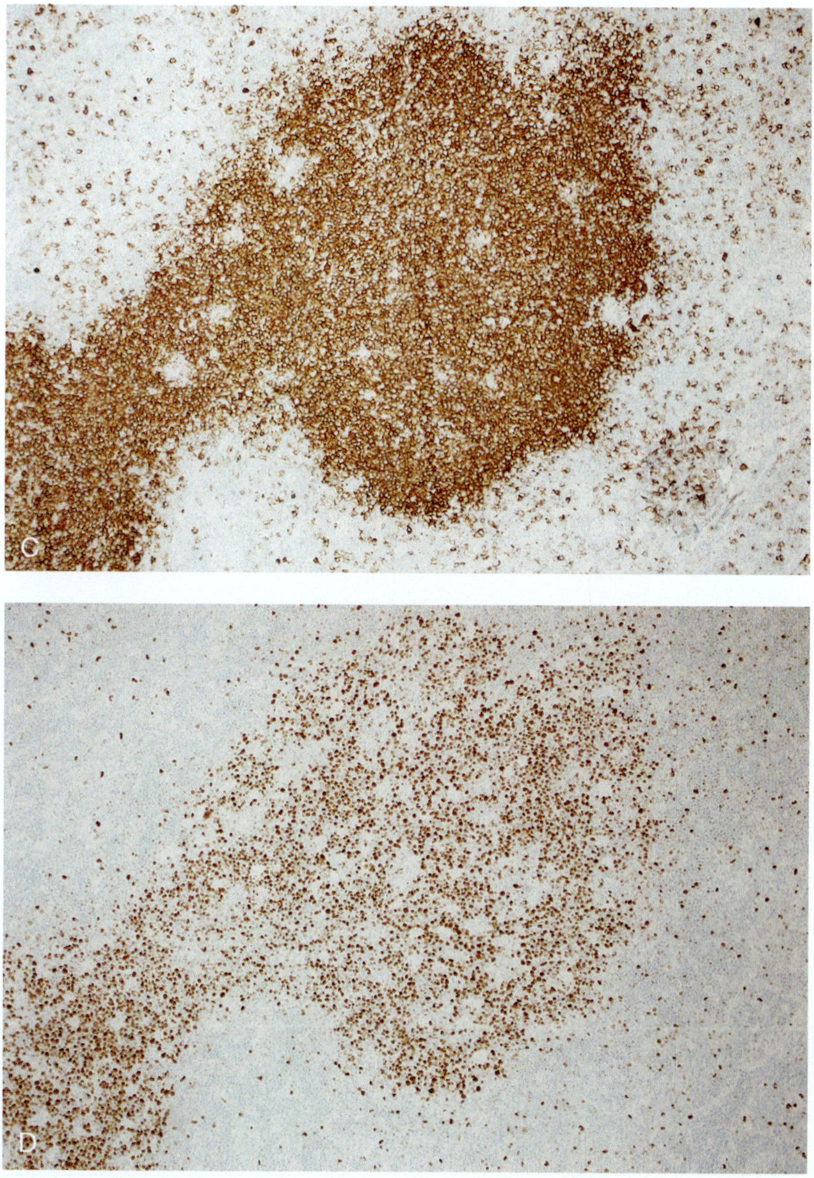

FIGURE 5.14 (*Continued*)

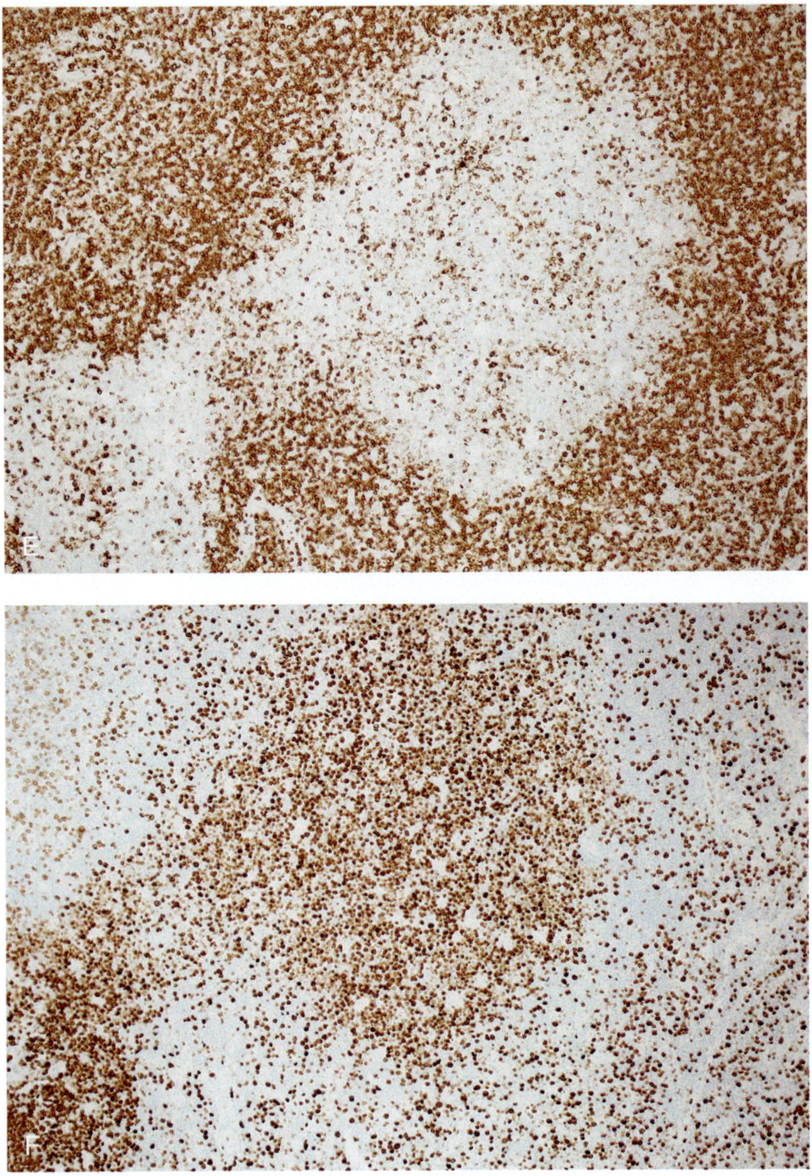

FIGURE 5.14 A, High power of pediatric-type follicular lymphoma showing predominantly intermediate-sized cells and abundant tingible body macrophages. B, CD20 is expressed in the neoplastic follicles, as well as (C) CD10 and (D) BCL6. E, Immunohistochemical staining pattern in pediatric type follicular lymphoma. BCL2 is typically negative in the neoplastic follicles. F, Ki-67 shows a high proliferation index.

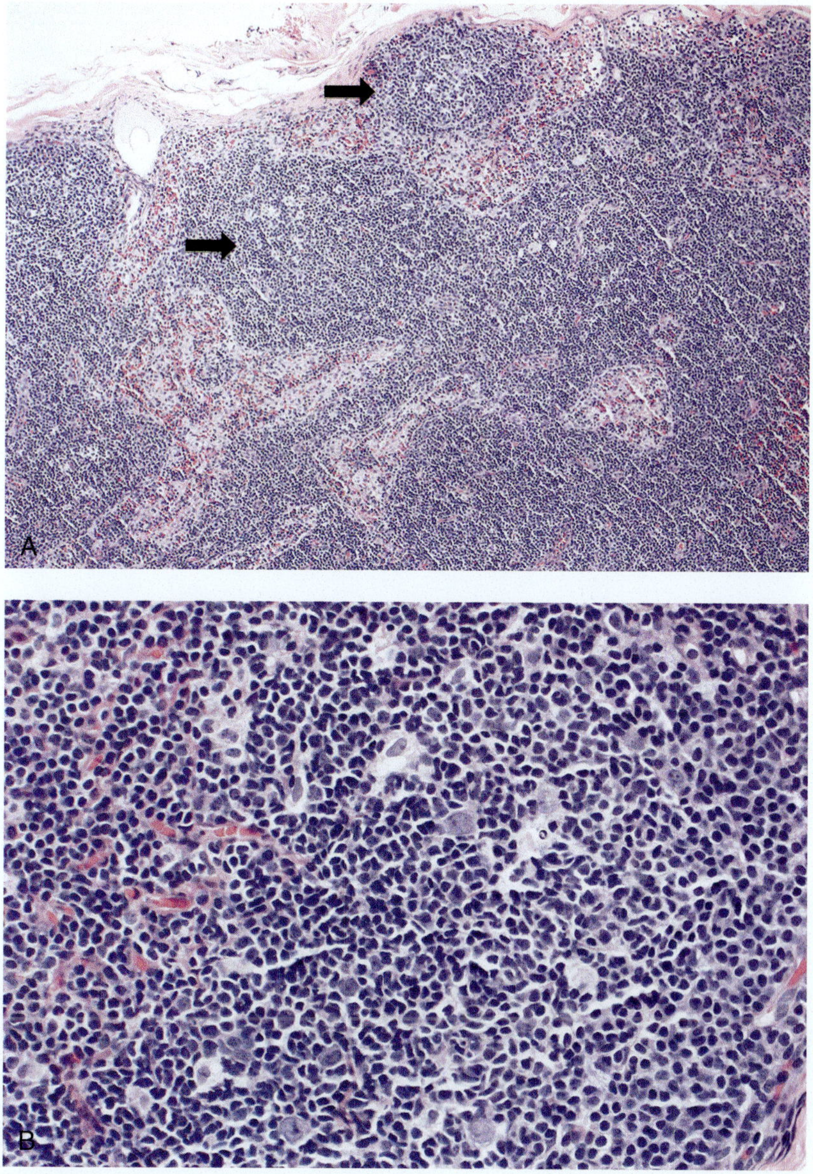

FIGURE 5.15 A, Low power of a reactive-appearing lymph node with subtle in situ follicular neoplasia (arrows). B, High power of in situ follicular neoplasia showing a germinal center composed predominantly of centrocytes. Immunohistochemistry is needed to confirm this finding.

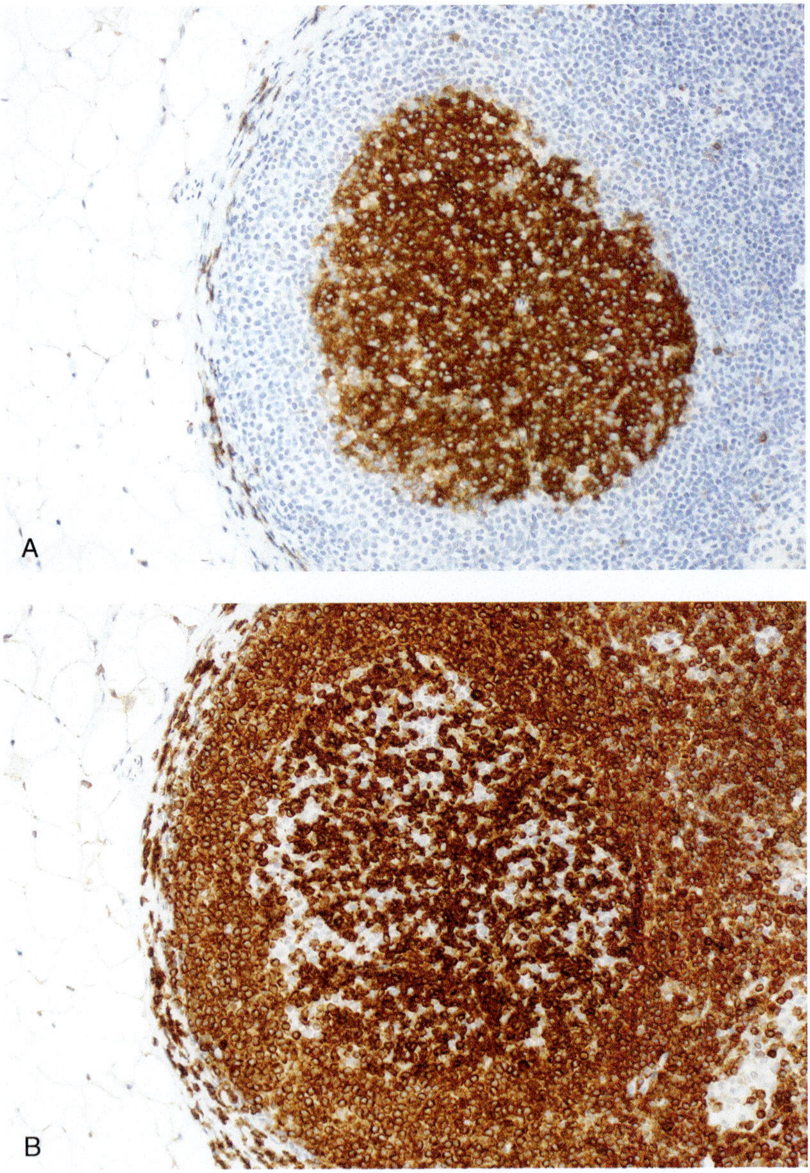

FIGURE 5.16 (*Continued*)

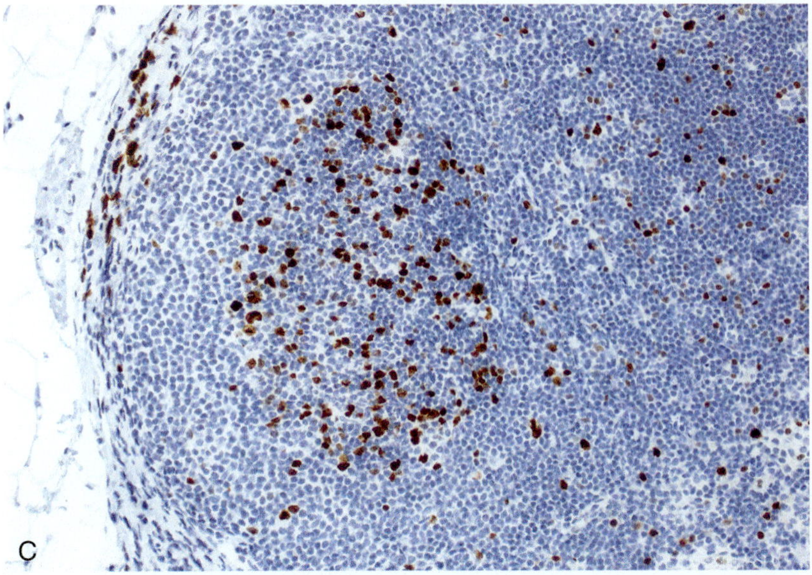

FIGURE 5.16 **In situ follicular neoplasia.** CD10 brightly stains a normal-appearing germinal center (A). B, Aberrant expression of BCL2 (bright) is seen within the germinal center. C, Ki-67 shows an aberrantly low proliferation index within the neoplastic follicle providing a clue to the neoplasia.

lymphoid tissue) challenging. Since the scope of this book encompasses nodal biopsies, the remaining discussion will focus on diagnosis of NMZL in the lymph node. However, morphologic and phenotypic features can be similar between the three MZL types, and the pathologist is not always privy to the clinical history. As such, in a lymph node biopsy a diagnosis of "MZL" without specifying subtype is acceptable, and often preferred in practice.

Morphology

In a classic MZL, the expanded compartment is that of the marginal zone B cells, leading to an interfollicular or perifollicular infiltrate with variably intact germinal centers and mantle zones in the background (Figure 5.17). NMZL can have variable growth patterns, and may grow in a completely diffuse pattern, a partially diffuse and partially nodular pattern, or even a nodular pattern mimicking FL. In addition, MZL can colonize reactive germinal centers (follicular colonization), making distinction from FL even more of a challenge.

Cytologically the most classic feature of MZL is described as "monocytoid" because the B cells of MZL have abundant pink or clear cytoplasm and thus appear the way monocytes (which have more abundant cytoplasm than lymphocytes) do in tissue (Figures 5.18 and 5.19). Cases may

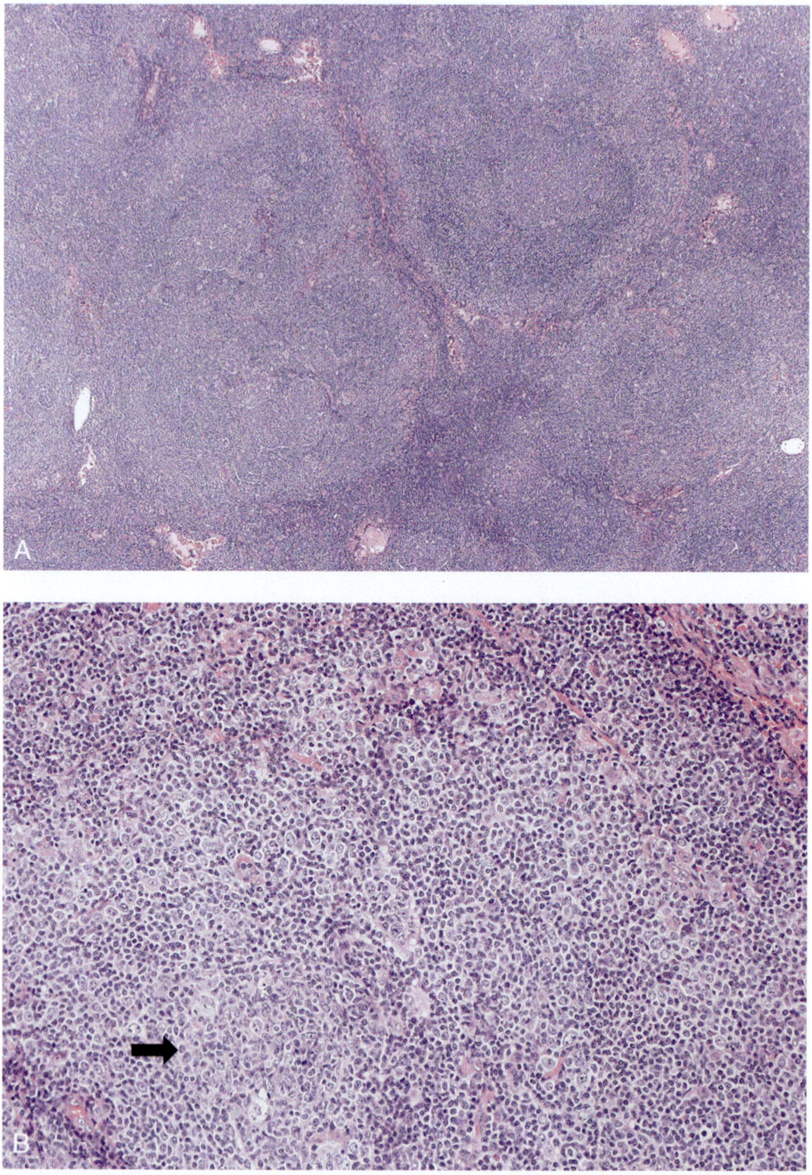

FIGURE 5.17 A, Nodal marginal zone lymphoma showing an expansion of marginal zones/interfollicular areas. Germinal centers and mantle zones are evident in the background. B, Small reactive germinal center (arrow) surrounded by marginal zone lymphoma.

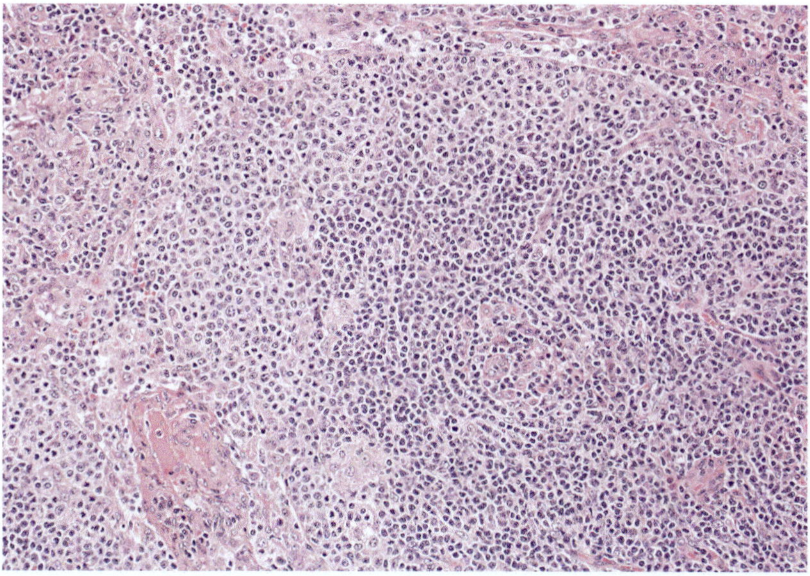

FIGURE 5.18 Marginal zone lymphoma with mixture of monocytoid cytology (left) and more bland small cell cytology (right).

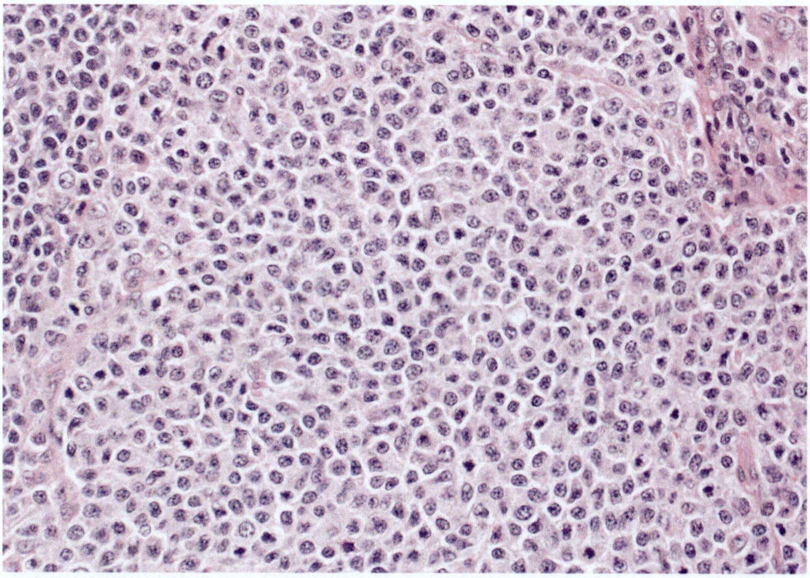

FIGURE 5.19 High-power appearance of monocytoid cytology in marginal zone lymphoma.

have areas of monocytoid cytology as well as areas with a more centrocyte-like or small round cell appearance. The size of the nuclei can be variable in MZL, and often is polymorphous within a single case. Recognition of the marginal zone pattern of growth, as well as the classic cytology, can be helpful to avoid misclassifying as DLBCL in this setting. Plasmacytic differentiation is common, although reactive polytypic plasma cells may also be seen in the background of MZLs and can mimic true plasmacytic differentiation.

Phenotype

MZL expresses pan B cell markers (CD20, CD19, PAX5, CD79a), and if plasmacytic differentiation is present may show a subset of mature plasma cells that are CD138+/MUM1+ and CD20-negative. MZL is typically negative for CD5, CD10, and BCL6, and may be a diagnosis of exclusion after other SBCLs are ruled out.[22] BCL2 is positive in the majority of cases, and as such this does not assist in the differential diagnosis between FL. However, evaluating for co-expression of CD10, BCL6 and BCL2 can be useful in the setting of a follicular-based process to distinguish between true FL and follicular colonization by MZL.[23] Kappa and lambda stains can be particularly useful to confirm clonality (Figure 5.20), especially if FCM is not performed. Although not the textbook rule, it is important in practice to acknowledge that up to 20% of MZLs can express CD5, CD23, and rarely they can express BCL6.[24] Cyclin D1, SOX11, and LEF1 should be negative. Newer markers IRTA1 and MNDA are not as widely utilized in routine practice, but in some studies have shown utility in helping distinguish MZL from FL since they are expressed in a high percentage of MZLs.[22]

In MZL, CD3 will often highlight abundant reactive admixed T cells (Figure 5.21). This phenomenon has been highlighted recently, as a pitfall to misdiagnosis of peripheral T-cell lymphoma (PTCL). Unlike in PTCL, T cells will be cytologically bland. Most express the T-follicular helper (TFH) marker PD1/CD279.[25] Since TFH lymphomas such as angioimmunoblastic T-cell lymphoma can have reactive B-cell infiltrates, it is critical to accurately distinguish these two processes. For this reason, as well as the nonspecific phenotype of MZL, definitive diagnosis on small or core biopsies can be more challenging than with the other SBCLs. In this setting, an excisional biopsy should be suggested.

Genetics

IgGR studies will reveal a clonal rearrangement in most cases and can be useful when the differential diagnosis is between reactive lymphoid hyperplasia and a noneffacing NMZL.

Genetic studies are primarily useful in MZL in order to exclude entities in the differential diagnosis. Trisomies of chromosomes 3 and 18 are

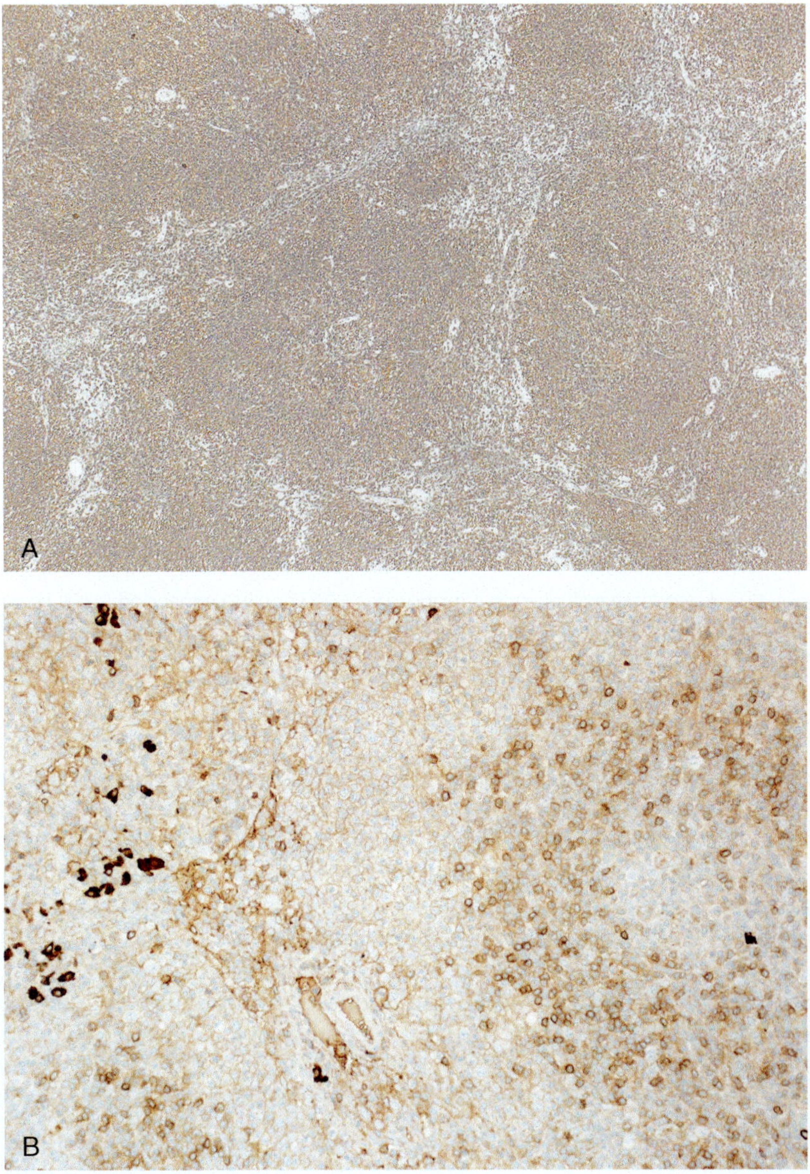

FIGURE 5.20 (*Continued*)

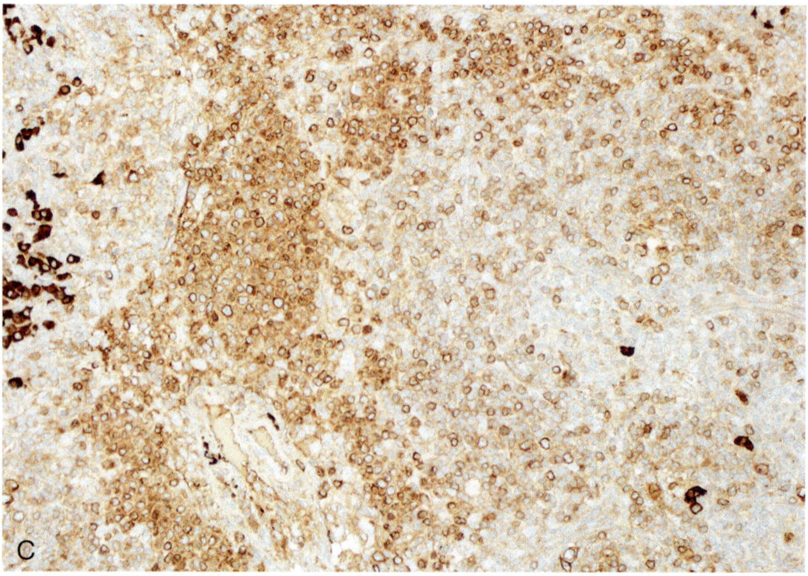

FIGURE 5.20 A, Nodal marginal zone lymphoma. CD20 showing expanded B-cell compartment. B, Kappa and (C) lambda show lambda restriction in the plasmacytoid component (dark cells, far left), as well as the B-cell component. Reactive polytypic mantle zones are also present and can make interpretation of light chain stains challenging.

common in MZL, but are not specific.[24] As discussed above, *BCL2* rearrangement (but not expression by IHC alone) supports FL over MZL.[23] The majority of the time FISH is not necessary in the workup of MZL.

Because of their frequency in LPL (see below) *MYD88* L265P mutations can be useful in distinguishing NMZL (usually negative) from LPL. However, *MYD88* mutations have been found in rare cases of NMZL and as such this testing should be used carefully in conjunction with clinicopathologic features (ie, IgM monoclonal gammopathy) in classifying cases.[26,27] Recent NGS studies have revealed numerous recurrent mutations in NMZL including *KMT2D*, *PTPRD*, *NOTCH2*, and *KLF2* as well as *BRAF*; however, utility of NGS testing in classification of SBCL is still evolving.[28,29]

PEDIATRIC NMZL

Currently recognized as a provisional entity by the 2022 ICC, there is a pediatric subtype of NMZL with distinct pathologic features.[1,2] Patients are typically young and skewed heavily toward males (20:1).[2,30] They present with localized lymphadenopathy in the head and neck. Histologically these cases tend to have a pattern of follicular hyperplasia and colonization that resembles reactive PTGC (Figure 5.22).[30] The phenotype is similar to adult-type MZL. Establishing light chain restriction (Figure 5.22)

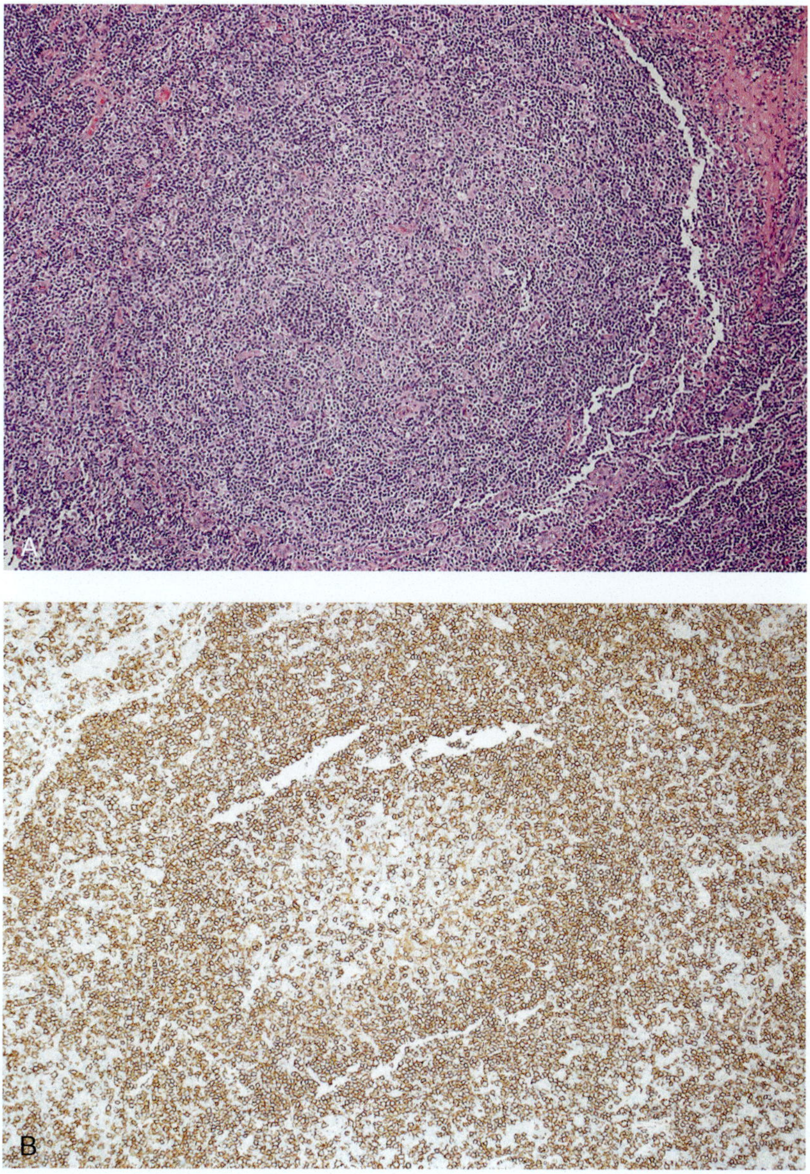

FIGURE 5.21 (*Continued*)

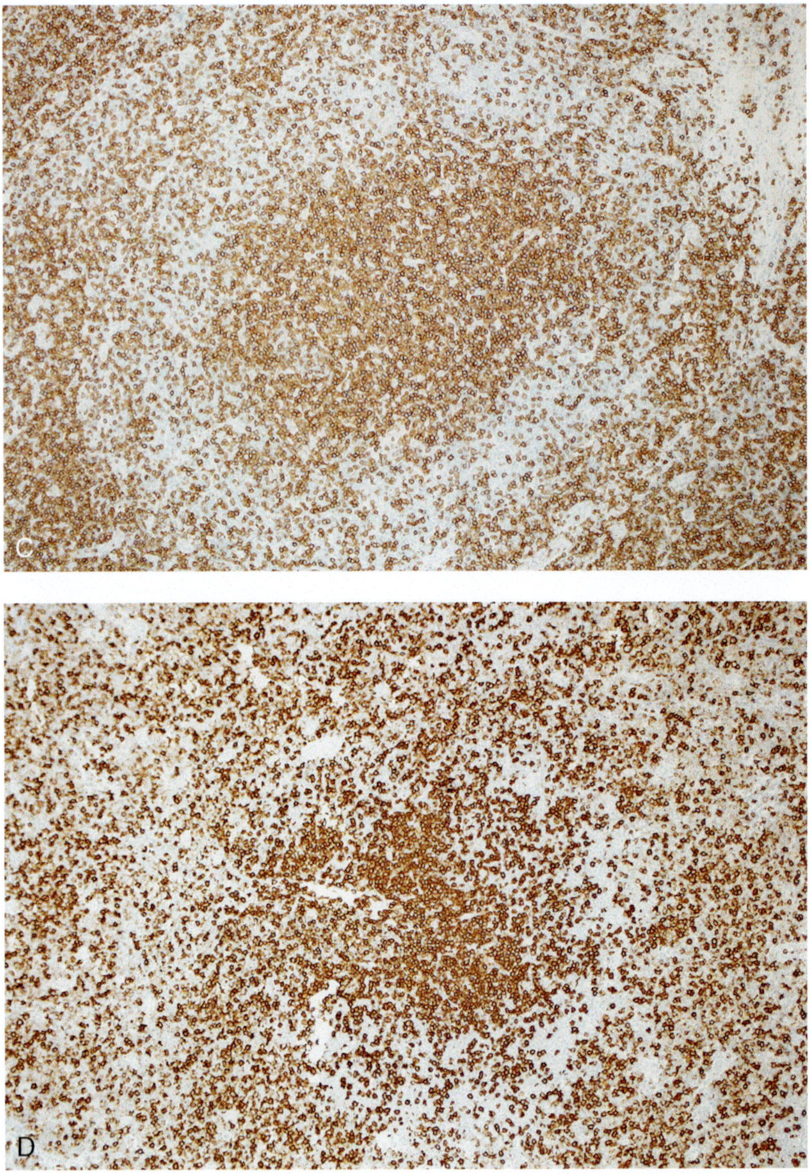

FIGURE 5.21 A, Marginal zone lymphoma with abundant admixed reactive T cells. B, CD20 stains the lymphoma cells, while (C) CD3 shows equal numbers of T cells. D, CD279 (PD1) stains the majority of the admixed T cells. This can result in a pitfall of misdiagnosis of T-cell lymphoma.

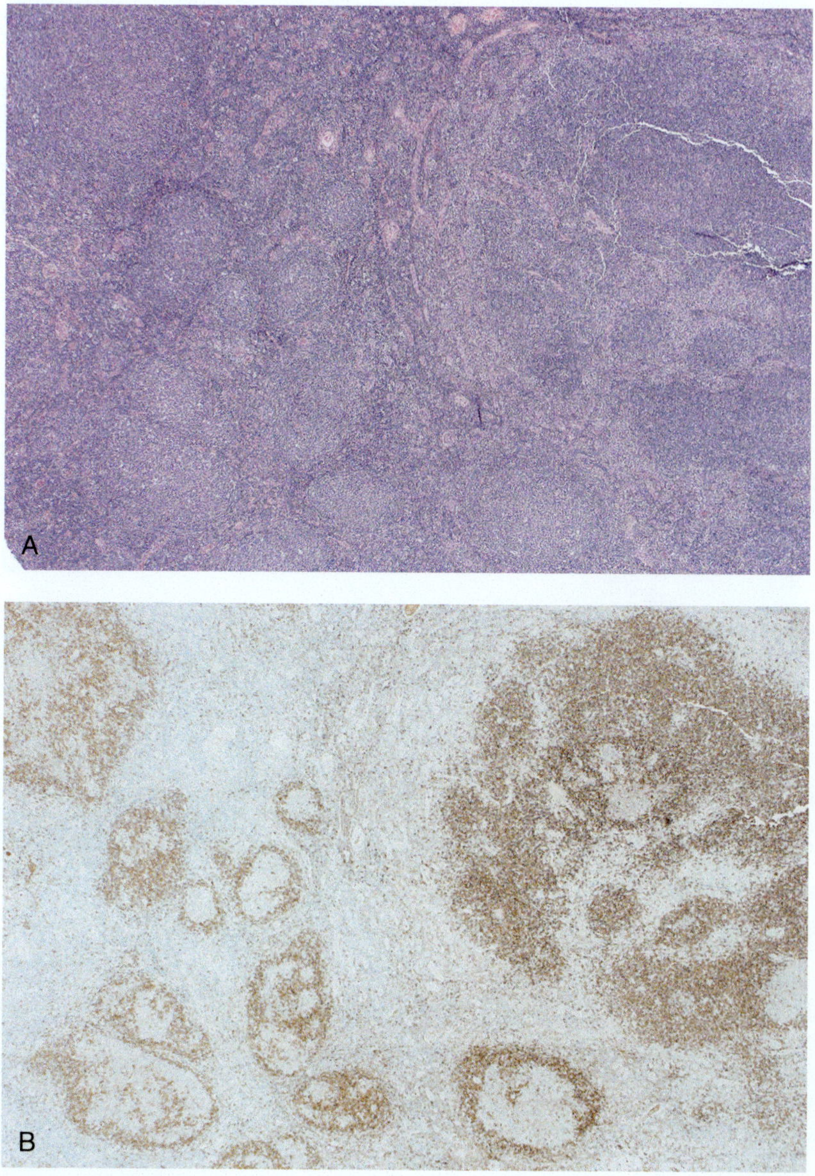

FIGURE 5.22 (*Continued*)

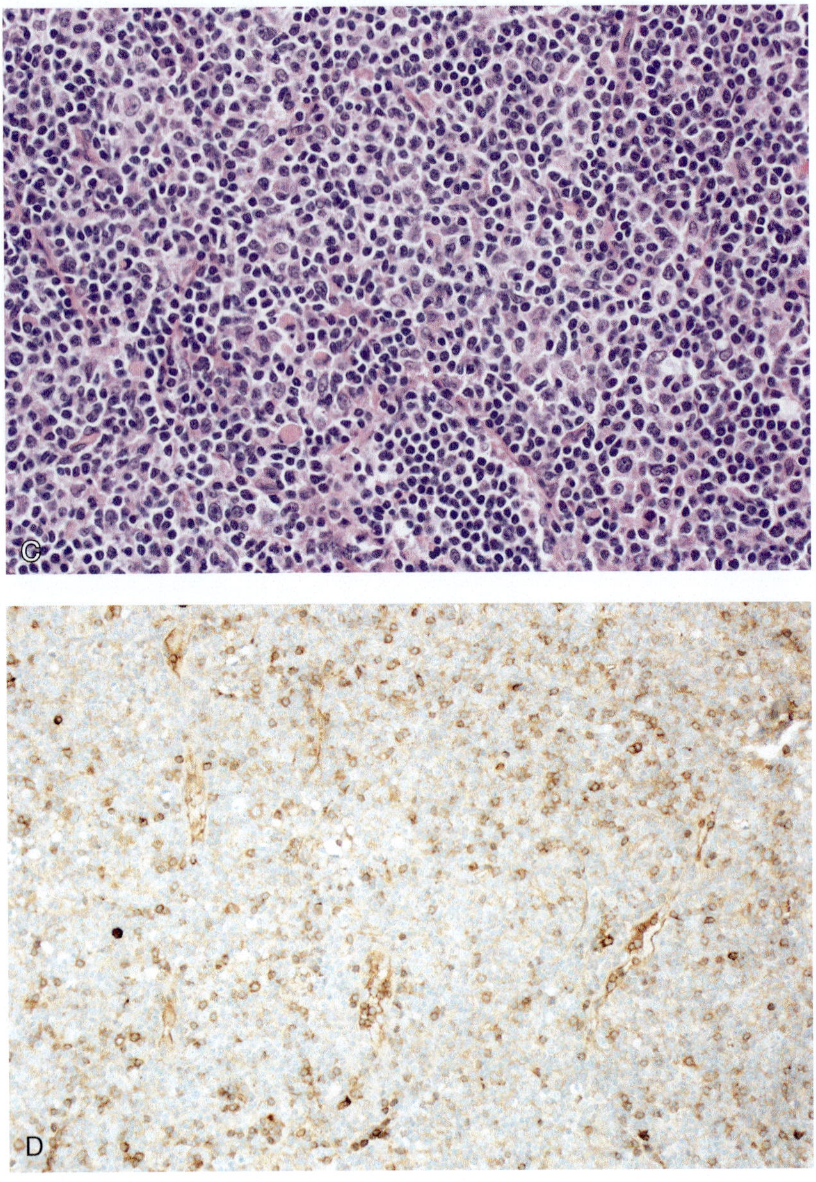

FIGURE 5.22 (*Continued*)

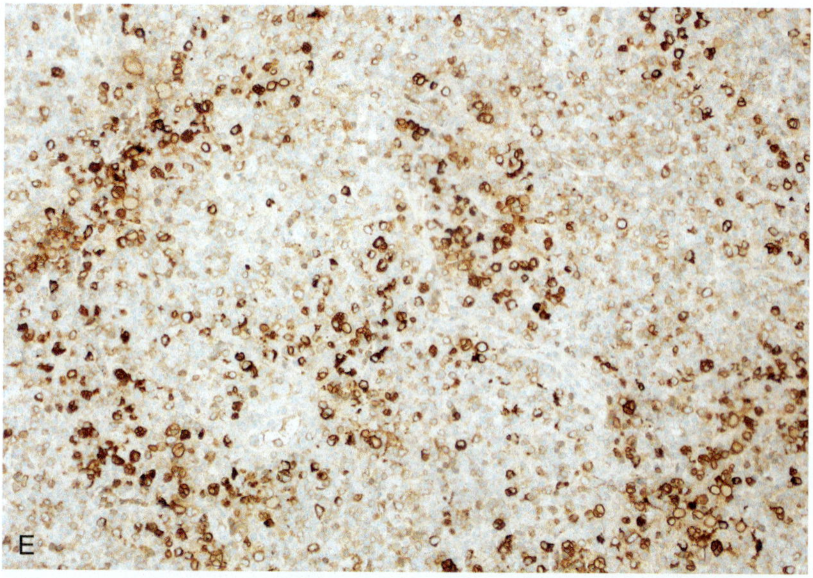

FIGURE 5.22 A, Pediatric nodal marginal zone lymphoma. B, A progressive transformation of germinal center–like pattern is often seen and can mimic reactive conditions and follicular lymphoma. IgD highlights the expanded reactive mantle zones creating progressive transformation of germinal center–like pattern. C, High-power magnification shows a cell composition of marginal zone lymphoma with small lymphocytes, monocytoid cells, and admixed mature plasma cells. A subset of plasma cells have abundant immunoglobulin inclusions in this case. D, Kappa and (E) lambda show lambda light chain-restriction.

and demonstrating a clonal IgGR is paramount in rendering a diagnosis of MZL in this setting because of reactive mimics. Specifically, atypical marginal zone hyperplasia is a light chain restricted (always lambda) but polyclonal reactive process that can morphologically mimic MZL.

MANTLE CELL LYMPHOMA

Mantle cell lymphoma (MCL) is unique among the SBCLs as it is not generally an indolent disease. However, with newer therapies and biologic insights, prognosis has improved for MCL patients over the past two decades. Recently, two biologic subgroups have been described, including a less aggressive form characterized by absence of nodal disease, SOX11 negativity, and IGVH-mutations.[1,31-34] In general, MCL presents in older patients (median age 60 years), and usually with widespread disease. Unlike with MZL and FL, MCL in children and young adults is exceedingly rare.

Morphology

MCL is a neoplasm of small, mature lymphocytes, classically resembling the cells residing in the normal mantle zone. They have round to ovoid (sometimes angulated) nuclei, condensed chromatin, and scant cytoplasm, and may resemble centrocytes of FL or the more rounded cells of CLL/SLL. They may grow in a mantle zone pattern (Figure 5.23), but more commonly show diffuse effacement of the nodal architecture.[2] Singly scattered epithelioid histiocytes may be present in the background, but in general the proliferation is rather monomorphous (Figure 5.24). Proliferation centers seen in CLL/SLL are absent.

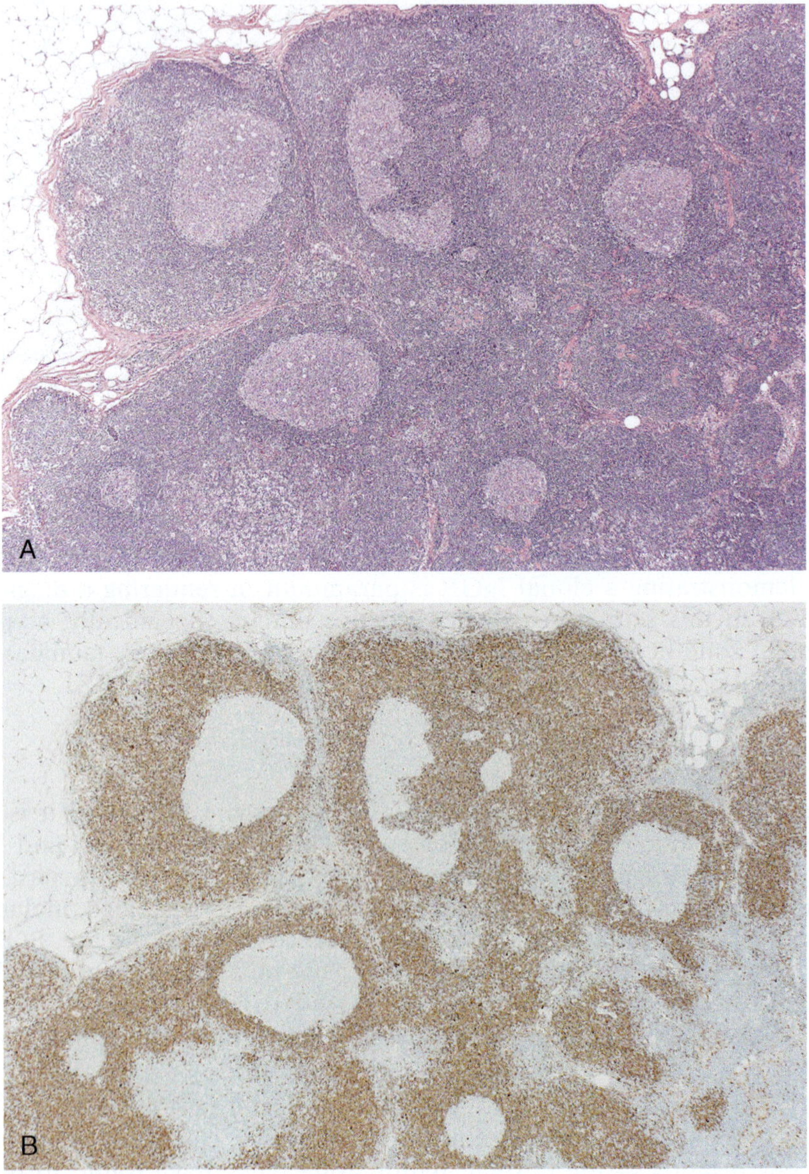

FIGURE 5.23 A, Mantle cell lymphoma, mantle zone pattern. B, Mantle zone pattern is highlighted with aberrant cyclin D1 staining.

Unlike the other SBCLs, MCL does not transform to DLBCL. However, a blastoid/pleomorphic variant of MCL is recognized, in which the cells have larger nuclei and may have more open, blastic chromatin (blastoid) (Figure 5.25) and/or a large cell lymphoma appearance with nuclear irregularity (pleomorphic). Blastoid/pleomorphic features are

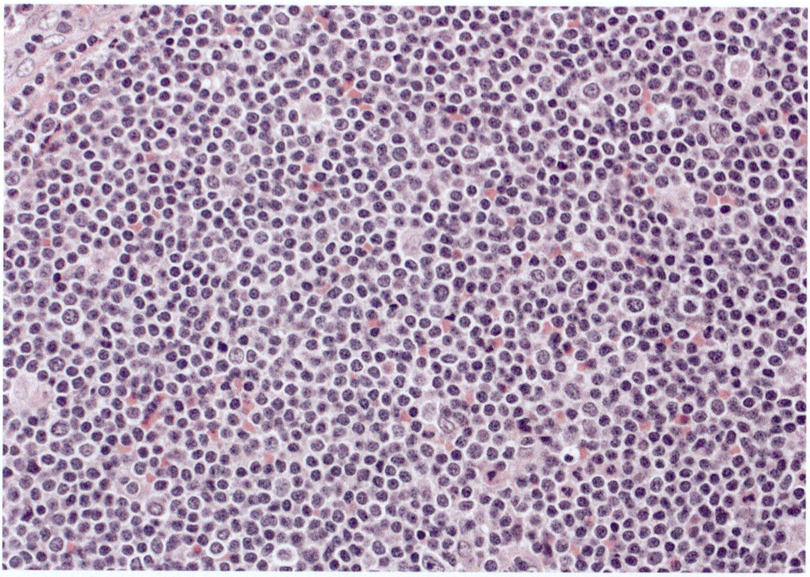

FIGURE 5.24 Monomorphic small lymphocytes in mantle cell lymphoma.

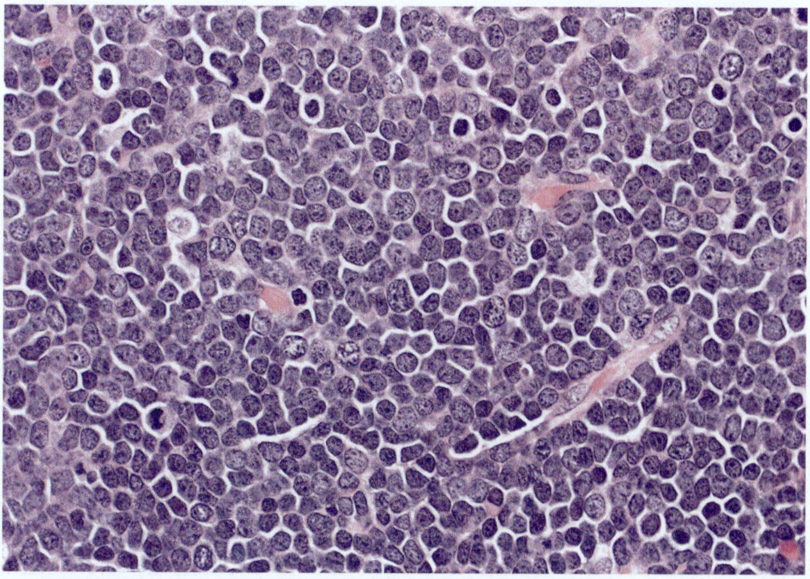

FIGURE 5.25 Blastoid/pleomorphic variant of mantle cell lymphoma in which the cells have large nuclei and open, blastic chromatin.

generally regarded as a marker of more aggressive disease along with increased Ki-67 (≥30%) and *TP53* mutation (discussed below).[1] In these cases, the differential diagnosis typically includes the more aggressive B-cell lymphomas, and pathologic workup should proceed accordingly.

Phenotype

MCL expresses pan B-cell markers (CD20, CD19, PAX5, CD79a) and typically shows aberrant coexpression of the T-cell marker CD5. In addition, there is expression of nuclear cyclin D1 in the neoplastic cells (Figure 5.26). SOX11 is a newer marker, which is also positive in the majority of MCLs and is specific within the SBCLs.[35] In contrast to CLL/SLL, which also is CD5 positive, MCL is CD23 and LEF1 negative, and CD200 negative-to-dim. In addition, while CLL/SLL is characterized by dim CD20 expression, MCL typically has moderate to bright CD20, most evident by FCM. BCL2 is uniformly positive. Germinal center markers CD10 and BCL6 are usually negative, although exceptions do occur. As mentioned above, a subset (<10%) of MCL will be SOX11-negative and this does not preclude the diagnosis. Nonnodal, leukemic MCLs are frequently SOX11-negative and may be indolent. However, absence of SOX11 alone should not be used to indicate indolent disease.

MCL is the only SBCL in which Ki-67 proliferation index has been well established as a prognostic marker. Ki-67 greater than 30% is associated with a poor prognosis.[36,37] As such, Ki-67 should be performed in all cases of MCL.

Genetics

MCL is characterized by the translocation t(11;14)(q13;q32), which places the *CCND1* gene in regulatory control of the *IGH* promoter leading to the characteristic overexpression of cyclin D1. Given the high sensitivity and specificity of cyclin D1 expression in a lymphocyte population, FISH is not usually necessary for MCL diagnosis.

Very rare cases of cyclin D1-negative MCL do exist, and generally fall into two scenarios: (1) *CCND1* rearrangement is present but the protein is not expressed or detected by IHC, or (2) *CCND1* rearrangement is not present.[38] In some of these instances, rearrangements of *CCND2,* or *CCND3* (although the latter appears to be less specific), can be found by FISH.[39] A diagnosis of *CCND1*-negative MCL should only be rendered on a well-fixed, excisional biopsy in which the morphology, phenotype, and genetics support the diagnosis, and in which FISH for both *CCND1* and *CCND2* rearrangements has been performed. CD5 positivity in other SBCLs (such as MZL, LPL, etc.) is far more common than *CCND1*-negative MCL.

TP53 mutations in MCL correlate with poor prognosis[40]; assessing for *TP53* mutation status in MCL is now essential per clinical guidelines. Although FISH for 17p deletion frequently is present in the setting of *TP53* mutation, del17p by FISH has not shown the strong correlation with

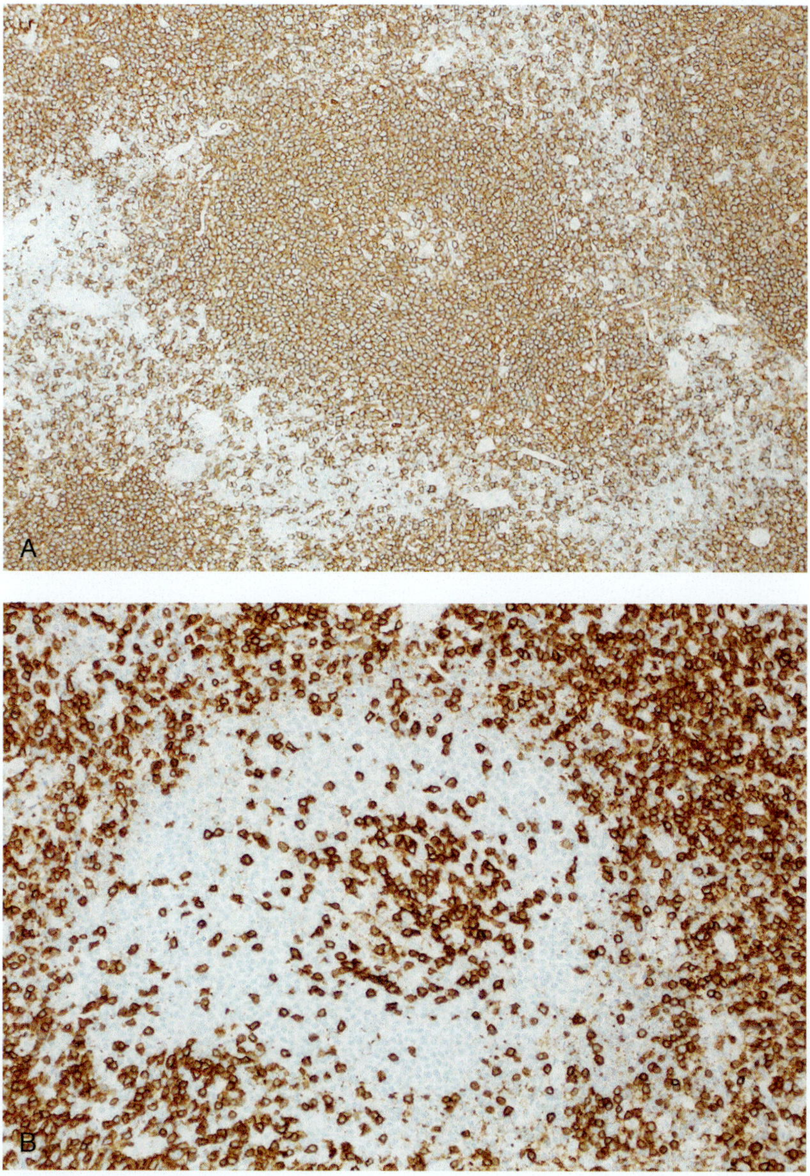

FIGURE 5.26 (*Continued*)

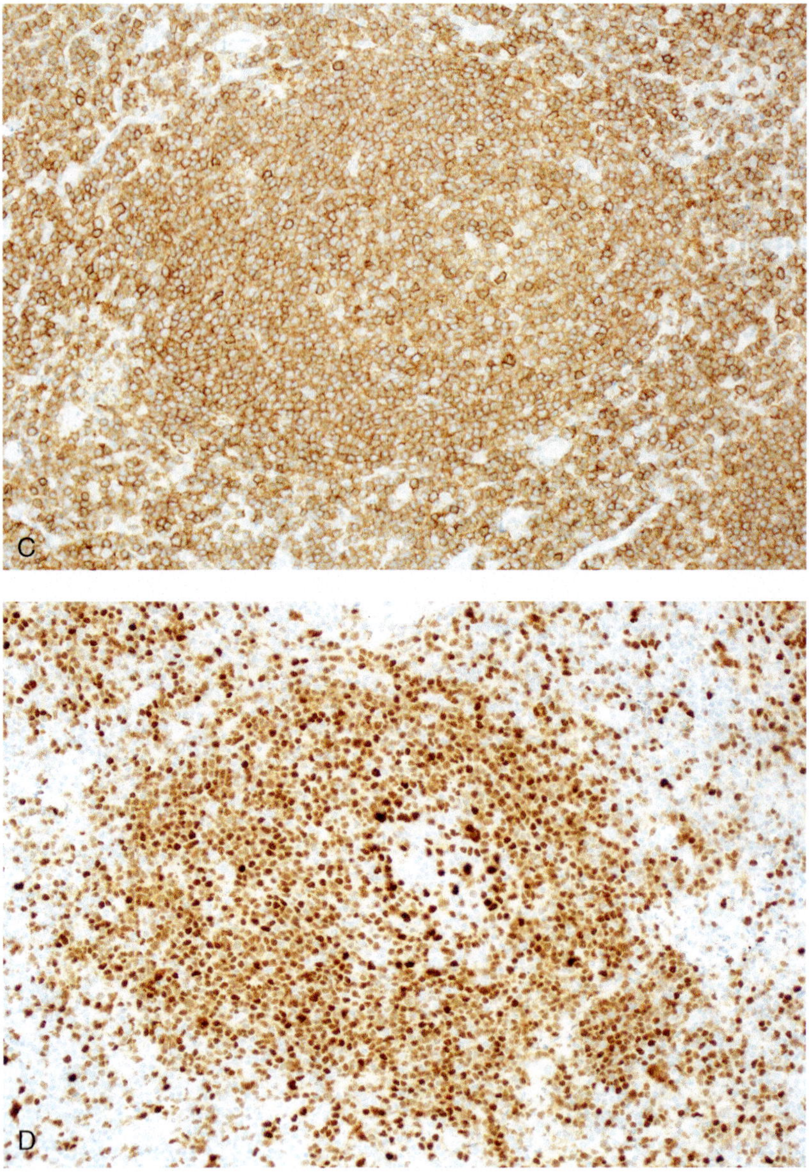

FIGURE 5.26 (*Continued*)

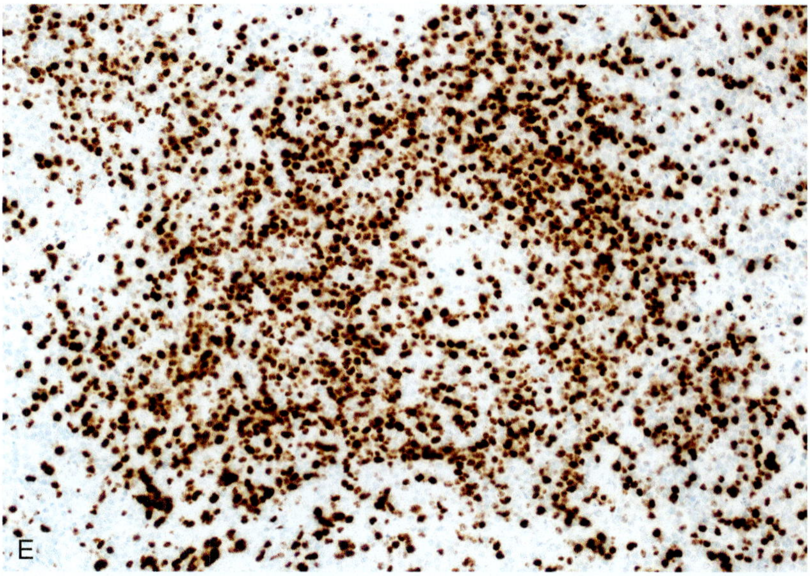

FIGURE 5.26 **Immunohistochemical staining pattern in mantle cell lymphoma.** A, CD20 stains the lymphoma. B, CD3 stains background T cells. C, CD5 compared to CD3 shows staining in T cells as well as aberrant staining in B cells. D, Cyclin D1 is positive in the lymphoma. E, SOX11 is positive in the lymphoma.

prognosis that mutation status has.[40,41] As such, it is recommended that *TP53* be assessed by sequencing in MCL, although FISH is still sometimes used as a surrogate.

Up to one-third of MCL will have somatic mutation of the *IGHV* gene, correlating with the lack of SOX11, nonnodal disease, and more indolent course.[31-34] As such *IGHV* sequencing may be requested in some MCL cases.

In Situ Mantle Cell Neoplasia

Similar to ISFN, there are rare clonal mantle zone proliferations, which harbor the *CCND1*-IGH rearrangement, but do not efface tissue architecture and have been termed in situ mantle cell neoplasia (ISMCN) (Figure 5.27). CD5 and SOX11 are variably positive. Importantly, any extension of the cyclin D1-positive cells outside of the confines of a normal-appearing mantle zone supports a diagnosis of MCL with a mantle zone pattern rather than ISMCN. The clinical significance of ISMCN is variable, with some patients progressing to MCL and some having an indolent course. When reporting ISMCN, the pathologist should acknowledge this uncertainty in a diagnostic comment.

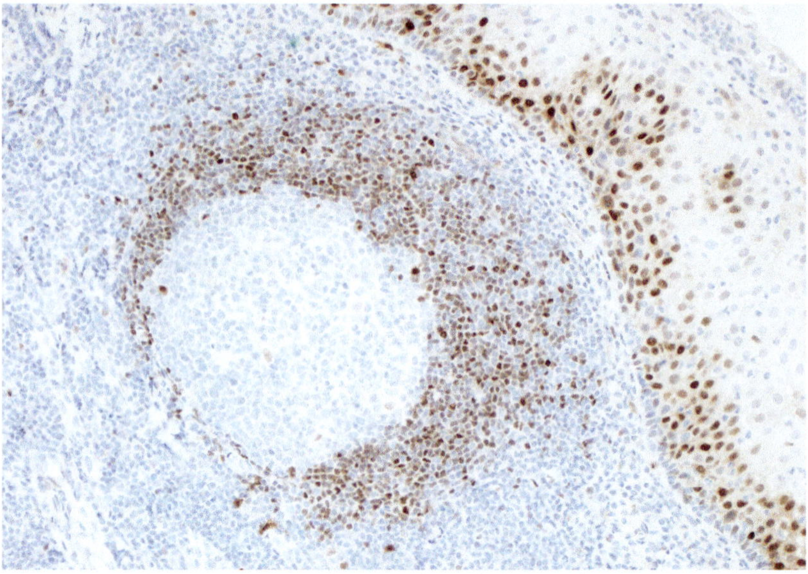

FIGURE 5.27 **In situ mantle cell neoplasia showing aberrant cyclin D1 expression within an otherwise normal-appearing mantle zone.** Note the retained polarization of the mantle zone.

LYMPHOPLASMACYTIC LYMPHOMA

Lymphoplasmacytic lymphoma (LPL) is an SBCL that is more often bone marrow-based but can involve lymph nodes as well. Patients are generally in a similar age range to the other SBCLs. They often have an associated IgM paraprotein (ie, Waldenstrom macroglobulinemia [WM]), but this is not required for the diagnosis of LPL. WM itself is not a pathologic diagnosis and to avoid confusion should not be used interchangeably with LPL by the pathologist. Diagnosing LPL in a lymph node biopsy can be challenging, due to the overlap with other SBCLs, especially MZL. In some instances, a diagnosis of "low-grade B-cell lymphoma with plasmacytic differentiation" may be rendered when the pathologic features cannot be fully resolved between LPL and MZL. Frequently, excisional biopsy is needed in this setting, and correlation with bone marrow findings and serum protein findings is recommended.

Morphology

LPL is a tumor of small lymphocytes, lymphoplasmacytoid cells, and mature plasma cells, and can have various proportions of these cell types in a given case. In the lymph node, the infiltrate generally appears monomorphous on a low-power, and sinuses are characteristically open within the infiltrated node. Infiltration outside the lymph node capsule, but sparing the intact subcapsular sinus, can be a helpful clue if present (Figure 5.28). If there are significant admixed large cells, or a prominent monocytoid-appearing population, MZL should be favored over LPL.

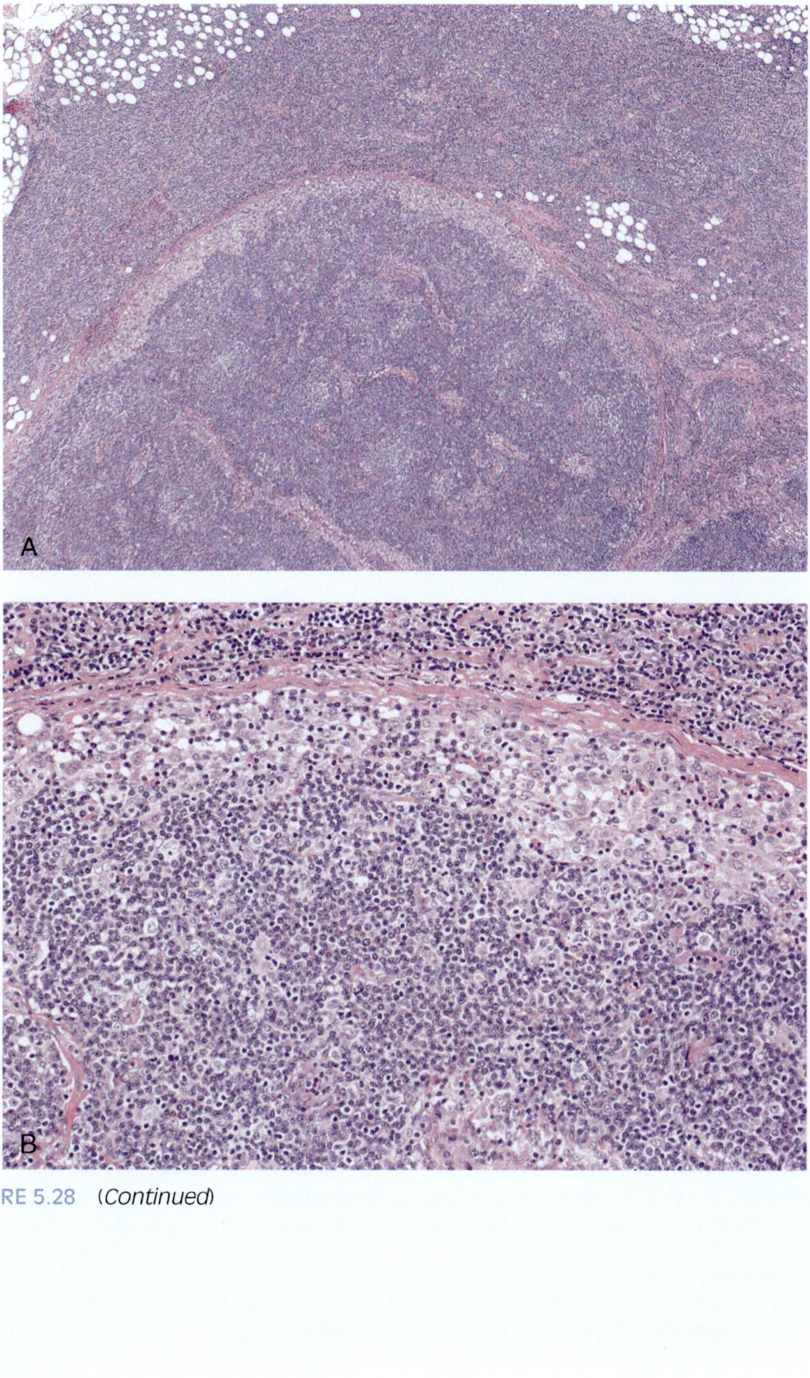

FIGURE 5.28 (*Continued*)

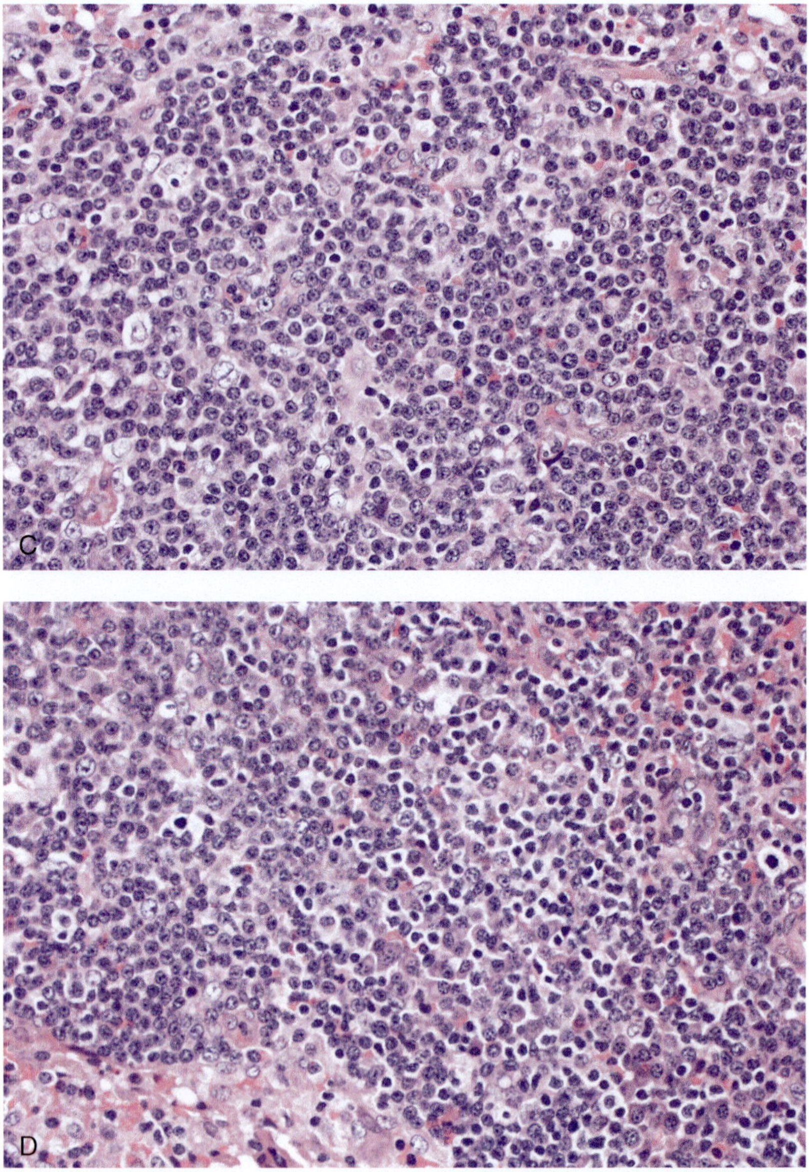

FIGURE 5.28 A, Lymphoplasmacytic lymphoma showing extension outside the lymph node with sparing of the subcapsular sinus. B, Lymphoplasmacytic lymphoma—high-power view of infiltrate and retained subcapsular sinus. C, The cytologic composition of lymphoplasmacytic lymphoma is typically small lymphocytes and mature plasma cells, with intermediate plasmacytoid lymphocytes (difficult to see on tissue sections). D, Lymphoplasmacytic lymphoma with areas showing more abundant mature plasma cells.

Phenotype

The B-cell component of LPL expresses pan-B-cell markers (CD20, CD19, PAX5, CD79a). Admixed plasma cells, which can be present in varying proportions, express typical plasma cell markers (CD38, CD138, MUM1), are light chain restricted (Figure 5.29), and more often

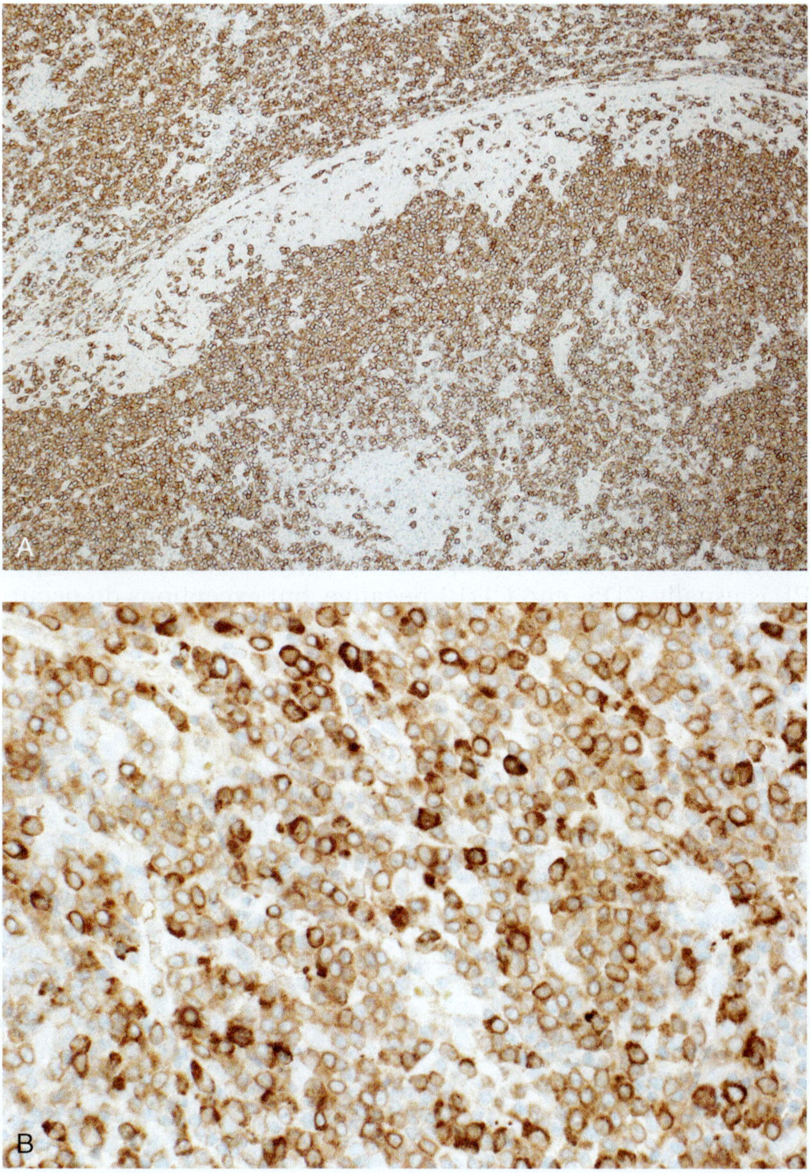

FIGURE 5.29 (*Continued*)

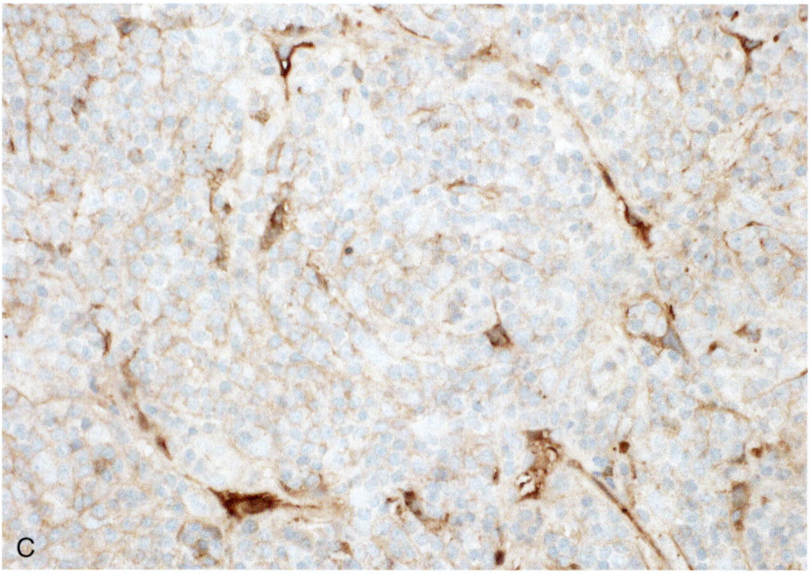

FIGURE 5.29 **Immunohistochemical staining pattern in lymphoplasmacytic lymphoma.** A, CD20 stains the majority of the tumor cells. B, Kappa and (C) lambda show kappa restriction in B cell and plasmacytic components of the tumor.

retain expression of CD19 and CD45 than in multiple myeloma. IgM is expressed by the clone in most cases, although a small subset can express class-switched heavy chains or light chain-only.[1,42] The B-cell component of LPL is usually CD5- and CD10-negative, but exceptions do occur and CD5 is expressed in as many as 20% of cases.[43] LEF1, cyclin D1, SOX11, and CD23 are negative.

Genetics

MYD88 L265P mutations are present in at least 90% of cases of LPL, and testing should be performed on a lymph node biopsy in which LPL is a consideration.[44,45] While not 100% sensitive and specific, in the appropriate morphologic and immunophenotypic context described here, the presence of a *MYD88* mutation can enable a confident diagnosis of LPL in the lymph node biopsy.[26] In cases negative for *MYD88* mutation, LPL may still be a consideration, but MZL may be more likely. As mentioned in their respective sections, occasional cases of MZL and CLL/SLL can harbor *MYD88* mutations, so caution is advised if the pathologic features are not conclusive. *CXCR4* mutations are present in 30% of LPL, and presence of both, *MYD88* and *CXCR4* mutations may add further specificity to a diagnosis of LPL, in addition to providing prognostic and therapeutic information.[44,45]

CHRONIC LYMPHOCYTIC LEUKEMIA/SMALL LYMPHOCYTIC LYMPHOMA

Chronic lymphocytic leukemia/small lymphocytic lymphoma (CLL/SLL) is one disease with two clinical manifestations: CLL in the blood/bone marrow, and SLL in lymph nodes and tissues. CLL is the most common adult leukemia in Western countries, and many patients will have concomitant SLL, while isolated SLL is rare. Median age of diagnosis is 70 years. A diagnosis of CLL requires at least 5×10^9/L clonal B cells in the peripheral blood assessed by FCM.[2] Clones below that threshold are considered as a separate, precursor "monoclonal B-cell lymphocytosis" (MBL).

CLL/SLL is a complex disease with myriad prognostic markers, some of which are pathologically and genetically based and which the hematopathologist must be familiar with. However, since the scope of this book focuses on lymph node-based disease, our discussion here will focus primarily on recognition of SLL. For most biopsies, the diagnosis rendered on a lymph node specimen should be "CLL/SLL" since the pathologist may not know in detail the absolute B-cell count in the patient's peripheral blood.

Morphology

The cells of CLL/SLL are classically small with round nuclei, condensed chromatin, and scant cytoplasm. In lymph nodes, the infiltrates are monomorphous, and effacement of the lymph node is frequently complete with a diffuse or vaguely nodular pattern (Figure 5.30). Areas of the infiltrate containing increased numbers of medium-sized cells, with either a single central nucleolus (prolymphocytes) or multiple nucleoli (paraimmunoblasts), are termed "proliferation centers." Their presence can lead to a sort of vague nodularity to the infiltrate from low power (Figure 5.30). The presence of proliferation centers is unique to CLL/SLL, but they can be challenging to distinguish from other features such as monocytoid areas or abnormal germinal centers in some cases. Cases in which lymph nodes are less than 1.5 cm with preserved nodal architecture and a subtle infiltrate of CLL/SLL-like cells without proliferation centers may represent a nodal variant of MBL, but correlation with clinical features is essential.[46] However, care should be taken in these settings to exclude other SBCLs and correlate with the peripheral blood findings.

Like other SBCLs, CLL/SLL can transform to overt DLBCL, frequently referred to as "Richter transformation." However, CLL/SLL can also exhibit morphologic changes associated with more aggressive disease, but which do not meet criteria for DLBCL.[47] This is more frequent in the setting of genetic features such as del17p and is usually termed "CLL/SLL with prominent proliferation centers."[47] Current guidelines define prominent proliferation centers as "broader than a 20× field and confluent"[2] but in practice it can be difficult to know the precise threshold. It is important not to overdiagnose confluent proliferation centers as transformation, the pitfall which more commonly occurs on a limited needle core biopsy.

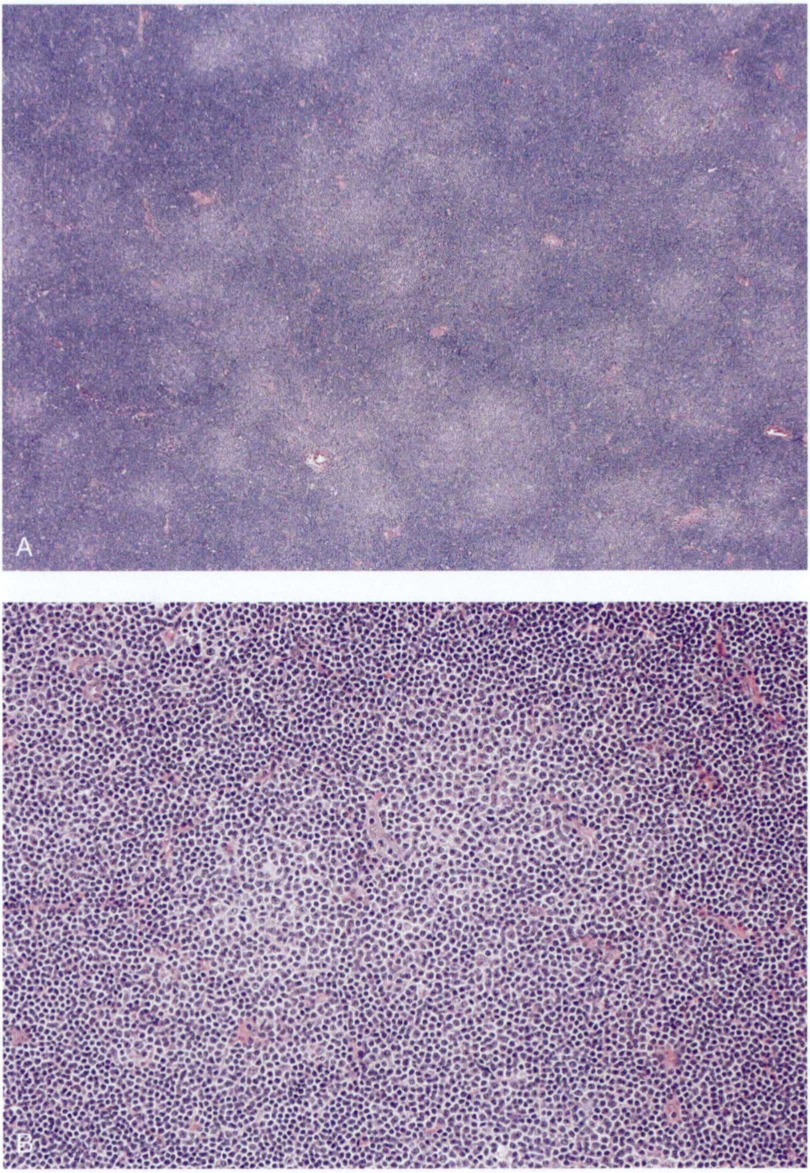

FIGURE 5.30 (*Continued*)

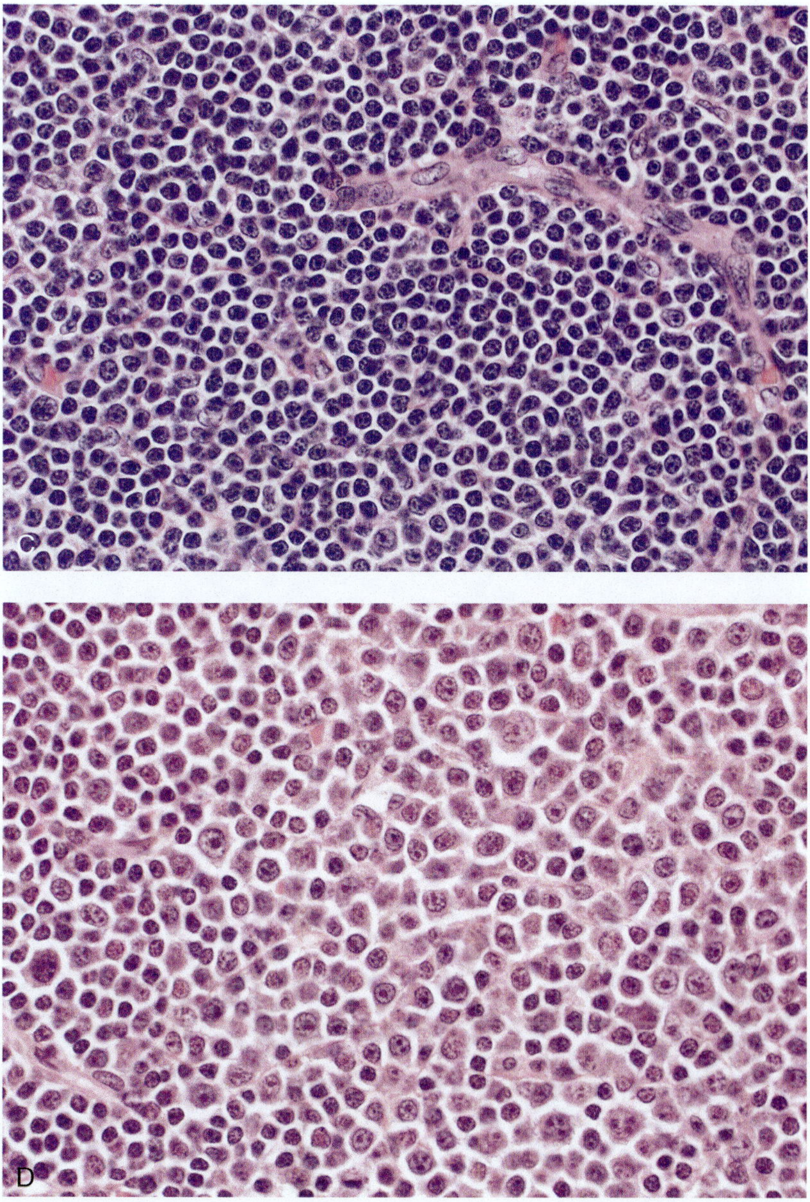

FIGURE 5.30 A, Chronic lymphocytic leukemia/small lymphocytic lymphoma showing a mottled appearance on low power. The pale areas represent proliferation centers. B, Proliferation center in chronic lymphocytic leukemia/small lymphocytic lymphoma. C, Chronic lymphocytic leukemia/small lymphocytic lymphoma. High-power magnification of typical small, round cell cytology. D, High-power view of a proliferation center (right) composed of prolymphocytes and paraimmunoblasts adjacent to the smaller lymphoma cells on the left.

CLL/SLL may also have Reed-Sternberg (RS)-like cells in two settings (Figure 5.31): (1) overt transformation to classic Hodgkin lymphoma (CHL) and (2) RS-like cells in a CLL background without the characteristic inflammatory milieu of CHL.[48,49] Both often show Epstein-Barr virus (EBV)-encoded small RNA (EBER) positivity within the RS cells. Distinction between these two can be challenging, and the clinical significance of the

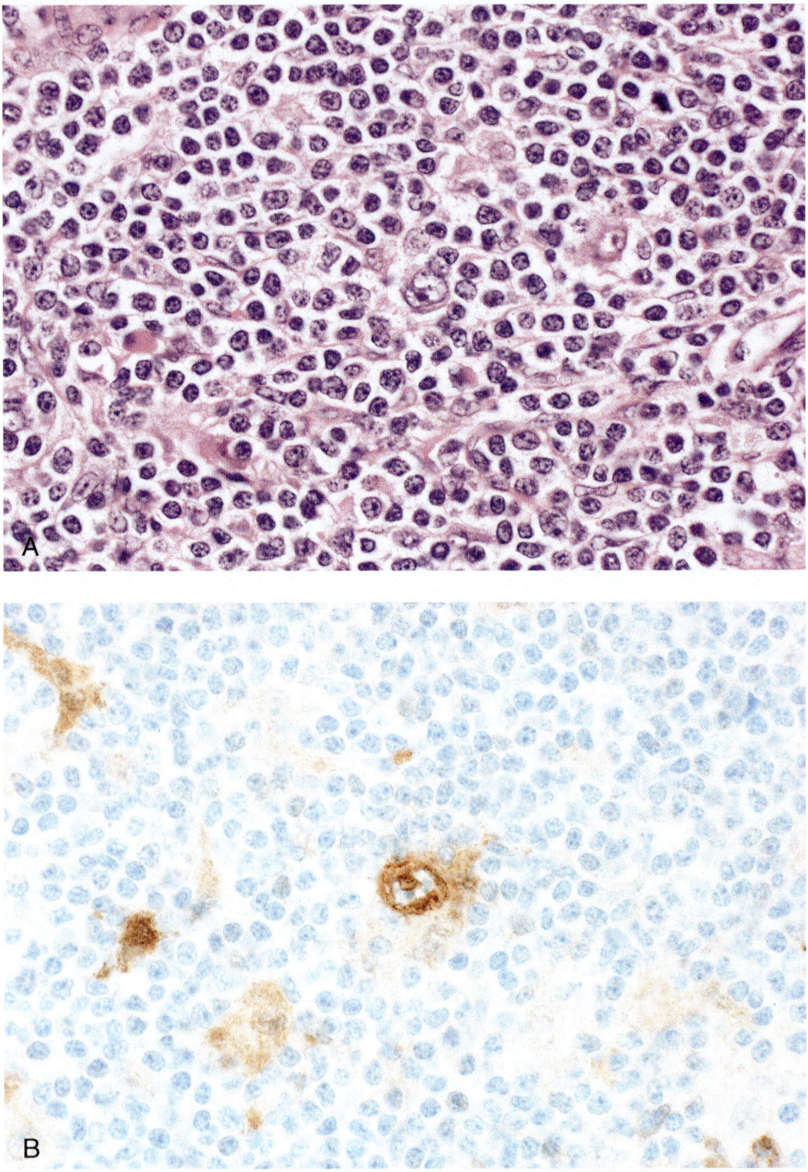

FIGURE 5.31 A, Chronic lymphocytic leukemia/small lymphocytic lymphoma with scattered Reed-Sternberg-like cells, which are staining with CD30 (B).

distinction remains uncertain. However, per current guidelines, the diagnosis of CHL transformation of CLL/SLL should only be made when there is a distinct inflammatory milieu in the background of the RS cells.[2]

Phenotype

Like the other SBCLs, CLL/SLL expresses pan B-cell markers (CD20, CD19, PAX5, CD79a), although expression of CD20 is characteristically dim compared to normal B cells. This along with dim expression of light chain (kappa or lambda) and coexpression of CD5 and CD23 are the hallmark phenotypic features of CLL/SLL (Figure 5.32). Diagnostically, the importance of the dim expression of light chain and CD20 makes FCM particularly useful in the diagnosis of CLL/SLL. CLL/SLL is typically negative for germinal center markers CD10 and BCL6. CD200 and LEF1 are markers positive in CLL/SLL and may help distinguish it from other CD5 positive SBCLs. Cyclin D1 and SOX11, which stain MCL but are negative in CLL/SLL, may also help in this regard. However, one important pitfall to be aware of is that proliferation centers in CLL/SLL can show dim and variable staining for Cyclin D1 (Figure 5.33). SOX11 and/or FISH to exclude a *CCND1*-IGH rearrangement (both negative in CLL/SLL) can be used in this setting if the morphologic and phenotypic features are not conclusive.

Genetics

FISH using a panel of commonly encountered abnormalities is routinely performed for prognostic purposes in CLL/SLL (Table 5.2). However, importantly there are no cytogenetic abnormalities that are diagnostic or specific for CLL/SLL and FISH should not be used to confirm a diagnosis of CLL/SLL. The most common alterations, and those typically assessed by FISH, include del 13q14.3, trisomy 12, del 11q22-23, del 17p, and del 6q. The frequency of these findings in CLL is well established, but less well documented in SLL.[50]

Additional genetic testing frequently performed for prognosis in CLL/SLL patients is *IGHV* mutation status and *TP53* mutation analysis (Table 5.2).[51-53] *TP53* mutations are associated with poor prognosis and poor response to chemotherapy. Mutated *IGHV* genes correlate with more favorable prognosis. Most often these will be performed on peripheral blood or bone marrow, rather than lymph node samples. Overall, prognostication in CLL/SLL relies on a combination of clinical and pathologic/genetic features.[54]

Other Small B-cell Neoplasms Involving Lymph Nodes

The entities discussed above cover the majority of the SBCL cases the pathologist will encounter in the lymph node biopsy. Rarely, lymph nodes can be involved by predominantly extranodal lymphomas, splenic lymphomas, or plasma cell neoplasms (PCNs).

Extranodal MZLs and splenic MZLs can sometimes exhibit regional lymph node involvement. In this setting, the morphologic and phenotypic

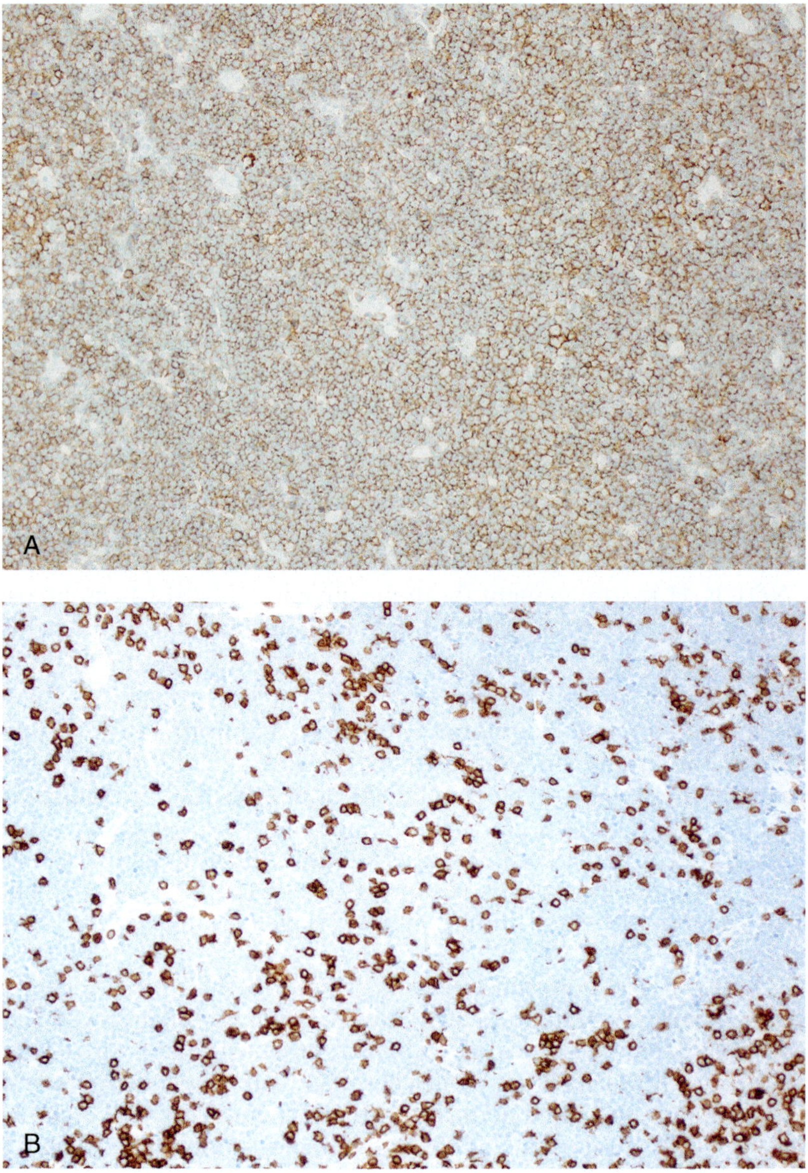

FIGURE 5.32 (*Continued*)

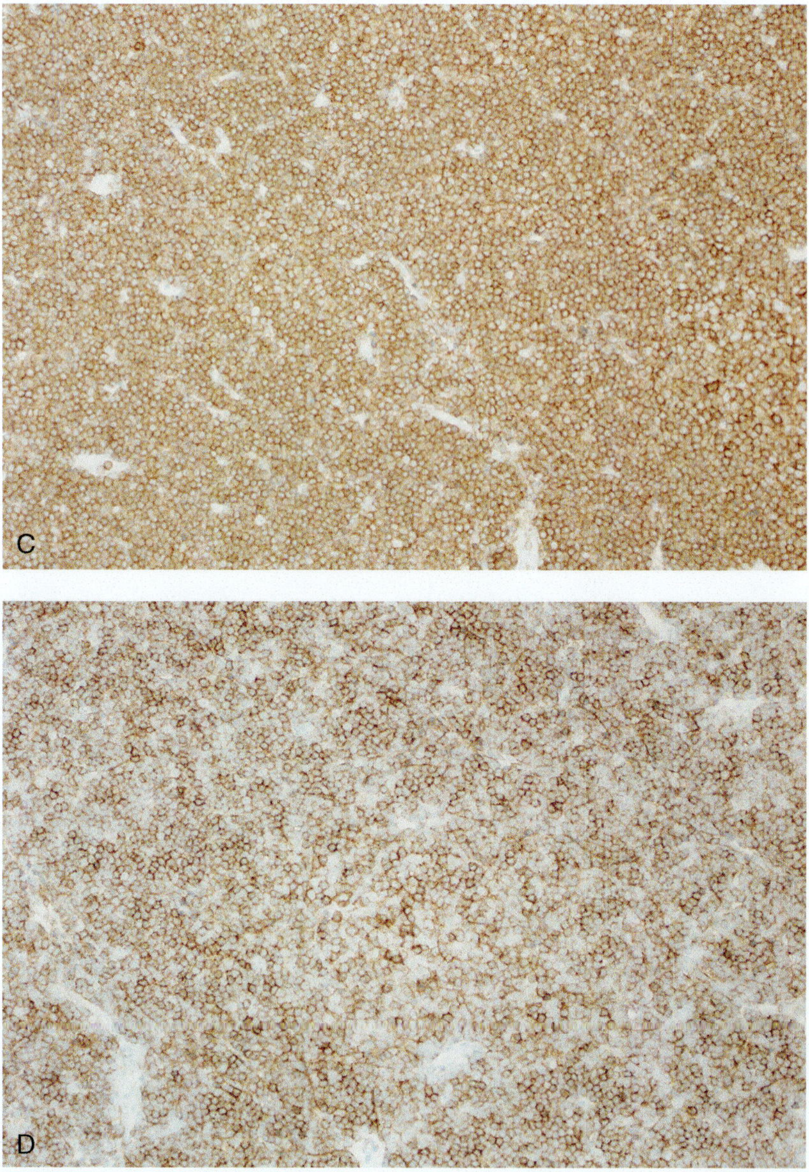

FIGURE 5.32 *(Continued)*

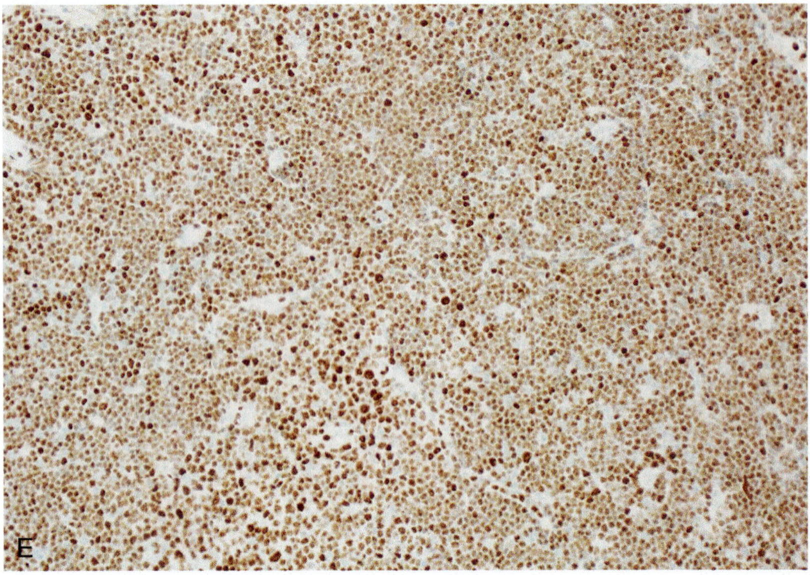

FIGURE 5.32 **Immunohistochemical stain pattern in chronic lymphocytic leukemia/small lymphocytic lymphoma.** A, CD20 shows diffuse, but dim, staining in the tumor cells. B, CD3 stains background T cells. C, CD5 shows aberrant expression in the tumor cells and is positive in background T cells. D, CD23 is positive in the tumor cells. E, LEF1 is positive in the tumor cells and background T cells.

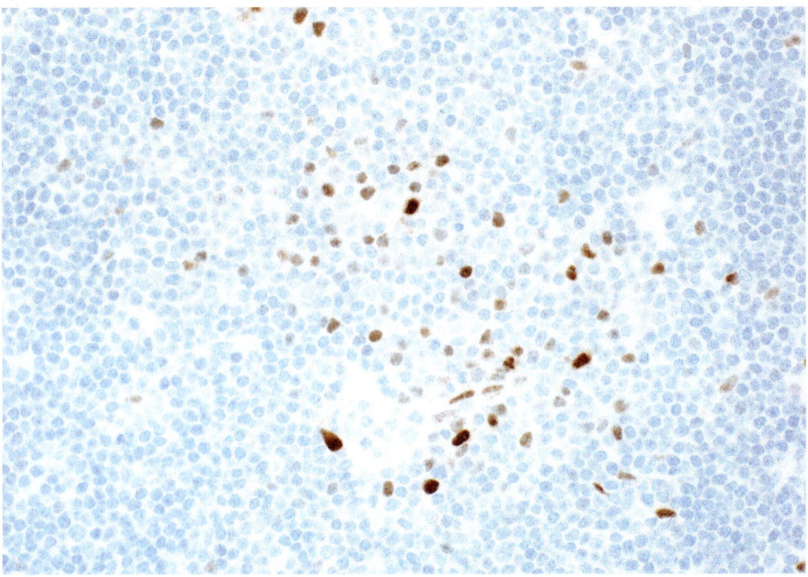

FIGURE 5.33 **Chronic lymphocytic leukemia/small lymphocytic lymphoma.** Cyclin D1 can show dim staining of a subset of cells within proliferation centers. This must be distinguished from mantle cell lymphoma.

TABLE 5.2 Prognostic Genetic Findings in Chronic Lymphocytic Leukemia/Small Lymphocytic Lymphoma

Genetic Alteration	Prognosis
Interphase FISH	
del 11q	Unfavorable
del 17p	Unfavorable
Normal	Neutral
Trisomy 12	Neutral
del 13q	Favorable
Karyotype[a]	
≥3 unrelated chromosome abnormalities in more than one cell	Unfavorable
Molecular	
TP53 mutation	Unfavorable
Mutated *IGHV* > 2%	Favorable
Mutated *IGHV* ≤ 2%	Unfavorable

[a]Refers to results of conventional karyotype of stimulated CLL cells.

features will be similar to what is seen in the primary site, and difficult to distinguish from NMZL as discussed above. As mentioned, these lymph node biopsies may be best diagnosed as "MZL" if there is concern that the node may not be the primary site of disease.

Hairy cell leukemia (HCL) is a mature B-cell lymphoma, which typically involves spleen, bone marrow, and blood. Lymph node involvement is rare but can occur in advanced cases (Figure 5.34). In the absence of a history of HCL, phenotypic features may provide the best clue to consider HCL in the differential diagnosis. HCL has a characteristic immunophenotype including expression of bright CD20, CD11c, CD103, CD25, CD123, TBET, Annexin A1, and CD200. In addition, cyclin D1 is dimly but uniformly expressed (in the absence of *CCND1-IGH* rearrangement seen in MCL). *BRAF*V600E mutations are found in close to 100% of HCL, and IHC for this mutation can also be useful in this setting to support HCL, since this mutation is not seen in other SBCLs.

PCNs, including plasmacytoma and multiple myeloma, can rarely involve lymph nodes. Again, clinical history is essential in arriving at the correct diagnosis. The differential diagnosis in this setting typically rests between LPL, MZL, and a PCN (Figures 5.35 and 5.36). Establishing the presence of the clonal B-cell component can sometimes be challenging. Retained plasma cell expression of CD45 and CD19 in this setting may support a lymphoma over PCN. *MYD88* mutation supports lymphoma

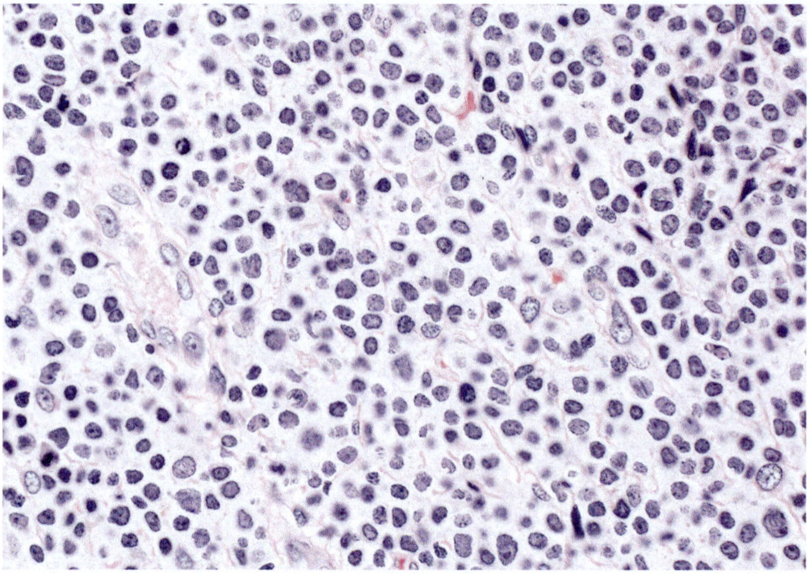

FIGURE 5.34 **Hairy cell leukemia involving a lymph node.** Typical cytology with oval nuclei and abundant pale or clear cytoplasm.

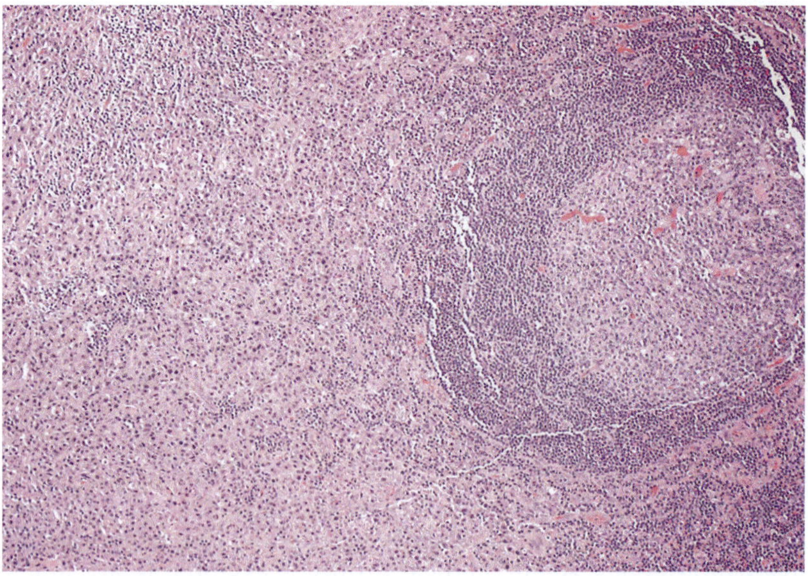

FIGURE 5.35 **Plasmacytoma involving a lymph node surrounding a reactive follicle.** This morphology can overlap with lymphomas that have plasmacytic differentiation.

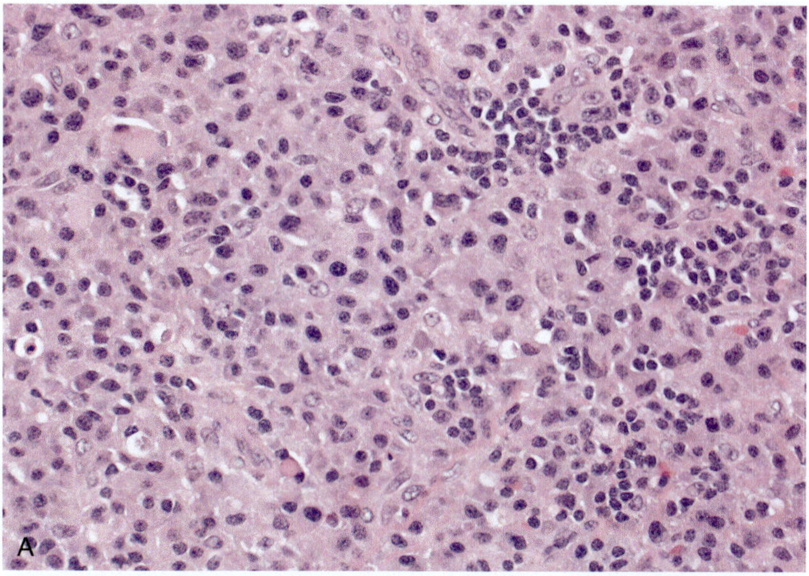

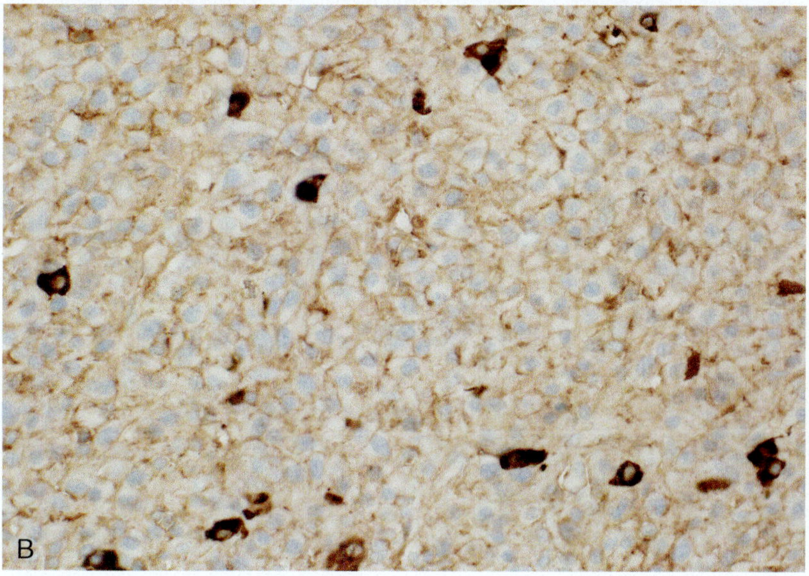

FIGURE 5.36 (*Continued*)

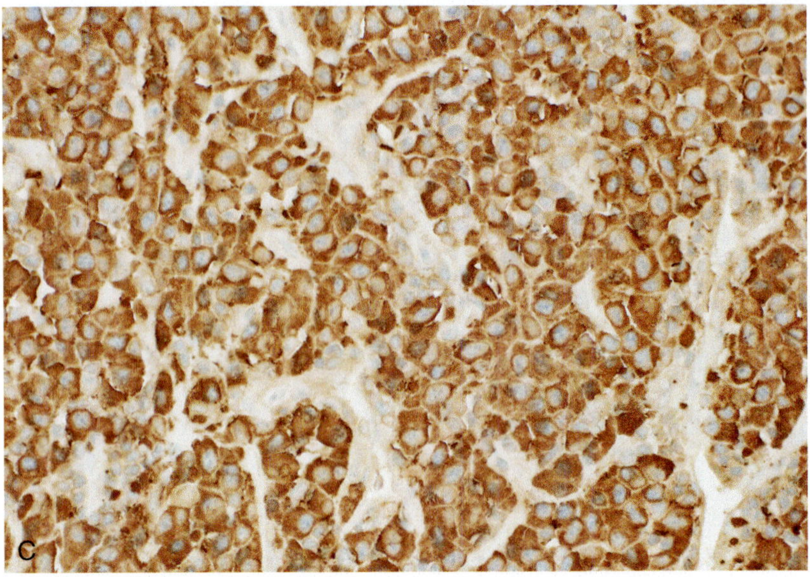

FIGURE 5.36 A, High power of plasmacytoma involving a lymph node showing sheets of mature plasma cells. Kappa (B) and lambda (C) show lambda light chain restriction.

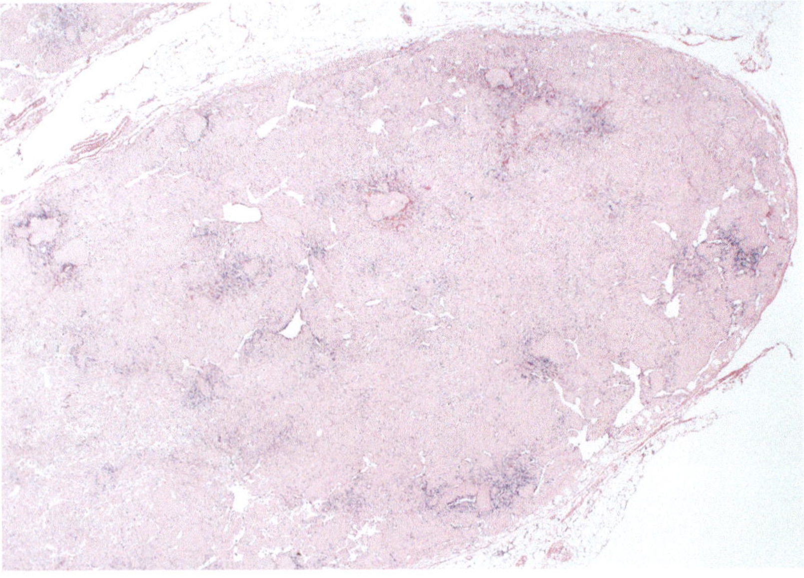

FIGURE 5.37 **Amyloid replacing lymph node parenchyma.**

as this is not seen in PCN. However, in many instances, correlation with overall clinical findings, laboratory, and bone marrow studies is essential and the diagnosis must reflect the differential diagnostic considerations acknowledging the rarity of nodal plasmacytomas.

Amyloid can be found in lymph nodes and is often associated with low-grade B-cell lymphomas with plasmacytic differentiation. Amyloid deposition may be extensive and replace the parenchyma with only minimal evidence of the clonal process (Figures 5.37 and 5.38). Mass spectrometry to subtype the amyloid is essential in this setting, as non-light chain amyloid can also involve lymph nodes.[55,56]

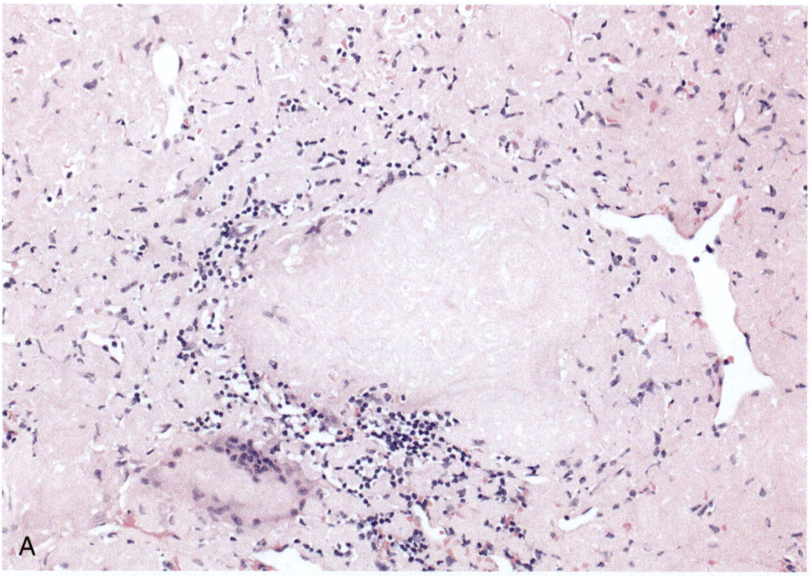

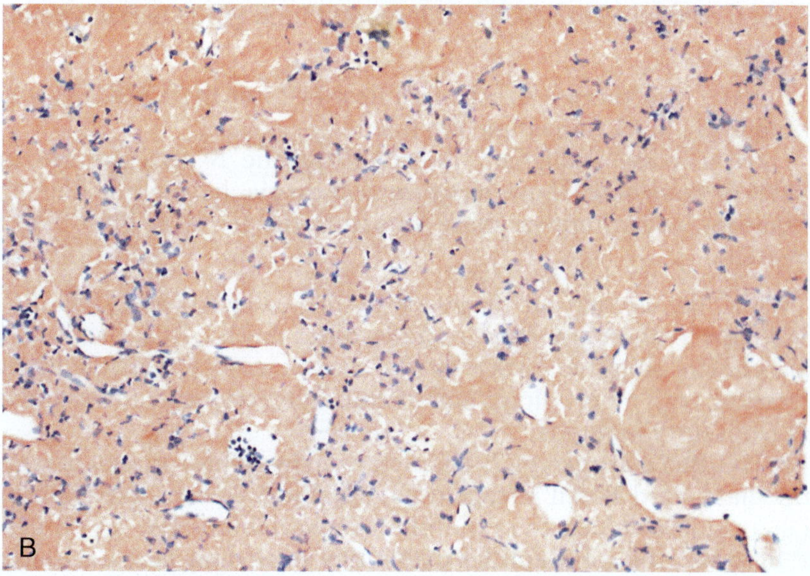

FIGURE 5.38 (*Continued*)

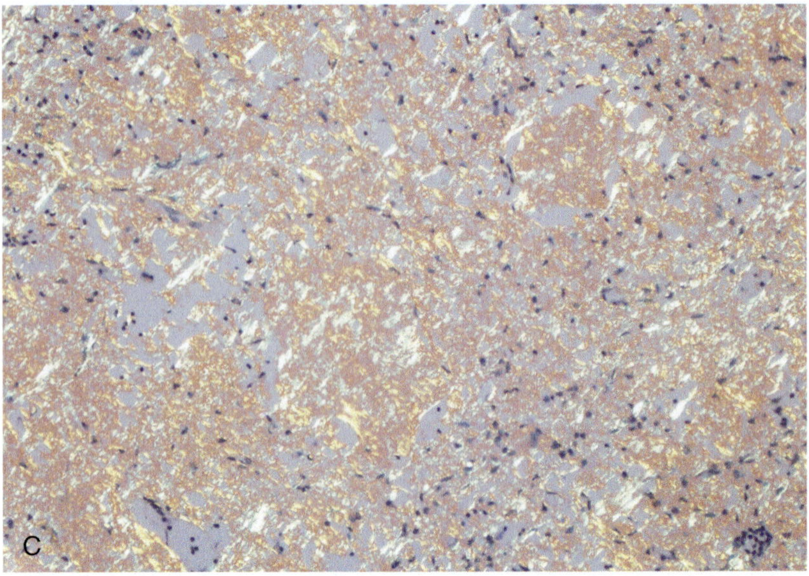

FIGURE 5.38 **Amyloid involving a lymph node.** A, Infiltrates of lymphocytes and/or plasma cells may be seen but are often sparse. Multinucleated giant cells can be associated with the amyloid deposits. B, Congo red stain is positive and shows an apple-green birefringence under polarized light (C).

LARGE AND HIGH-GRADE B-CELL LYMPHOMA

In general, compared to SBCL, the large and high-grade B-cell lymphomas (L/HG BCL):

- Behave in a more aggressive clinical fashion than SBCL, generally requiring more immediate treatment.
- Have a more "malignant" morphology: the B cells are intermediate- or large-sized, have more nuclear atypia, have easily identifiable mitoses, and/or appear more immature (ie, are more blast-like) than SBCL.

While the archetypal diagnosis in the category of L/HG BCL is DLBCL, the pathologist must exclude other L/HG BCLs according to certain clinical situations (such as site, disease course, possible immunosuppression, etc), morphologic and immunophenotypic features, and additional laboratory methods.

L/HG BCLs are generally characterized by diffuse growth of large- or intermediate-sized B-cell lineage cells, usually in a sheet-like pattern, but with a considerable degree of morphologic variability. We say "B-cell lineage" here because some entities within this group may lack CD20 expression and show an immunophenotype more characteristic of plasma cells than true B cells (eg, plasmablastic lymphoma [PBL], ALK-positive large B-cell lymphoma, or HHV8-positive DLBCL), but still remain within the lineage of B cells.

In general, the neoplastic cells of all L/HG BCLs will have one of five cytologies: (1) centroblastic (large cells with vesicular chromatin and multiple membrane-bound nucleoli), (2) immunoblastic (large cells with round nuclei and single, large central nucleoli), (3) plasmablastic (similar to immunoblastic but with more abundant, often eccentric cytoplasm), (4) anaplastic/pleomorphic (large to very large, pleomorphic cells, often with prominent nucleoli, variably shaped, frequent Hodgkin-like forms or multinucleate forms), and (5) high-grade (medium/intermediate-sized cells, often with fine chromatin and inconspicuous nucleoli or blastoid appearance) (Figure 5.39).

Determining cell size is a critical aspect of L/HG BCL assessment and is inherent to current classification schemes. It is important to remember that cell size refers actually to nuclear size, as cells with abundant cytoplasm such as in MZL can appear large when stained with membranous stains. It can be helpful to compare the size of the tumor nuclei with those of an internal ruler such as a histiocyte/macrophage nucleus or a vascular or lymphatic endothelial cell nucleus. If the neoplastic cells show nuclei that are, on average, larger than a histiocyte nucleus, the entity is classified as "large cell." If they are the same size as the histiocyte nucleus, they are deemed "intermediate-sized." Burkitt lymphoma (BL) is the prototypical lymphoma with intermediate-sized cells, although high-grade B-cell lymphoma, not otherwise specified, is also definitionally composed of intermediate-sized (not large) cells. Another common internal ruler is a background small lymphocyte nucleus: on average, large cells show nuclei that are over twice the size of background resting lymphocytes.

Immunophenotyping of L/HG BCLs is critical for diagnosis and has some therapeutic and prognostic implications in many lymphoma subtypes. FCM has less utility in L/HG BCL than in SBCL as the larger cells of L/HG BCL can aggregate or lyse and occasionally produce false negatives.[57] Additionally, the benefit of establishing clonality by FCM is often unnecessary in L/HG BCL given the atypical, more obviously malignant morphology. For this reason, it is recommended that IHC be performed for immunophenotyping in all cases, with or without FCM. A typical IHC panel for the workup of an L/HG BCL (such as DLBCL) would start with CD3 and CD20 to assess underlying immunoarchitecture and confirm B-cell lineage, but would also include determining the cell of origin via algorithmic approach (ie, CD10, BCL6, MUM1), determining the expression status of BCL2 and MYC by IHC, with or without assessing underlying follicular dendritic cell meshworks by CD21 and/or CD23. A panel may expand to include additional markers based on clinical or morphologic parameters such as Burkitt-like morphology (Ki-67, CD43), primary mediastinal large B-cell lymphoma (MAL, PD-L2, CD23, CD30),

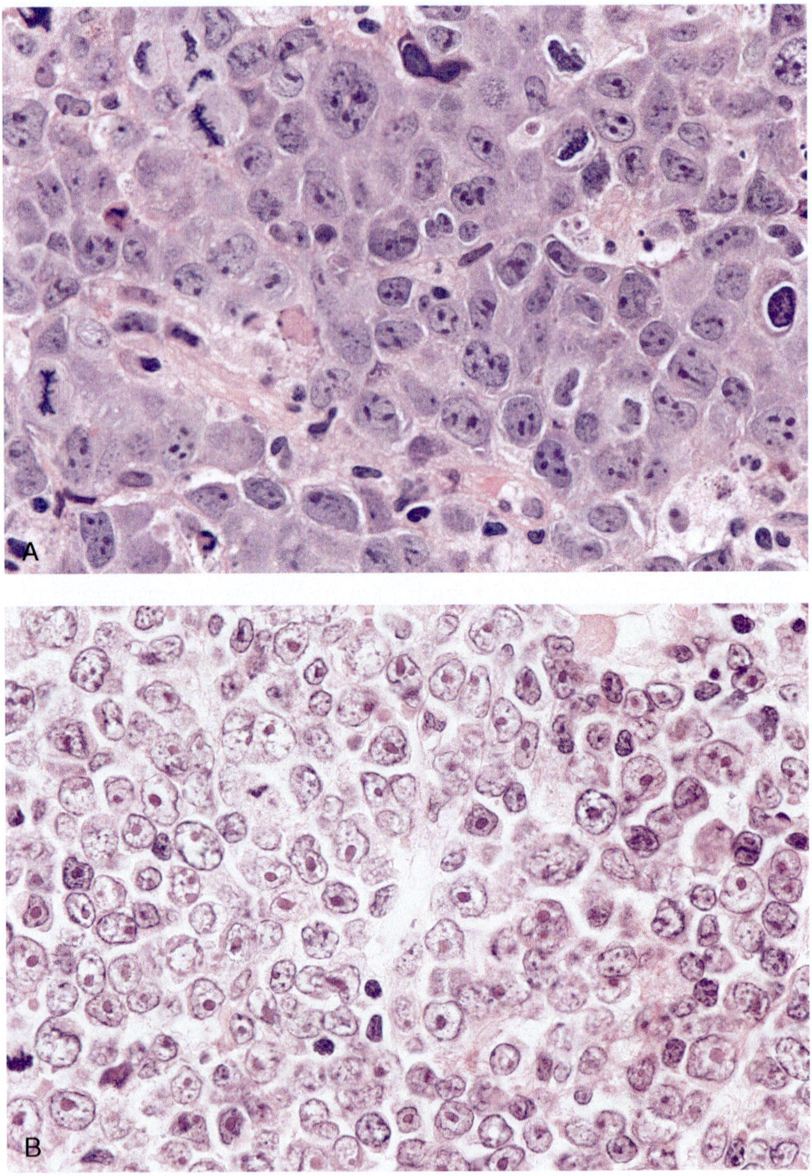

FIGURE 5.39 (*Continued*)

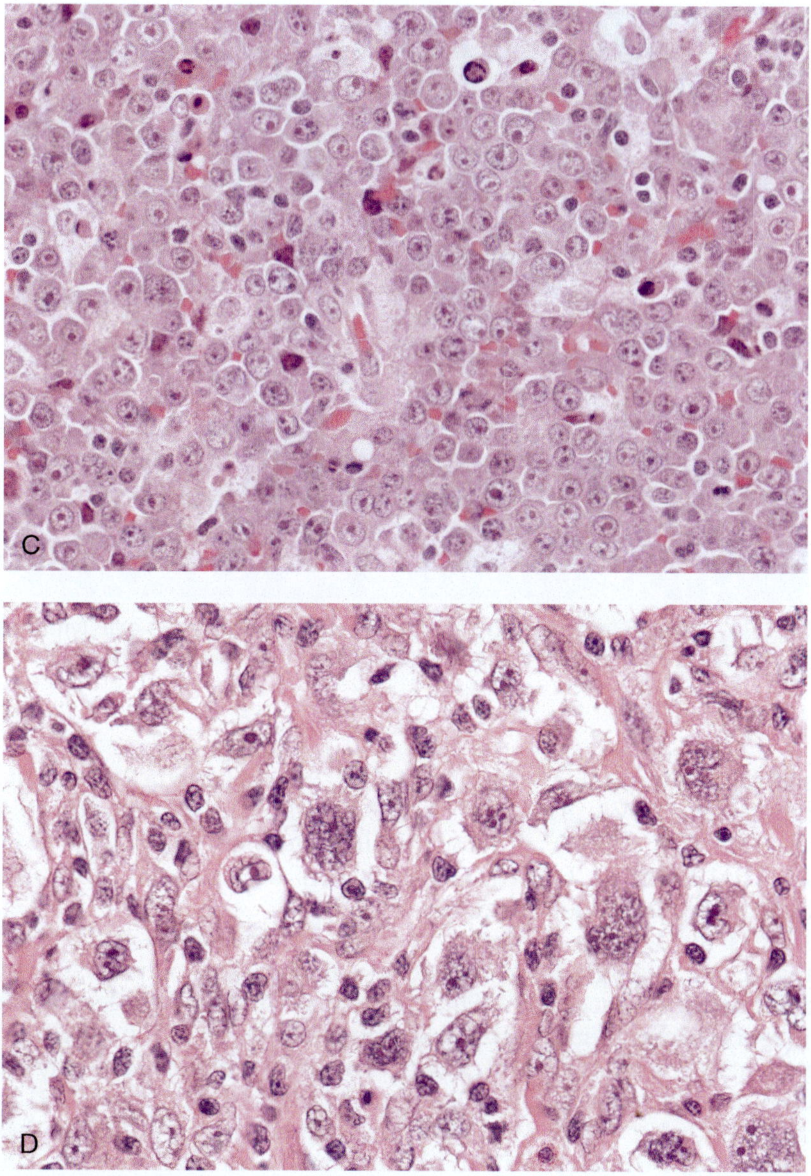

FIGURE 5.39 (*Continued*)

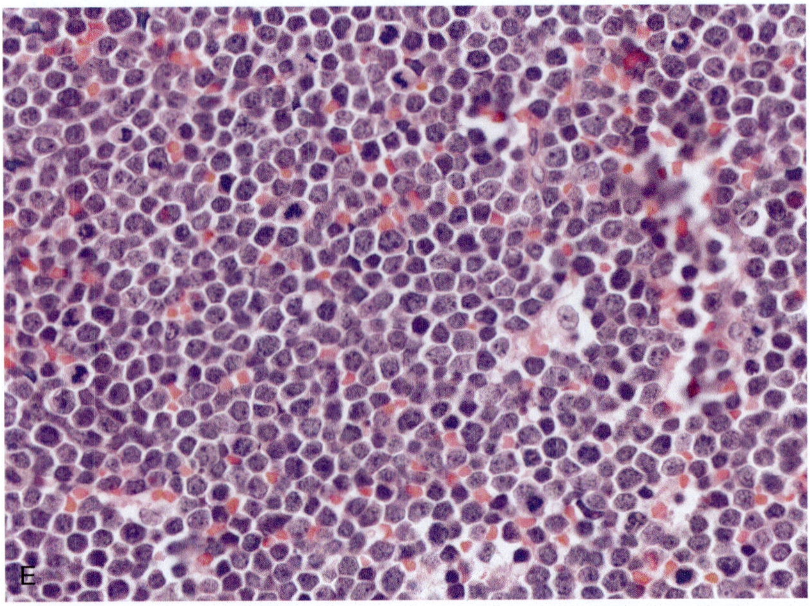

FIGURE 5.39 **Varying morphology in large and high-grade B-cell lymphomas.** A, Centroblastic; B, immunoblastic; C, plasmablastic; and D, anaplastic. (E) High-grade B-cell lymphoma morphology. Cells are intermediate in size, often with fine or blastoid chromatin.

plasmablastic morphology (PAX5, CD138, kappa/lambda IHC or in situ hybridization, HHV8, ALK, CD19, CD45, EBER), blastoid morphology (cyclin D1, TdT, CD34), or Hodgkin-like morphology (CD30, BOB.1, OCT-2, CD19, CD79a, EBER). These markers are discussed below in conjunction with the relevant diagnoses.

FISH for *MYC* is indicated in every new diagnosis of L/HG BCL with large cell, high-grade, or Burkitt-like morphology, when tissue quantity and quality are acceptable. This testing is performed in order to exclude the diagnosis of high-grade B-cell lymphoma with *MYC* and *BCL2* rearrangements or with *MYC* and *BCL6* rearrangements (colloquially called "double hit lymphoma" [DHL]), even in cases with otherwise DLBCL-like morphology.[58] While *MYC* rearrangements may be seen in other L/HG BCLs (eg, PBL, blastoid MCL), these cases currently remain in their respective diagnostic categories if criteria are met, and "double-hits" in these entities are rare.[58]

In order to exclude *MYC* rearrangements, we recommend interphase FISH as it can be performed on formalin-fixed, paraffin-embedded tissue (FFPE) and has an acceptable sensitivity and turnaround time. However, because *MYC* breakapart probes alone can produce a false negative result in at least 4% of cases,[59] we also recommend doing simultaneous (or reflexive) testing using an additional dual fusion probe for *MYC/IGH*, to avoid missing DHL. Once a *MYC* rearrangement is detected, additional FISH testing for *BCL2* and *BCL6* rearrangements can be reflexively performed. This algorithmic approach changes when the diagnosis of BL is in the differential, especially in a younger person (see below).

DIFFUSE LARGE B-CELL LYMPHOMA, NOT OTHERWISE SPECIFIED

The archetypal L/HG BCL is also the most common lymphoma in Western countries, as DLBCL, not otherwise specified (NOS) accounts for over 30% of all non-Hodgkin lymphomas.[60] Clinically, DLBCL can arise in both nodal and extranodal locations, with the gastrointestinal tract (stomach and ileocecal region) being the most common extranodal site.[58] Approximately 40% of cases will have exclusively extranodal disease on presentation.[61] When bone marrow is involved by lymphoma (seen in a quarter to half of cases), the process is termed "concordant" if DLBCL is present, and "discordant" if a low-grade B-cell lymphoma is present in the bone marrow.[62,63] More common in older adults (median age is in the seventh decade), DLBCL can also occur in younger adults and even in children.[61] DLBCL may arise in the setting of a preexisting SBCL such as FL or CLL/SLL (called "transformed" or secondary DLBCL) or, more commonly, arise without a history of other lymphoma (termed de novo). DLBCL is a heterogeneous disease, with various groupings and subclassifications by morphologic, immunophenotypic, clinical, and molecular characteristics, discussed in the following pages.

Morphology

Aptly named, DLBCL is defined by a proliferation of large-sized (on-average) B cells in a diffuse growth pattern.[58] Lymph node architecture shows total effacement in most cases, but partial or interfollicular growth is possible. Cells should be classified as large in most cases, as cases with more medium-sized cells need extensive correlation with ancillary testing to exclude high-grade lymphomas, extramedullary leukemias, or BL. As discussed above, DLBCL can have centroblastic, immunoblastic, plasmablastic, or anaplastic/pleomorphic cytology. The several other cellular morphologies that do exist (eg, myxoid stroma, fibrillary matrix, spindle-shaped, etc) are exceedingly rare or only focally present within DLBCL lesions. DLBCL is often associated with a noticeable mitotic rate, with evident apoptotic bodies and occasional areas of necrosis.

Phenotype

The immunophenotyping of DLBCL starts with demonstrating the expression of pan-B-cell markers, namely strong CD20 or PAX5. If the patient has received prior rituximab therapy, the expression of CD20 might be diminished or absent, so demonstration of B-cell lineage may require PAX5 or other pan-B-cell markers such as CD19, CD79a, or CD22. After establishing B-lineage in a diffuse proliferation of large atypical cells, a diagnosis of "large B-cell lymphoma" can be rendered, but until a DHL has been excluded, a definitive diagnosis of DBLCL should not be made.

Cell of Origin

Gene expression profiling (GEP) studies have demonstrated that DLBCLs fall into three subgroups, which resemble normal B-cell counterparts: those derived from a GCB, those derived from a cell just exiting the germinal center, the so-called "activated B-cell" (ABC) subtype, and a third unclassifiable type. GCB and ABC represent two biologically distinct subsets of DLBCL and have been an important prognosticator in the "R-CHOP era": ABC has a slightly worse prognosis than GCB and has shown differing responses to certain therapies.[64,65]

To practically determine cell of origin in the clinical setting, many IHC algorithms have been developed, the most established of which is the Hans algorithm using CD10, BCL6, and MUM1.[66] Because the algorithm only approximates the ABC group, and does not include an unclassifiable group, the two outcomes of the algorithm are referred to as GCB and non-GCB. Although it is important to note the Hans algorithm struggles with reproducibility among pathologists, and shows variable prognostic value, it has become standard of care in DLBCL (Figure 5.40).[67] Newer GEP assays are clinically available for FFPET, and are acceptable substitutes for the Hans algorithm although they have not been widely adopted by most practices.[68,69]

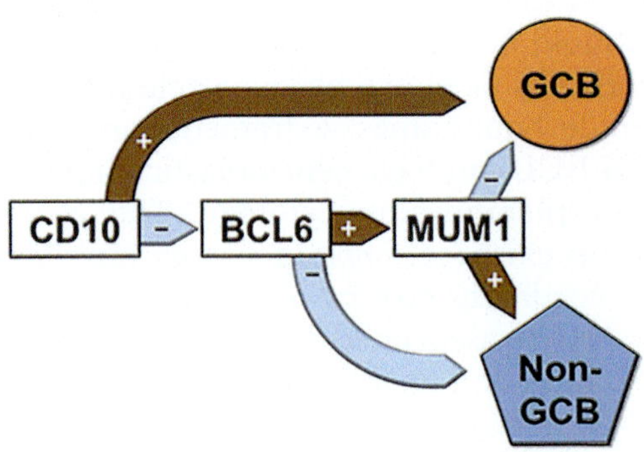

FIGURE 5.40 **Flow chart representation of the Hans algorithm cell-of-origin determination by immunohistochemistry with CD10, BCL6, and MUM1.** A cutoff of 30% positivity of tumor cells is used for each stain. GCB, germinal center B cell.

Dual Expression of BCL2 and MYC by IHC

The expression status of BCL2 and MYC is an immunohistochemical prognosticator in DLBCL, but with weaker prognostic significance than DHL. When the DHLs are removed, cases found to be expressers of both proteins (using the cutoff of 50% expression for BCL2 and 40% expression for MYC in most studies) have a slightly worse prognosis compared with those that lack expression.[70-72] It is also important to note that, while dual protein expression may be more likely to have a *MYC* rearrangement and may be reclassified as DHL, approximately 25% of DHLs do not have corresponding dual protein expression.[73] Thus, dual protein expression is not an acceptable screening method for DHL or substitute for FISH. Utility of the double-expresser data is still an open question, and these stains may not be required for definitive diagnosis depending on the clinical setting.[1]

Genetics

Even when morphologic and immunophenotypic criteria are satisfactory for the diagnosis of DLBCL, a DHL must be excluded in every case. Specifically, this means excluding a *MYC* rearrangement by FISH testing in every new diagnosis of DLBCL by the methods discussed above. The relative frequency of *MYC*, *BCL2*, and *BCL6* rearrangements in DLBCL is 8% to 14%, 20% to 30%, and up to 30%, respectively.[58,73] Therefore, of cases that morphologically resemble DLBCL, approximately 4% to 8% of cases will be reclassified as DHL.[73,74]

Beyond testing for *MYC*, *BCL2*, and *BCL6* rearrangements, additional genetic testing is usually not performed on typical DLBCL. This is certainly not for a lack of genetic heterogeneity in DLBCL, but for practical purposes. Although the mutational landscape of DLBCL is diverse and subclassification by molecular groups is possible,[73,75] it remains an active area of research. A transition to molecular classification of DLBCL may arise in the future.

Subtypes of DLBCL

There are several important subtypes of DLBCL that are recognized as distinct entities by the current classifications, which sometimes show significant morphologic and immunophenotypic overlap with DLBCL, NOS. Primary DLBCL of the central nervous system (CNS) has a distinct immunophenotypic and molecular profile and presents in the brain, spinal cord, leptomeninges, or eye, and primary DLBCL of the testis shares some of the same features arising in immune-privileged sites.[76] Primary cutaneous DLBCL, leg type presents in the skin. These subtypes are beyond the scope of this text, which encompasses nodal disease. Several other subtypes of DLBCL, which are given separate diagnostic names, are discussed next.

T-CELL/HISTIOCYTE-RICH LARGE B-CELL LYMPHOMA

A unique lymphoma that shows scattered large B cells within a background of T cells and histiocytes, T cell/histiocyte-rich large B-cell lymphoma (TCHR-LBCL) differs from most of the other large B-cell lymphomas in that there is neither confluent growth nor aggregates of large B cells present. Given the paucity of tumor cells, TCHR-LBCL has many features in common with nodular lymphocyte predominant B-cell lymphoma (NLPBL), discussed in detail in Chapter 7. While TCHR-LBCL and NLPBL can be distinguished by their overall architecture and microenvironment, it may be impossible to distinguish between the two on small core biopsies and a diagnosis of TCHR-LBCL should not be rendered on such biopsies. These cases should be diagnosed as "large B-cell lineage lymphoma" and a differential given.

Two imperfect ways to conceptualize TCHR-LBCL could be a "paucicellular DLBCL" or an "NLPBL without nodules." If you observe a confluence of large B cells, consider DLBCL; and if you see macronodular growth instead of diffuse, consider NLPBL instead of TCHR-LBCL.

TCHR-LBCL is an uncommon lymphoma, far outnumbered by DLBCL, NOS with a prominent inflammatory reaction. These usually nodal lymphomas affect a wide age range (12-61 years of age) and 75% of cases occur in men.[58] Most cases present at a high clinical stage at diagnosis, with bone marrow, spleen, and liver being commonly involved.

Morphology

TCHR-LBCL is defined by a diffuse infiltrate composed predominantly of histiocytes and small T cells with scattered large atypical B cells, which effaces the lymph node architecture (Figure 5.41). Diffuse growth is typical, with rare cases showing vague nodularity; distinct macronodule formation must be absent.[77] The large tumor cells should be singly scattered and should not form sheets or aggregates, typically comprising 10% or less of the total cellular volume. The tumor cells can mimic centroblasts or have more atypical features that resemble Hodgkin or RS cells.[78]

The background cells present within the infiltrate help to define TCHR-LBCL. These should consist predominantly of bland histiocytes and small T-lymphocytes. The presence of abundant small B cells, plasma cells, or eosinophils in the background should raise concern for an alternate diagnosis. Patients with a history of NLPBL, or with NLPBL elsewhere in a lymph node, should not be diagnosed with TCHR-LBCL and may have so called "TCHR-LBCL-like growth pattern of NLPBL"[74] (see Chapter 7).

Phenotype

Typical of other large B-cell lymphomas, the large tumor cells of TCHR-LBCL should demonstrate strong pan-B-cell markers such as CD20 (Figure 5.41), PAX5, and CD19, usually without expression of CD30,

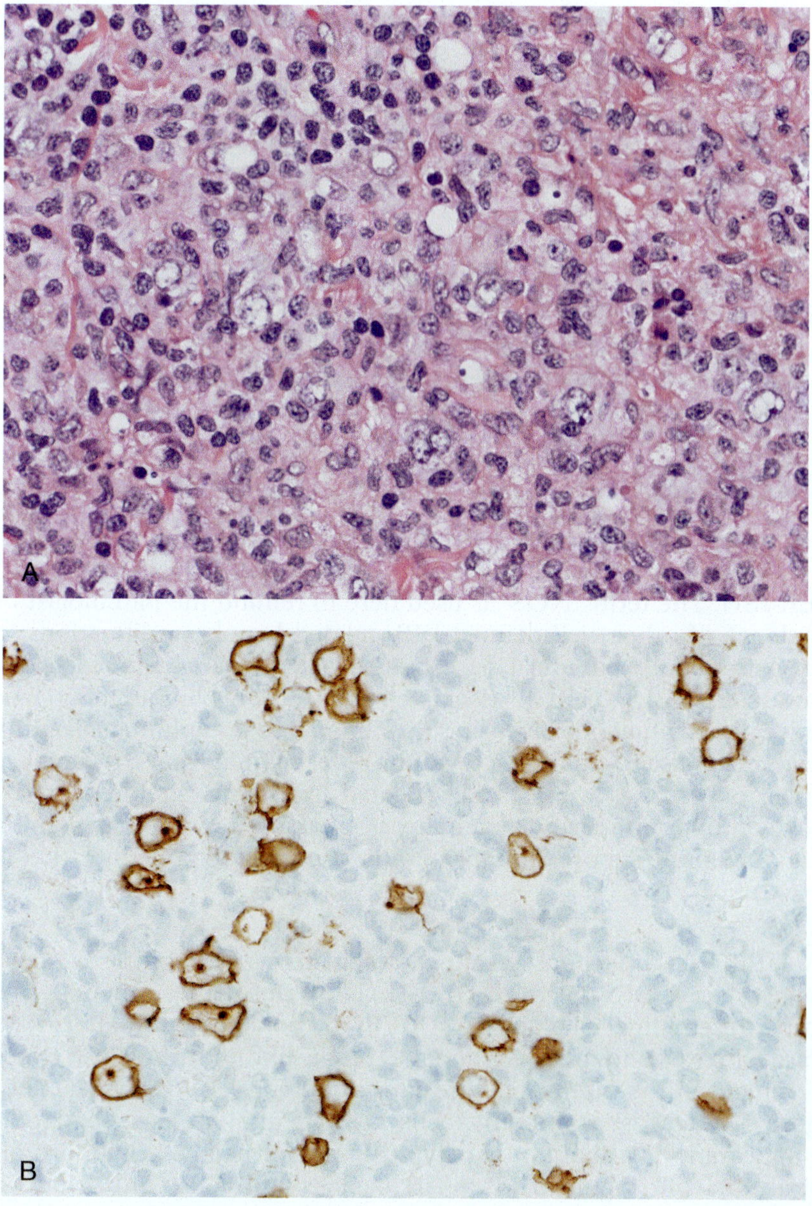

FIGURE 5.41 A, T cell/histiocyte-rich large B-cell lymphoma. Large tumor cells are singly scattered within a background of small lymphocytes and histiocytes. B, CD20 staining highlights large tumor cells singly scattered in a background that is devoid of small CD20-positive B cells.

CD15, or CD138.[58] The tumor cells usually also express BCL6 an immunophenotype similar to tumor cells seen in NLPBL. The background should be composed of CD68/CD163-positive histiocytes and CD3-positive small T cells, with a mixture of both CD4- and CD8-positive T cells, usually with a cytotoxic CD8-predominance.[79,80] Small CD20-positive B cells should be absent.

Genetics

Beyond a clonally rearranged immunoglobulin gene, there are few, if any, genetic features helpful in the differential for TCHR-LBCL. GEP studies suggest that these tumors may exist on a spectrum with NLPBL,[74] but this continues to be an evolving area of research. Routinely, no additional cytogenetic or molecular studies are performed. DHL with this morphology are rare.

EBV-POSITIVE DLBCL, NOS

EBV-positive DLBCL, NOS is defined as a large B-cell lymphoma effacing lymph node architecture that shows greater than 80% positivity for EBV by EBER-ISH. The term "NOS" is used here to remind the pathologist of the abundance of other well-defined EBV-related lymphoproliferations (most often extranodal) that must be excluded using various clinicopathologic features (eg, PBL, DLBCL associated with chronic inflammation, EBV-positive mucocutaneous ulcer, and lymphomatoid granulomatosis). Initially considered a disease exclusive to adults older than 50 years, it can occur in younger patients, as well.[81-83] EBV-related lymphoma should always raise consideration for underlying immune suppression; however, an identifiable cause of immune suppression may not be found in all patients.

Morphology

EBV-DLBCL is morphologically heterogeneous, exhibiting a spectrum between that of EBV-negative DLBCL, NOS (monomorphic pattern) and features resembling CHL or TCHR-LBCL (polymorphic patterns). Only a third of cases show conventional DLBCL-like morphology.[84] Necrosis is common and is often a clue to an underlying EBV-related lymphoma (Figure 5.42). Most commonly, cells take an immunoblast- or Hodgkin-like appearance, with abundant atypical transformed cells with prominent central nucleoli (Figure 5.43).[58] The background cells can include small lymphocytes, plasma cells, histiocytes, and eosinophils.[83,84]

Phenotype

In general, EBER staining should be considered in large B-cell lymphomas that exhibit any of the following features: (1) necrosis, (2) RS-like cytology, and (3) a prominent lymphohistiocytic background. Any patient with a history of immune suppression should also have EBER testing in the setting of any type of lymphoma or lymphoproliferation. EBER is

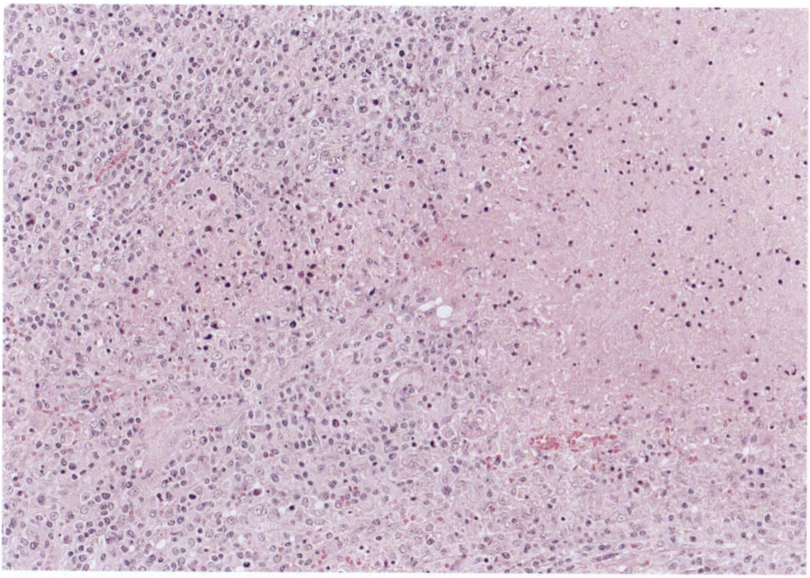

FIGURE 5.42 Epstein-Barr virus–positive diffuse large B-cell lymphoma frequently shows areas of necrosis.

strongly expressed in >80% of tumor cells (Figure 5.43). EBV latent protein expression pattern is usually latency type II (which includes EBNA1, LMP1, and LMP2), but occasionally shows latency type III (full spectrum of latent proteins expression).[82,85] In practice, demonstrating latent protein expression by IHC can help confirm the diagnosis in some cases, as approximately 90% of cases express LMP1 and 7% to 36% of cases express EBNA2 (latency type III).[58] Latency III pattern should prompt particular evaluation for underlying immunodeficiency.

Tumor cells may express pan-B-cell antigens, but more commonly show loss of these antigens than DLBCL, NOS. They usually have a non-GCB phenotype.[86] EBV-DLBCL can express CD30 and sometimes CD15, making distinction from CHL challenging.[84] In the differential with EBV-positive CHL, EBV-DLBCL should express more and/or stronger B-cell antigens (Figure 5.43).[87] In this setting, a comprehensive panel of B-cell antigens is recommended including CD20, CD79a, OCT-2, BOB.1, and CD19. CD45 expression may also be useful in excluding CHL, although it may be lost in EBV-DLBCL as well.

Genetics

No specific diagnostic genetic alterations for EBV-DLBCL are reported.[58] FISH is generally recommended to exclude a DHL if sufficient tissue is present. In the presence of a *MYC* rearrangement, however, PBL should also be excluded.[83]

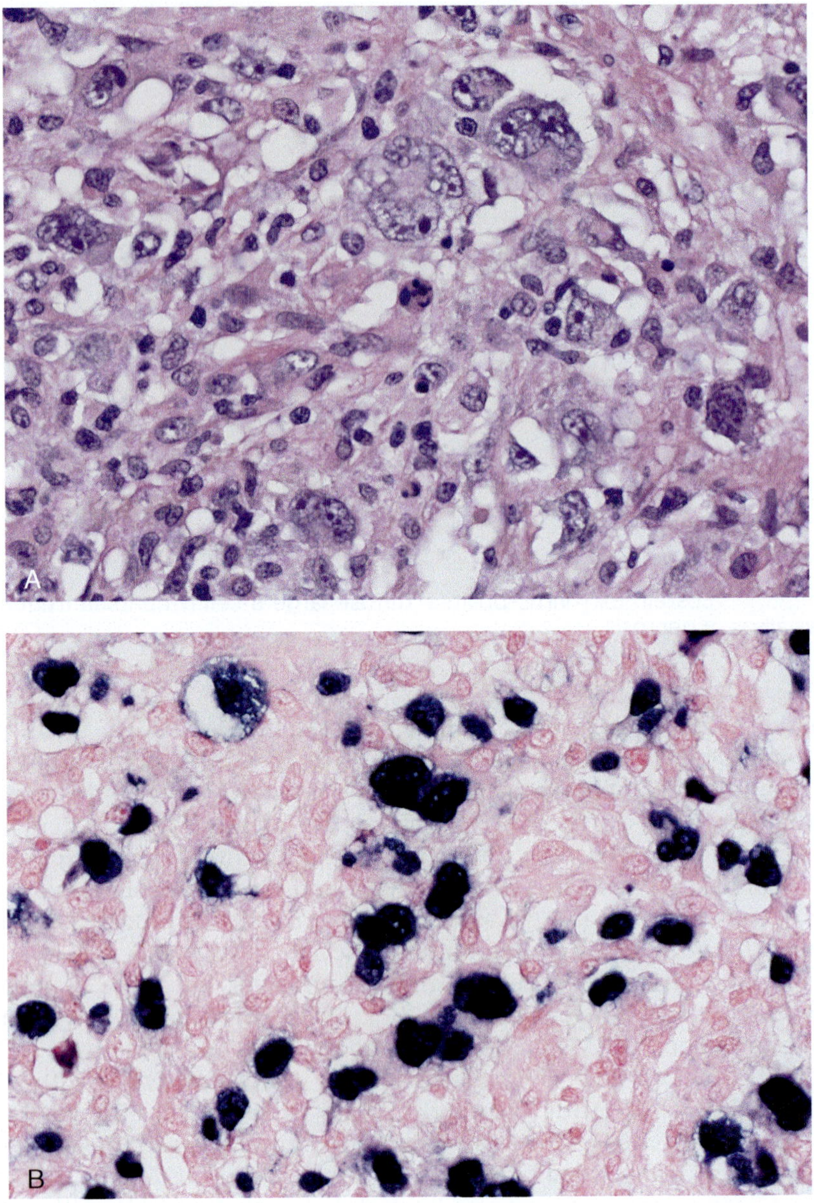

FIGURE 5.43 (*Continued*)

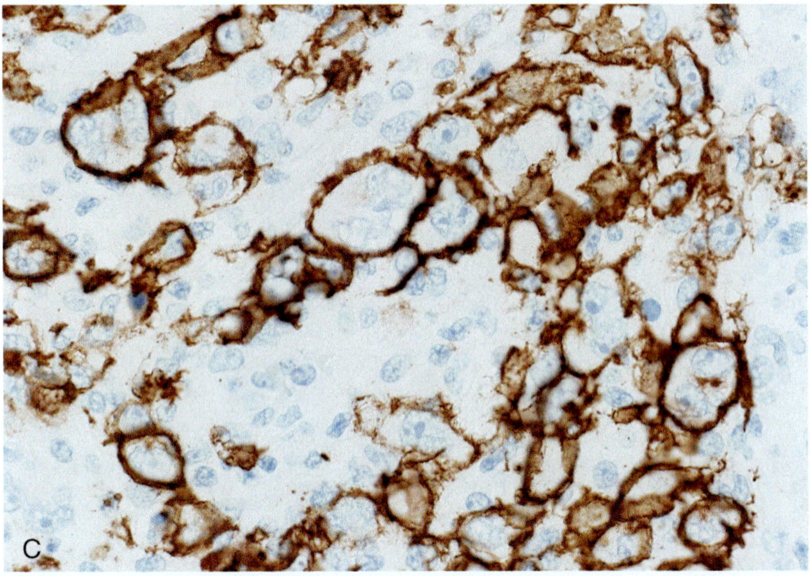

FIGURE 5.43 A, Epstein-Barr virus (EBV)-positive diffuse large B-cell lymphoma, polymorphic pattern. B, In situ hybridization for EBV-encoded small RNA showing strong positivity in virtually all tumor cells of EBV-positive diffuse large B-cell lymphoma. C, CD20 stain shows strong membranous staining in EBV-positive diffuse large B-cell lymphoma. Strong expression of CD20, while not always seen in EBV–diffuse large B-cell lymphoma, helps to exclude classic Hodgkin lymphoma in this case.

PRIMARY MEDIASTINAL (THYMIC) LARGE B-CELL LYMPHOMA

Primary mediastinal (thymic) large B-cell lymphoma (PMBL) is an aggressive B-cell lymphoma thought to arise from a thymic B cell, giving it a somewhat unique immunomorphology and genetic makeup. The majority of PMBL present with a large (>10 cm) anterior mediastinal mass at low disease stage (I-II).[88] Patients may present with superior vena cava syndrome, a finding that is more common in PMBL than CHL. The absence of extensive peripheral lymph node and bone marrow involvement can help distinguish PMBL from systemic DLBCL, NOS involving the mediastinum, though this differential can sometimes present a challenge. Hilar lymph nodes and even cervical lymph nodes are commonly involved in PMBL, and the pathologist should consider this diagnosis in the appropriate clinical setting with biopsies of these sites. The typical patient demographic for PMBL is also unique compared with other DLBCL: young adults (median age 35) with a 2:1 female predominance.[89,90]

Morphology

PMBL typically shows large centroblastic cells with clear cytoplasm and background compartmentalizing fibrosis (Figure 5.44), but there is

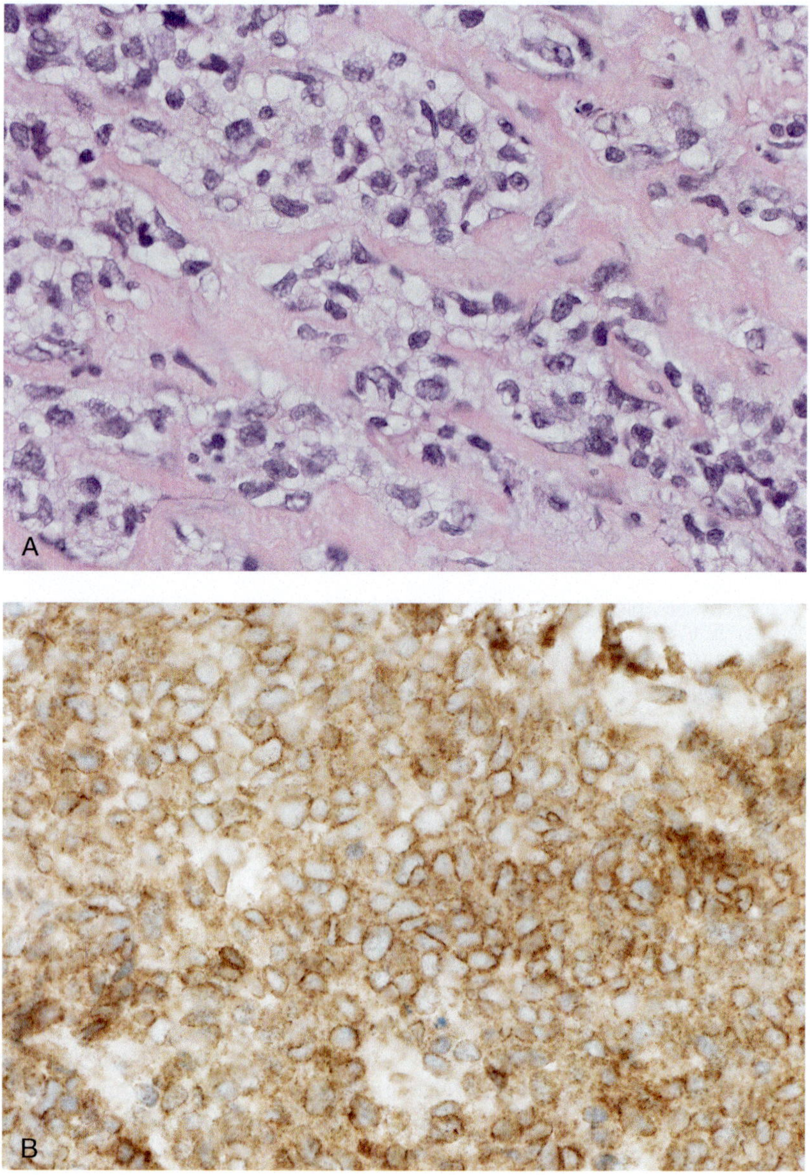

FIGURE 5.44 *(Continued)*

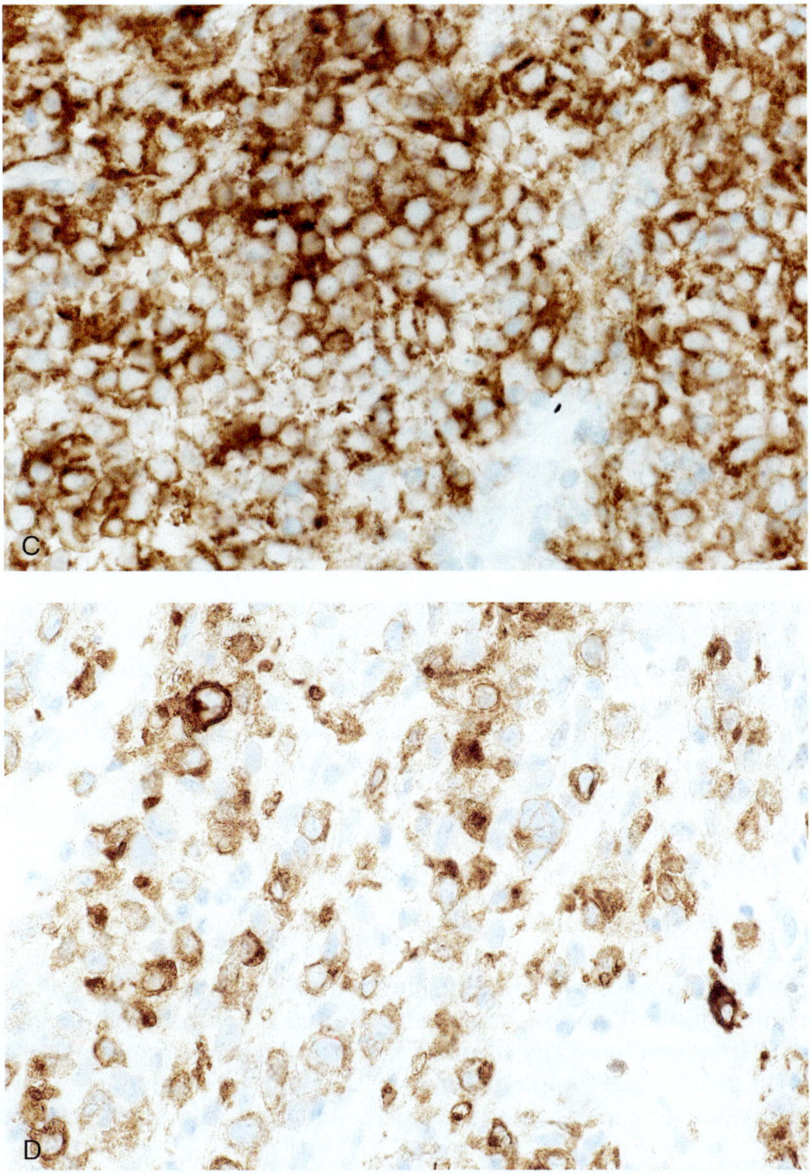

FIGURE 5.44 A, Primary mediastinal large B-cell lymphoma (PMBL). Large tumor cells show abundant clear cytoplasm and characteristic compartmentalizing fibrosis. By immunohistochemistry PMBL is positive for MAL (B) and PDL2/CD273 (C); these stains in combination are helpful in diagnosing PMBL. D, CD30 shows a typical heterogeneous staining pattern in PMBL.

significant morphologic variability.[91,92] Cases with a more Hodgkin-like morphology may occur, making distinction from mediastinal gray zone lymphoma (MGZL) (discussed below) challenging.

Phenotype

Pan-B-cell antigen expression (CD20, CD79a, PAX5) is present, but surface immunoglobulin is often absent.[92] CD30 expression is seen in the majority of cases, but usually in a more heterogeneous pattern than the strong, uniform staining pattern of CHL.[93] Most cases lack CD10 expression and are positive for MUM1. However, it is important to note that PMBL represents a significant component of the unclassifiable cases in the original DLBCL GEP studies, and actually has a GEP more closely resembling CHL.[68,94,95] As such the Hans algorithm does not apply to cases of true PMBL. Expression of additional unique markers, when used as a panel, including MAL, PD-L2 (CD273), CD30, and CD23, favor a diagnosis of PMBL over systemic DLBCL (Figure 5.44).[69,92,96,97]

Genetics

Unique gene expression profile studies and other somewhat-specific genetic events set PMBL apart from other DLBCL.[58] For example, constitutive activation in the NF-kappa B and JAK/STAT pathways show that PMBL is genetically more closely related to CHL than DLBCL.[94,95] Newer GEP assays can be used to help classify cases as PMBL and may be increasingly utilized in the future.[98] FISH to exclude DHL should be performed but is most commonly negative.[99]

ALK-POSITIVE LARGE B-CELL LYMPHOMA

A rare yet distinct type of large B-cell lymphoma (accounting for <1% of LBCL), ALK-positive large B-cell lymphoma (ALK-LBCL) should be in the differential diagnosis when dealing with a nodal large cell lymphoma with immunoblastic or plasmablastic features. Typically, younger male patients (median age 43) without a history of immunosuppression present with generalized lymphadenopathy and high clinical stage; however, a wide age range and extranodal involvement have also been reported.[100]

Morphology

These tumors show a diffuse effacement by large immunoblastic or plasmablastic cells, sometimes involving lymph node sinuses (Figure 5.45).

Phenotype

The tumor cells usually lack expression of standard pan-B-cell markers, CD20 and PAX5, and instead express MUM1, CD138, EMA, and light chain-restricted cytoplasmic immunoglobulin (Figure 5.45).[100,101] This

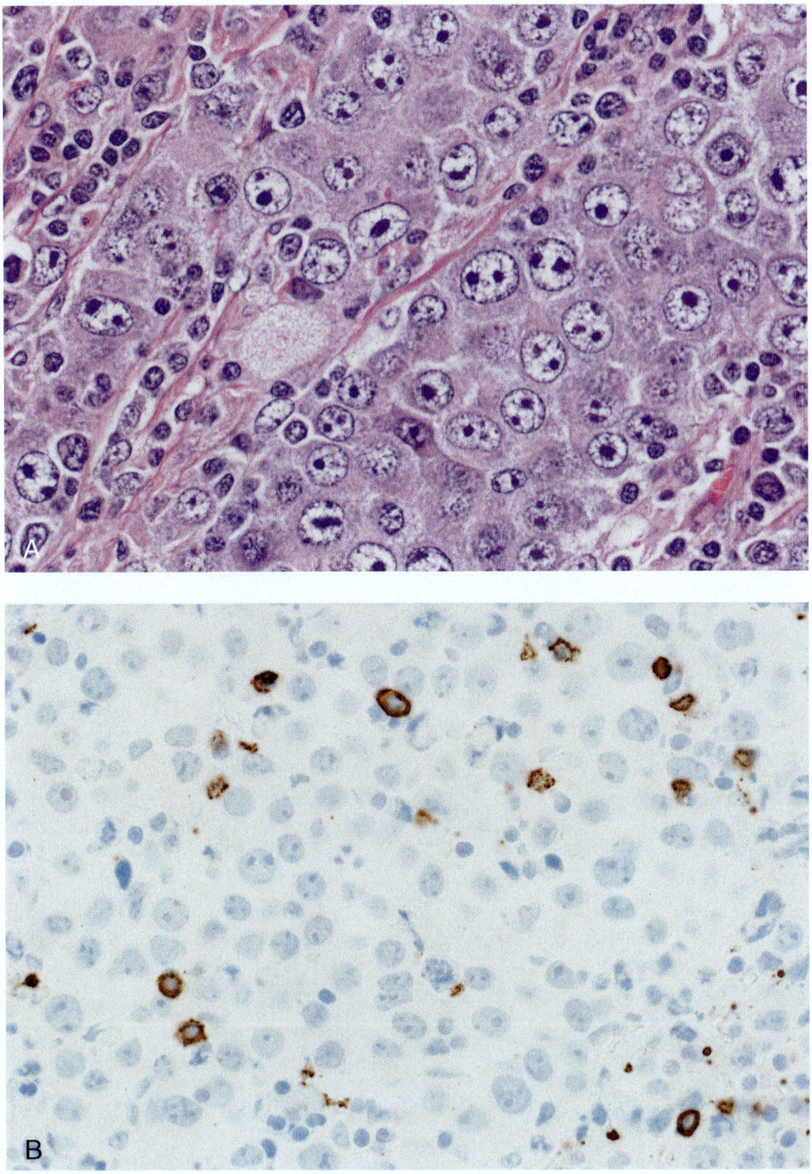

FIGURE 5.45 *(Continued)*

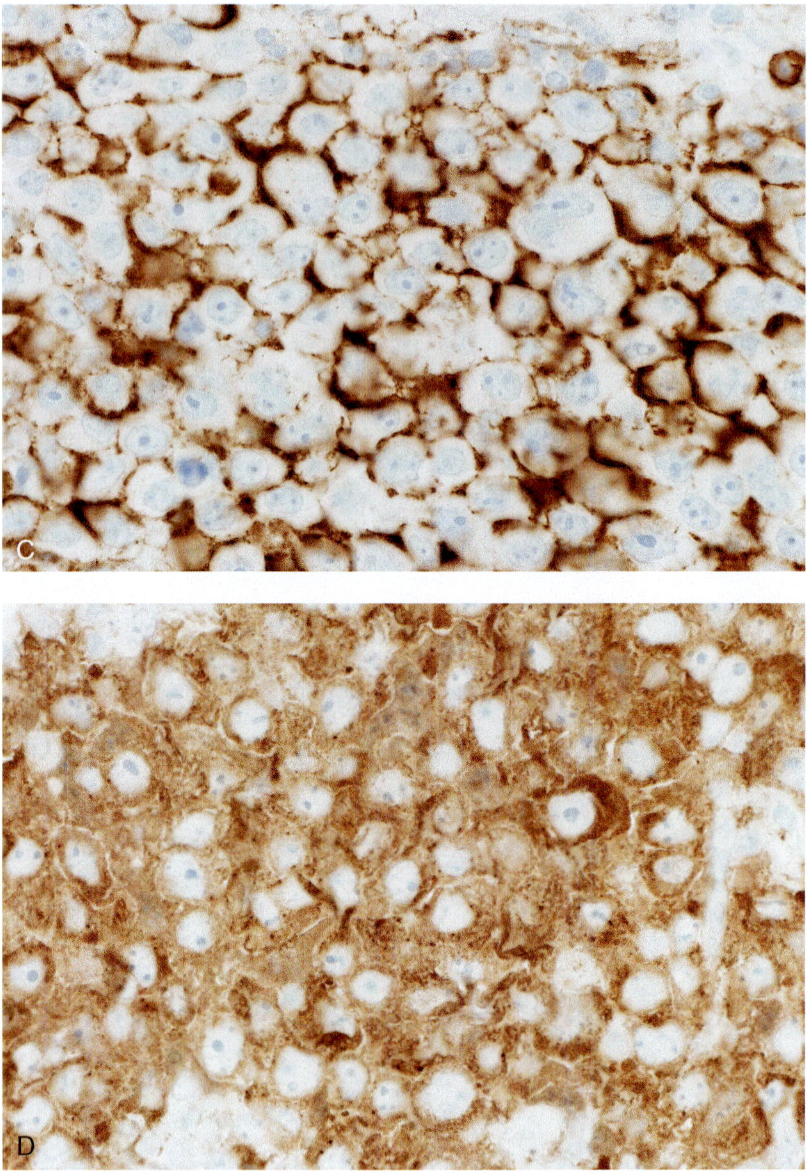

FIGURE 5.45 A, ALK-positive large B-cell lymphoma (ALK-LBCL). The cells show plasmablastic morphology (prominent nucleoli and abundant cytoplasm) as well as immunoblastic morphology (less cytoplasm). B, Lymphoma cells in ALK-positive large B-cell lymphoma are negative for CD20 and positive for (C) CD138. D, A granular cytoplasmic staining pattern for ALK, as seen here, is both sensitive and specific for the most frequent translocation seen in ALK-LBCL, the t(2;17)(p23;q23); *CLTC-ALK*

staining pattern, indicating terminal B-cell differentiation, is more typical of PCNs or PBLs. Of note, all cases of ALK-LBCL are negative for EBV and HHV8, helpful in the differential diagnosis. ALK IHC is positive, most commonly in a granular cytoplasmic pattern (Figure 5.45)[100] although any pattern can be seen including nuclear and/or cytoplasmic; however, CD30 is typically negative, or at most very focal and weak, assisting with excluding anaplastic large cell lymphoma.

Genetics

The most frequent translocation is a t(2;17)(p23;q23) creating a *CLTC-ALK* fusion protein.[100] This ALK translocation is different than the common t(2;5)(p23;q35) seen in ALK-positive anaplastic large cell lymphoma, although rare cases of ALK-DLBCL show the latter translocation.[102] FISH is typically not needed for diagnosis, as IHC is sensitive and specific.

PLASMABLASTIC LYMPHOMA

Plasmablastic lymphoma (PBL) is a rare, aggressive, immunodeficiency- and EBV-associated extranodal lymphoma that only occasionally involves lymph nodes.[103] It is most common in older adults (median age ~60 years), but can occur in young patients, especially with HIV. There is a male predominance (~4:1).[104] Most often presenting as a mass in extranodal regions such as the oral cavity or elsewhere in the head and neck, patients diagnosed with PBL commonly have concomitant immunosuppression from conditions such as HIV, autoimmune disease, organ transplant, and presumed immunosenescence.[83,105,106] When considering the diagnosis of PBL, special attention should be made to exclude plasmablastic or anaplastic transformation of plasma cell myeloma, which has a different clinical presentation including bone marrow involvement, associated paraprotein, and lytic bone lesions.

Morphology/Phenotype

Much like ALK-positive DLBCL, the morphologic and immunophenotypic features of PBL are that of a terminally differentiated B cell (CD20 and PAX5-negative; MUM1 and CD138-positive with light chain restriction) with immunoblastic/plasmablastic morphology, but lacking expression of ALK. Instead, around two-thirds of cases of PBL show positivity for EBER (Figure 5.46).[107] HHV8 is negative.

Genetics

Approximately 50% of cases of PBL demonstrate a *MYC* rearrangement.[108] Concurrent *BCL6* and/or *BCL2* rearrangements are uncommon.

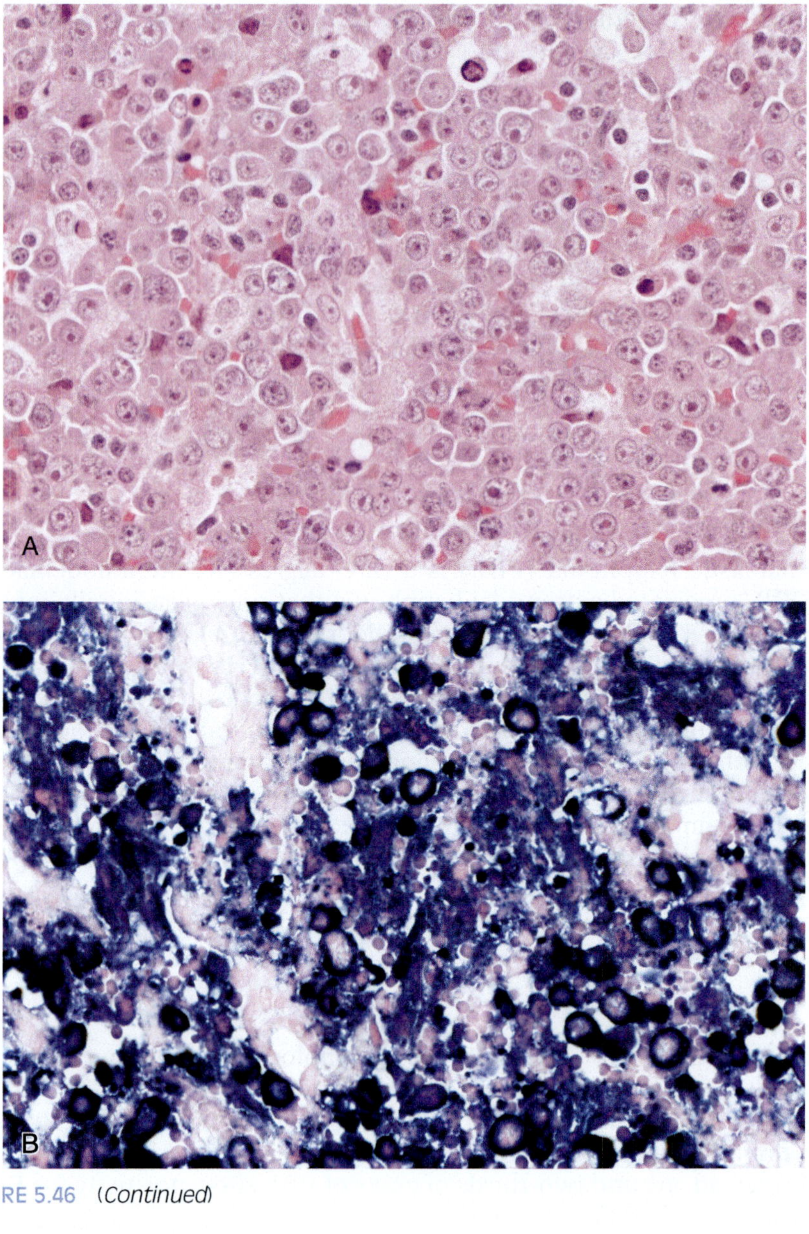

FIGURE 5.46 (*Continued*)

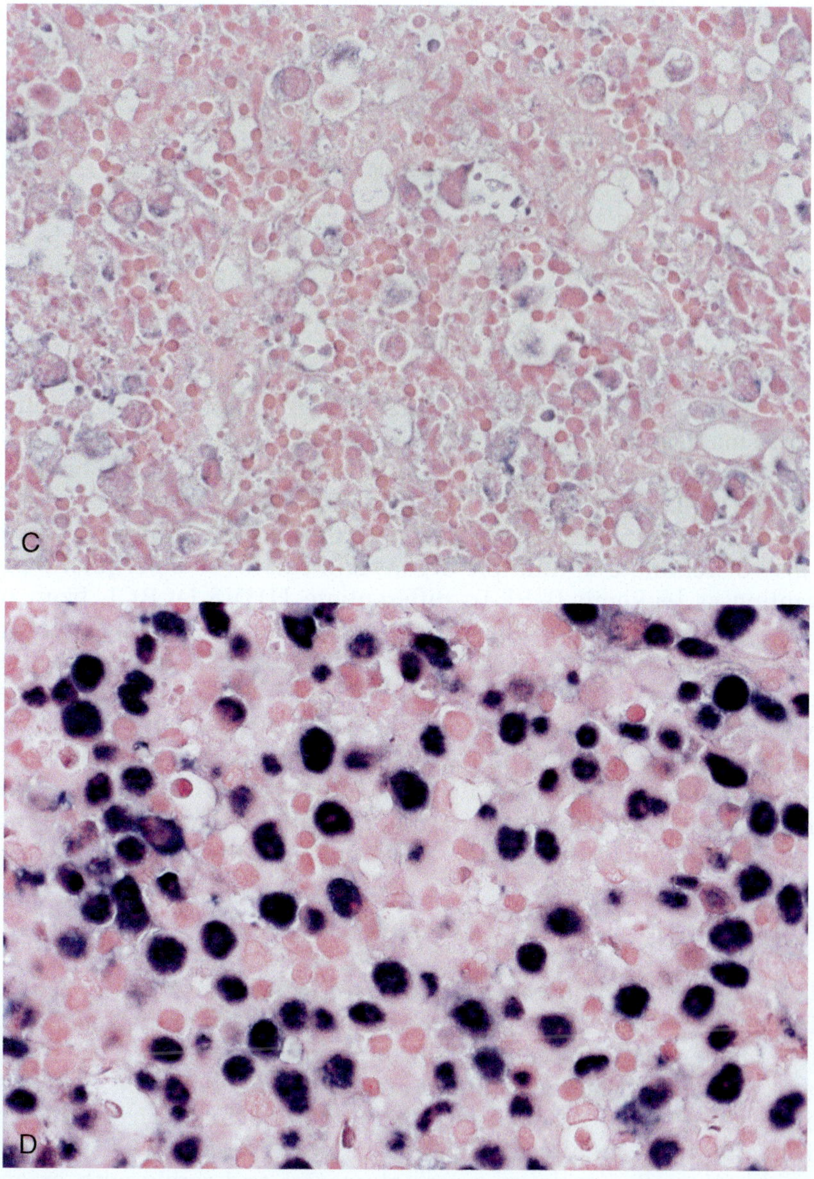

FIGURE 5.46 A, Plasmablastic lymphoma high-power magnification. in situ hybridization for immunoglobulin light chains kappa (B) and lambda (C) shows that lymphoma cells are kappa light chain-restricted. D, in situ hybridization for Epstein-Barr virus–encoded small RNA showing strong positivity, which is present in approximately two-thirds of cases of plasmablastic lymphoma.

HHV8-ASSOCIATED LYMPHOPROLIFERATIVE DISORDERS

HHV8 causes a spectrum of lymphoproliferative disorders with variable clinical presentation, pathologic features, and clonality. Most are seen in the setting of HIV or other immunosuppressed states.[109]

HHV8-positive Multicentric Castleman Disease

Discussed in more detail in Chapter 3, there is a subset of multicentric Castleman disease that is HHV8-associated.

HHV8-positive DLBCL, NOS

A third entity in the differential diagnosis of B-cell-lineage lymphomas with plasmablastic morphology and immunophenotype (along with PBL and ALK-positive DLBCL), HHV8-positive diffuse large B-cell lymphoma, NOS (HHV8-DLBCL) usually arises in HIV-infected patients with multicentric Castleman disease.[110] Typically a nodal lymphoma, tumor cells can also disseminate to multiple organs and can involve peripheral blood, presenting as leukemia.[110,111] To differentiate HHV8-DLBCL from other HHV8-positive lymphoproliferations, effacement of lymph node architecture should be prominent. While HHV8-DLBCL has plasmablastic morphology, a somewhat unique aspect of its phenotype is consistent expression of cytoplasmic IgM and lambda light chain restriction, while typically lacking expression of CD138. EBER and ALK should be negative. In the presence of dual positivity for HHV8 and EBER, an extracavitary primary effusion lymphoma (an extranodal lymphoma outside the scope of this book) should be considered.

HHV8-positive Germinotropic Lymphoproliferative Disorder

HHV8-positive germinotropic lymphoproliferative disorder is defined as monotypic HHV8/LANA1-positive plasmablasts, which partially or completely replace germinal center cells in otherwise-preserved lymph nodes (Figure 5.47). Interestingly, and despite tumor cells being also EBER-positive, there is no association with immunodeficiency or HIV infection. Lymph node architecture should be preserved, with HHV8-positive plasmablastic cells involving germinal centers and rarely with extension outside of the follicles.[112] Prognosis is usually good, with expected good response to chemotherapy and only rare progression to DLBCL.

BURKITT LYMPHOMA

An aggressive but often curable B-cell lymphoma with three unique epidemiological subtypes, BL requires rigid clinical, morphologic, immunophenotypic, and genetic criteria for diagnosis.[58]

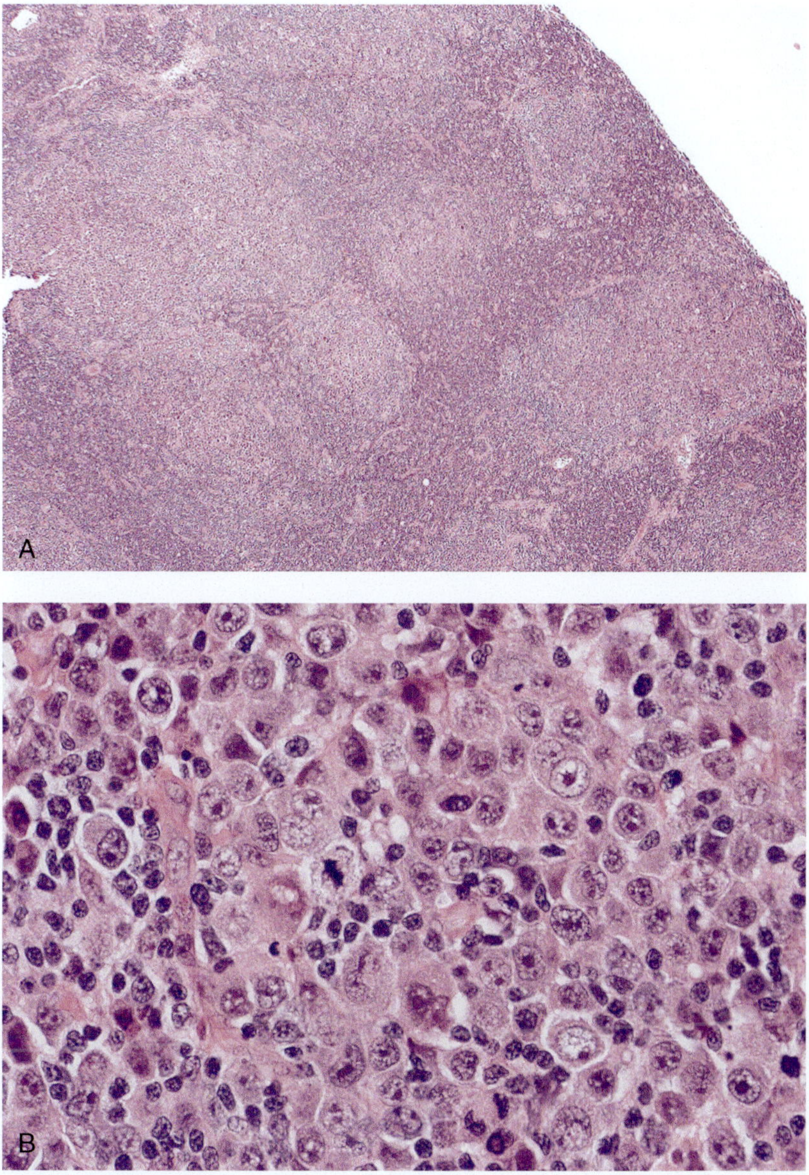

FIGURE 5.47 (*Continued*)

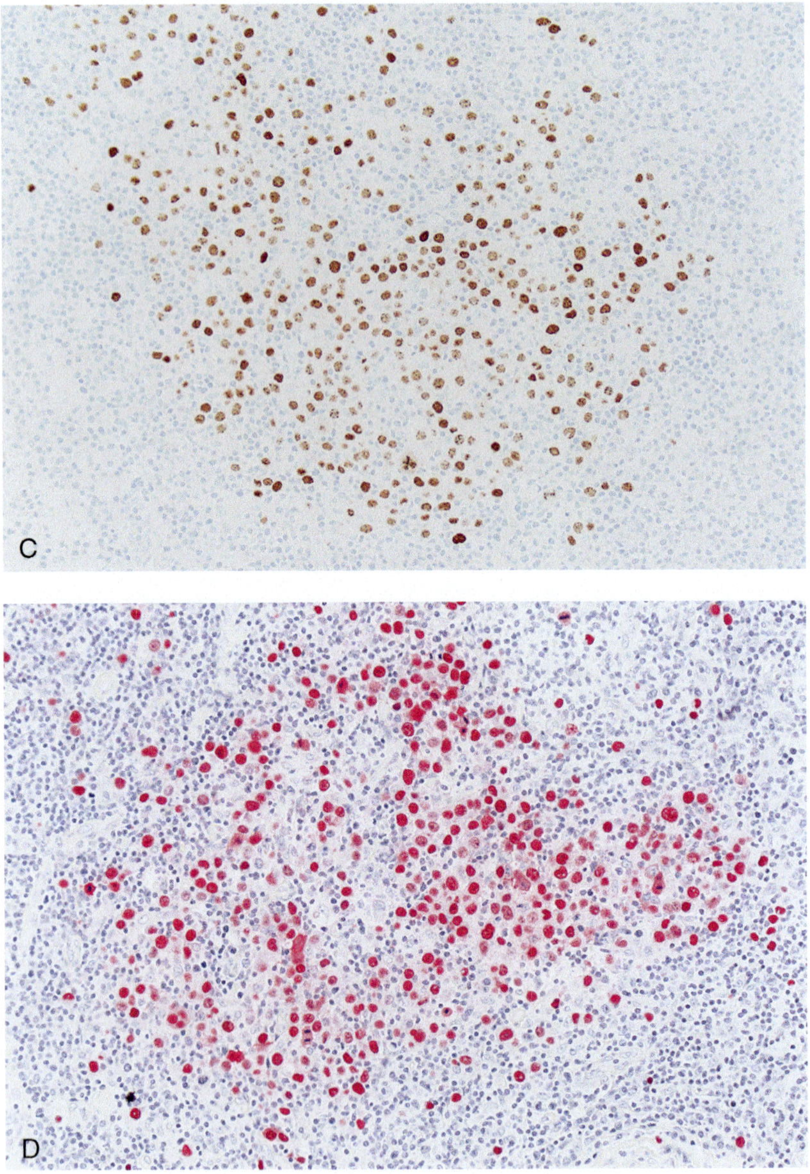

FIGURE 5.47 **HHV8-positive germinotropic lymphoproliferative disorder.** A, A low-power view showing intact nodal architecture with expanded germinal centers. B, High-power magnification highlights plasmablastic/immunoblastic morphology. C, HHV8/LANA1 immunohistochemistry is positive in the plasmablasts. D, Epstein-Barr virus–encoded small RNA is also positive, predominantly confined to the plasmablasts replacing the germinal centers.

Epidemiological Variants of BL

The three epidemiological variants include endemic, sporadic, and immunodeficiency-associated BL. Of these, lymph node and bone marrow involvement are most often seen in immunodeficiency-associated BL. This variant is usually associated with underlying HIV infection, but can be seen in other types of immunosuppression.[113] During HIV infection, the risk for BL is higher early in the disease when T-cell counts remain high, even with the modern HIV therapies.[114,115] EBV-positivity is seen in 25% to 40% of these cases.[58]

Endemic BL, as described by Dr. Denis Burkitt in 1958, follows a geographic distribution in equatorial Africa and Papua New Guinea (regions endemic to malaria caused by *Plasmodium falciparum*) and is almost always associated with underlying EBV infection and EBER-positivity in tumor cells. This variant affects the youngest age group (age 4-7 years) and typically involves extranodal sites including jaw or facial bones with systemic involvement of multiple abdominal organs being common.[116]

Sporadic BL has no geographic predilection and typically affects young adults (median age 30), accounting for 1% to 2% of all lymphomas in the United States.[58] EBV is present in only 20% to 30% of cases, and disease is more common in abdominal organs such as the ileocecal region, but not in the jaw or facial bones as seen in endemic BL. All three variants can show CNS involvement.

Morphology

The classic "starry sky" appearance of BL is due to the presence of diffuse sheets of intermediate-sized B cells effacing normal architecture with tingible body macrophages scattered throughout (Figure 5.48). Tumor cells are monotonous with fine chromatin and scant cytoplasm (Figure 5.49). Abundant mitoses and apoptotic figures from high cell turnover should be easy to identify. Cases with prominent background epithelioid histiocytes have been described and may have a more favorable prognosis.[117] On aspiration cytology, characteristic basophilic cytoplasm with lipid vacuoles is evident (Figure 5.50). Only rare cases deviate slightly from this classic morphology, showing greater nuclear pleomorphism or more prominent nucleoli.[113] The cases with so-called atypical morphology are more commonly seen in HIV positive patients. Specifically, cases with plasmacytoid morphology, and even some MUM1 expression, can occur in the HIV setting.[118]

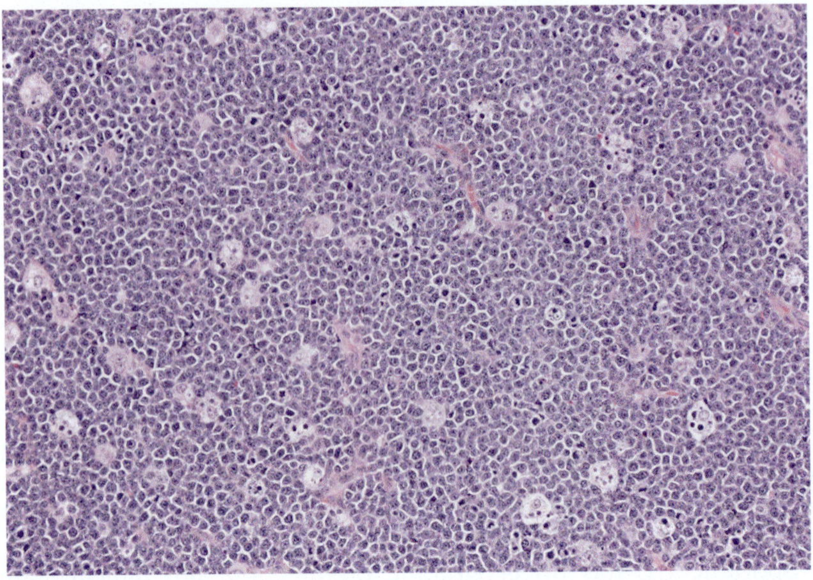

FIGURE 5.48 Burkitt lymphoma showing a "starry sky" pattern with scattered tingible body macrophages.

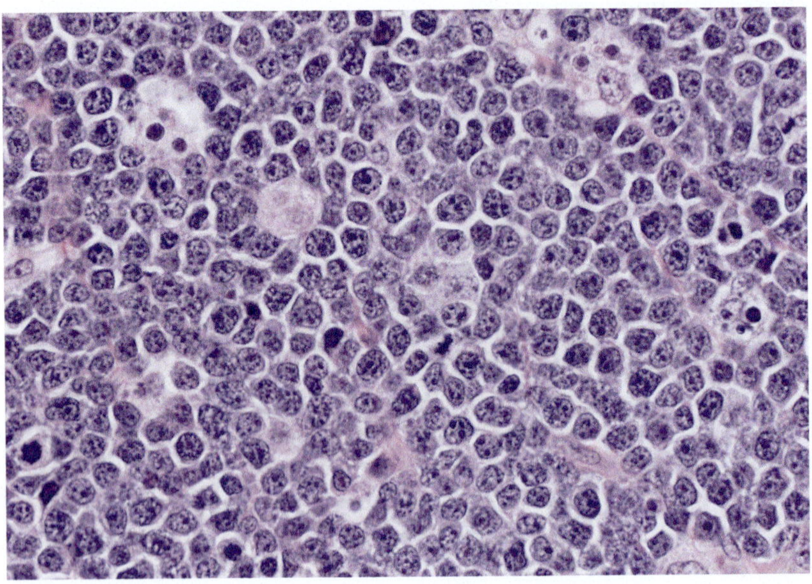

FIGURE 5.49 High-power magnification of Burkitt lymphoma showing intermediate-sized lymphoma cells with a high N:C ratio, more reminiscent of lymphoblastic lymphoma than some of the other aggressive B-cell lymphomas.

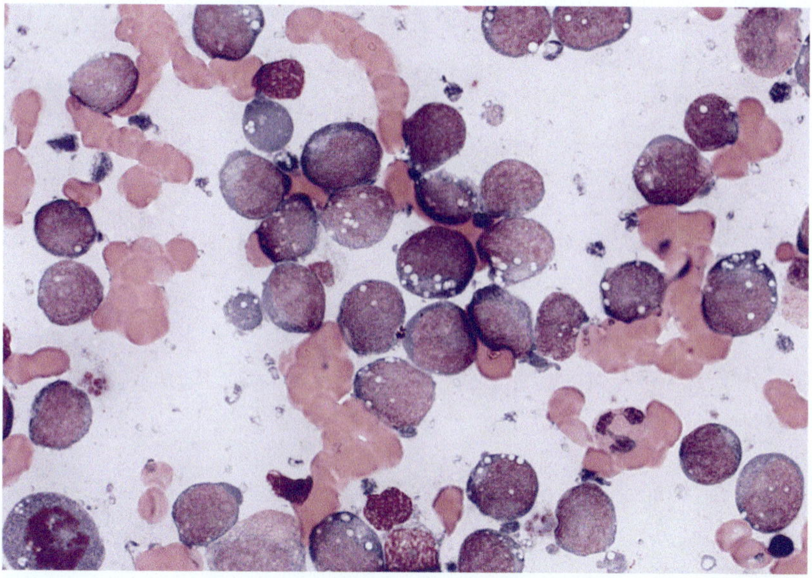

FIGURE 5.50 **Burkitt lymphoma aspirate cytology.** Note the blast-like morphology (reminiscent of lymphoblastic leukemia) with characteristic cytoplasmic vacuoles.

Phenotype

One should hesitate to diagnose BL without all of the following phenotypic hallmarks: strong pan-B-cell antigens, positive germinal center markers (CD10 and BCL6), lack of BCL2 co-expression, and very high expression of MYC and Ki-67 (nearly 100% of tumor cells) (Figure 5.51). Only rare cases of weak BCL2-positive, CD10-negative, or CD5-positive cases have been reported.[119] Surface immunoglobulin expression, usually IgM and light chain restriction, is also common. CD43 is expressed in 90% of BL and only 20% to 40% of other types of aggressive BCL.[120] Since B-lymphoblastic lymphoma is in the morphologic differential and commonly expresses CD10 and some B-cell markers, TdT and CD34 positivity should be excluded. Strong positivity for BCL2 excludes BL and raises the possibility of a DHL.

Genetics

A rearrangement of *MYC* at 8q24 with an immunoglobulin gene translocation partner is seen in virtually all cases of BL. Typically identified by FISH, the classic t(8;14) translocation, which juxtaposes *MYC* with the IGH gene at 14q32, is present in most cases. *MYC* translocations involving either kappa or lambda immunoglobulin light chain genes resulting in a t(2;8) (*IGK* at 2p12) or t(8;22) (*IGL* at 22q11) occur in the remainder of cases.[58] *BCL2* and *BCL6* rearrangements are absent.

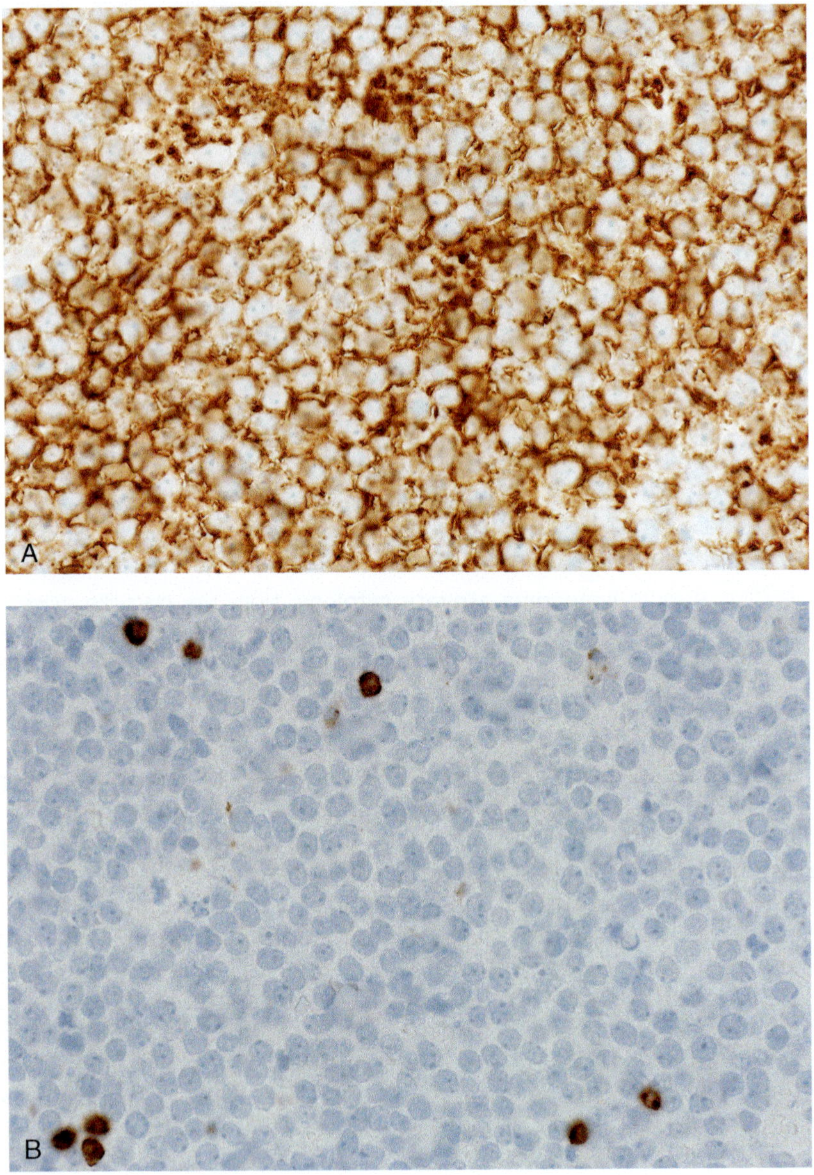

FIGURE 5.51 (*Continued*)

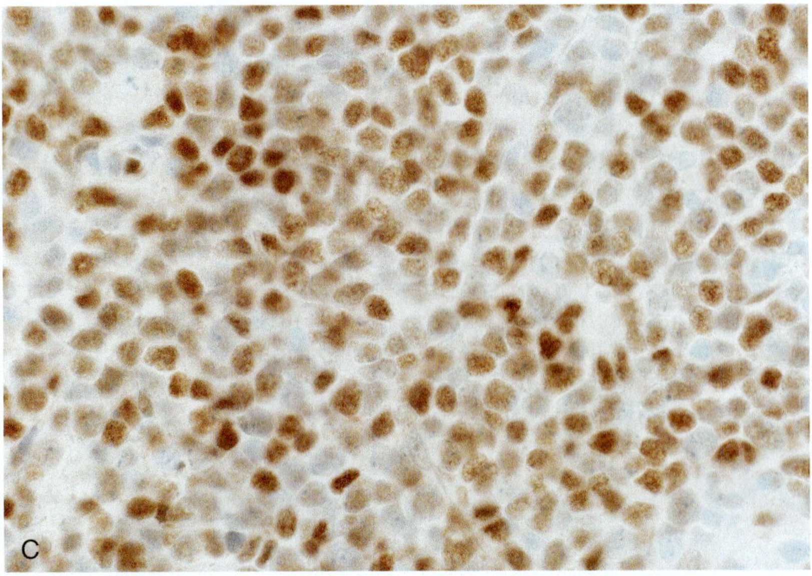

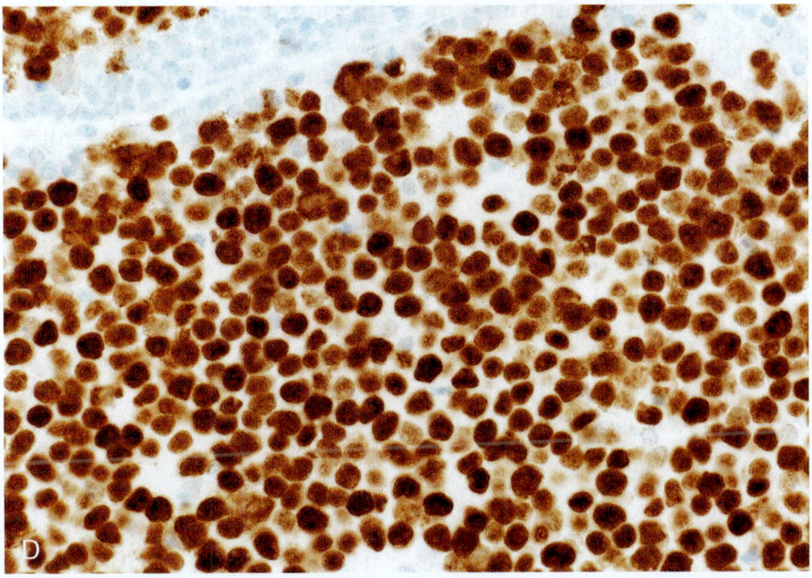

FIGURE 5.51 **Burkitt lymphoma immunohistochemistry.** A, Tumor cells are positive for germinal center markers CD10 as well as BCL6 (not shown). B, BCL2 is negative in tumor cells. C, MYC is highly expressed in tumor cells. D, Ki-67 proliferation index is typically 90% or higher.

LARGE B-CELL LYMPHOMA WITH 11q ABERRATION

This 2022 ICC provisional entity, formerly known as Burkitt-like lymphoma with 11q aberration, is a B-cell lymphoma, which can resemble BL both morphologically and immunophenotypically but can also rarely resemble otherwise typical DLBCL. Biologically, these are distinct from BL, hence the name change.[121,122] LBCL-11q, by definition, lacks a *MYC* rearrangement and instead shows proximal gains and distal losses of chromosomal material in the 11q region.[122] However, it is important to note that 11q aberrations are not specific and can be seen in *MYC* rearranged lymphomas. These cytogenetic aberrations can be detected using chromosomal microarray or FISH probes specific to those regions.[121] Some studies have shown similar clinical features to BL despite being biologically distinct although some cases do not behave as aggressively.

HIGH-GRADE B-CELL LYMPHOMA WITH *MYC* AND *BCL2* REARRANGEMENTS AND HIGH-GRADE B-CELL LYMPHOMA WITH *MYC* AND *BCL6* REARRANGEMENTS

The so-called "double hit lymphoma/triple hit lymphoma" is a high-grade B-cell lymphoma with the unique trait of being defined by its cytogenetics. Requirements for diagnosis include demonstrating a *MYC* rearrangement by FISH or equivalent technology (the "first hit"), along with either a *BCL2* rearrangement or *BCL6* rearrangement (the "second hit"), in a B-cell lymphoma with diffuse growth pattern and high-grade or large cell morphology.[58] Most present at a high stage and can arise both from transformation of low-grade lymphoma (usually FL) and de novo.[58,123] The 2022 ICC now separates high-grade B-cell lymphoma with *MYC* and *BCL2* rearrangements (DHL-*BCL2*) and high-grade B-cell lymphoma with *MYC* and *BCL6* rearrangements (DHL-*BCL6*) due to their distinct biology. The latter remains a provisional entity as less data are available regarding its biology and clinical significance. Cases with both *BCL2* and *BCL6* rearrangements are classified as DHL-*BCL2*.[121,124]

Morphology

DHL may have morphology that is indistinguishable from DLBCL, seen in approximately half of these cases.[58] The other half show a true "high-grade" morphology, with intermediate-sized cells with more finely dispersed chromatin, usually monomorphic with tingible body macrophages, but sometimes with areas showing more pleomorphism (these have been called "features intermediate between DLBCL and BL" in prior classifications) (Figure 5.52).[26] A small subset of DHL will show what is called blastoid morphology. These cases show intermediate-sized cells with fine chromatin and scant cytoplasm more akin to true lymphoblasts (Figure 5.53).[125] Because high-grade morphology may trend toward having

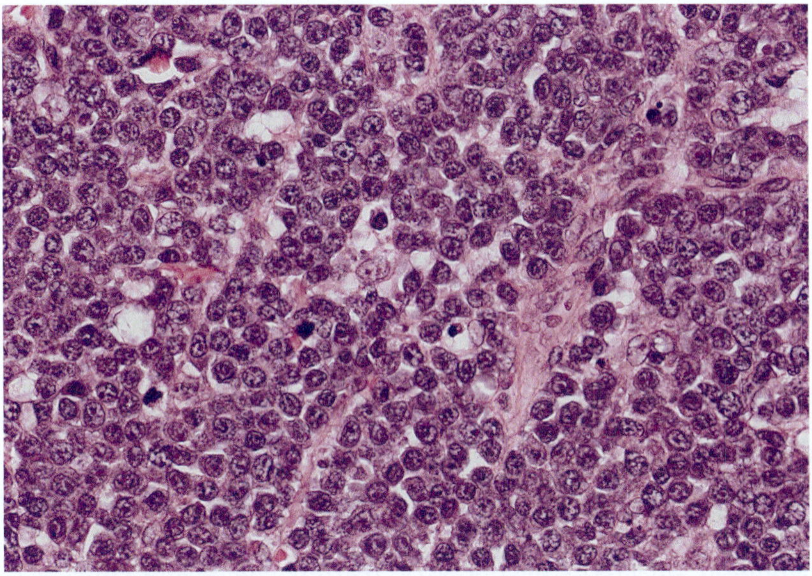

FIGURE 5.52 **High-grade morphology of lymphoma cells—intermediate-sized cells with a high nuclear-to-cytoplasmic ratio.** This morphology may be seen in approximately half of cases with a genetic "double-hit," and would be consistent with a diagnosis of high-grade B-cell lymphoma, not otherwise specified in the absence of a double-hit.

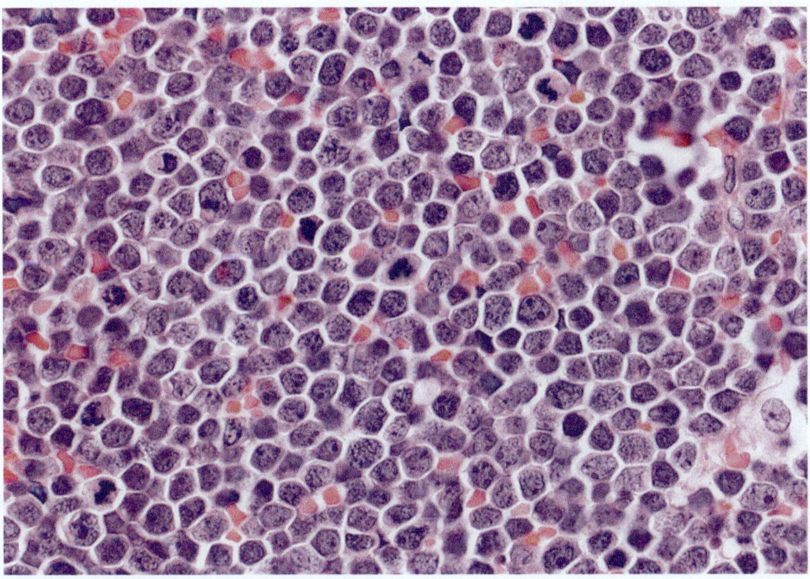

FIGURE 5.53 **High-grade B-cell lymphoma showing blastoid morphology.** Intermediate-sized cells with fine chromatin and high nuclear-to-cytoplasmic ratio, morphologically similar to lymphoblasts.

a worse prognosis when compared with DLBCL morphology,[55,126] the specific morphology present should be reported in cases of DHL.

Phenotype

DHL should show strong expression of pan-B-cell antigens. Essentially all DHL-*BCL2* have a GCB phenotype, whereas among DHL-*BCL6* 50% will have GCB and 50% ABC phenotype.[55,73] Ki-67 expression can vary widely unlike in BL. TdT expression was previously assumed to indicate an immature neoplasm; however, it is now known that DHL can express TdT and that these cases share genetic features with mature B-cell lymphomas and are distinct from lymphoblastic lymphomas.[127] Hence, expression of TdT in a DHL should be noted in the diagnostic line but should not prompt reclassification as lymphoblastic lymphoma.[1,127] CD34, in contrast, is negative in DHL.

Genetics

By definition, all DHLs have a *MYC* rearrangement and either a *BCL2* or *BCL6* rearrangement (or both). 80% to 90% of DHLs are DHL-*BCL2* (includes the THLs), while 10% to 20% are DHL-*BCL6*.[55,73,128] *MYC* is rearranged with an immunoglobulin gene in approximately 60% of cases, with the remaining 40% of cases showing a nonimmunoglobulin translocation partner; the significance of the *MYC* translocation partner is controversial, but presently classifications do not require identification of the *MYC* partner gene for diagnosis.[55,128,129]

The molecular characteristics of DHL are an evolving topic that is likely to impact diagnosis and classification in the future. Several groups have identified gene signatures of DHLs that identify both DHLs as well as cases of DLBCL that do not have the classic rearrangements but are predicted to behave aggressively.[130,131]

HIGH-GRADE B-CELL LYMPHOMA, NOS

A diagnosis of exclusion, high-grade B-cell lymphoma, NOS is defined as an aggressive B-cell lymphoma with high-grade morphologic features but which lacks a genetic "double hit."[58,125] This entity is somewhat subjective morphologically, and of unclear significance clinically. It is expected that these will behave more aggressively than DLBCL, NOS, but further studies are needed. Many of these cases will harbor single-hit *MYC* rearrangement without *BCL2* or *BCL6* rearrangements. Phenotypically they can be either non-GCB or GCB. Cases with large cell morphology should be classified as DLBCL, NOS. This diagnosis should be used sparingly and relies on morphologic examination in well-fixed tissue sections. This category should not be used for DLBCL with high proliferation index or fine chromatin.

MEDIASTINAL GRAY ZONE LYMPHOMA

In previous classifications, mediastinal gray zone lymphoma (MGZL) held an apt but lengthy name, which still helps to describe its diagnostic characteristics: "B-cell lymphoma, unclassifiable, with features intermediate between DLBCL and CHL.[58]" Notably, the "DLBCL" features of MGZL most closely resemble PMBL.[132] A typical presentation is a young male (age 20-40 years) with a bulky mediastinal mass. Although previously cases of nonmediastinal GZL were identified, these have now been shown to be genetically distinct from MGZL, emphasizing the importance of the thymic niche. A challenging diagnosis, as many as 60% of MGZL diagnoses are reclassified on consensus review.[133]

Morphology

MGZL may show morphology akin to a tumor-cell-rich CHL or to PMBL. Cases that show separate areas diagnostic of both CHL and DBLCL are termed "composite lymphomas" and are excluded from MGZL.[134] One hallmark of MGZL is the abundance of tumor cells. Otherwise-typical CHL with sparse, singly scattered tumor cells and CD20 expression should not be considered MGZL. On the other end of the spectrum, cases that resemble PMBL may have more pleomorphism than expected.

Phenotype

MGZL with a CHL-like morphology shows frequent CD30 and CD15 expression and lacks CD45 expression, but unexpectedly shows strong, consistent expression of multiple pan-B-cell markers (Figure 5.54). MGZL with PMBL morphology, instead, shows strong expression of CD30 and frequently CD15, but lacks significant B cell marker expression, more in keeping with the phenotype of CHL.

The vast majority of MGZL are EBV negative. EBV positivity, especially with disease outside the mediastinum, should prompt consideration for EBV-DLBCL.

Genetics

On GEP studies, MGZL shows expected overlap with, but remains distinct from, both PMBL and CHL[25,135] with emphasis on NFkB activation and alterations in JAK/STAT signaling.[127]

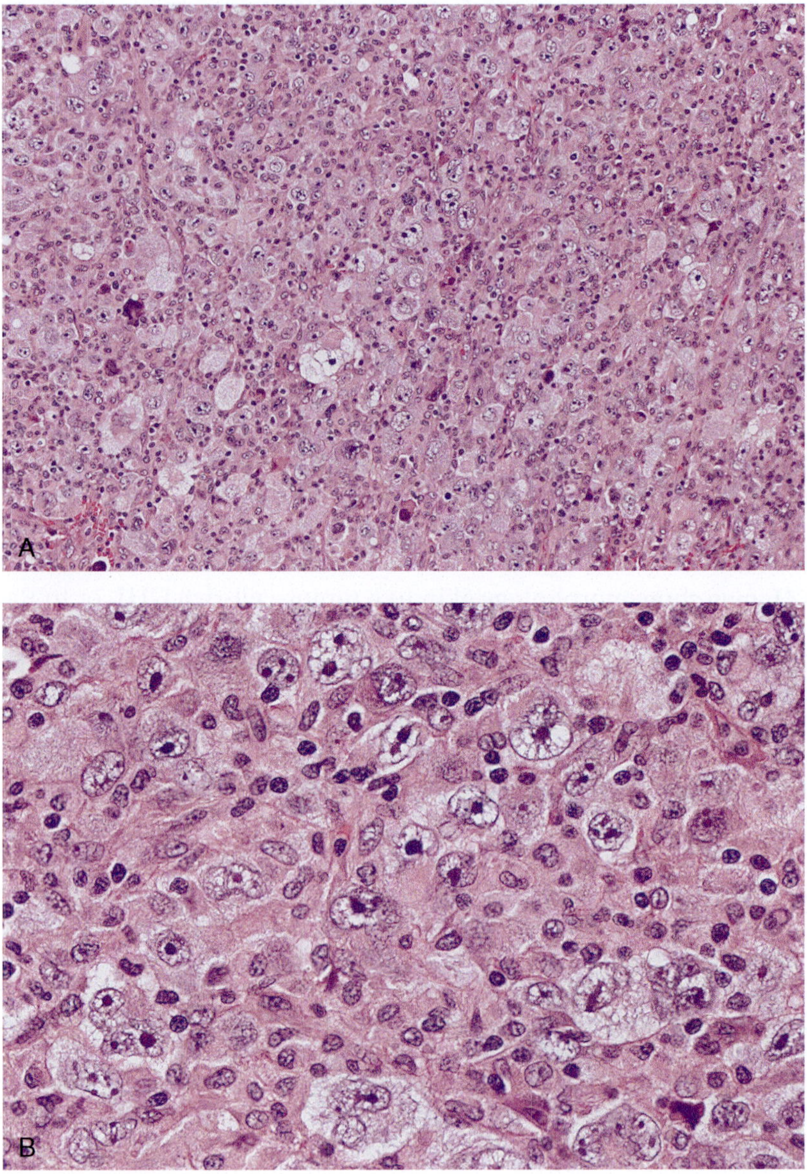

FIGURE 5.54 (*Continued*)

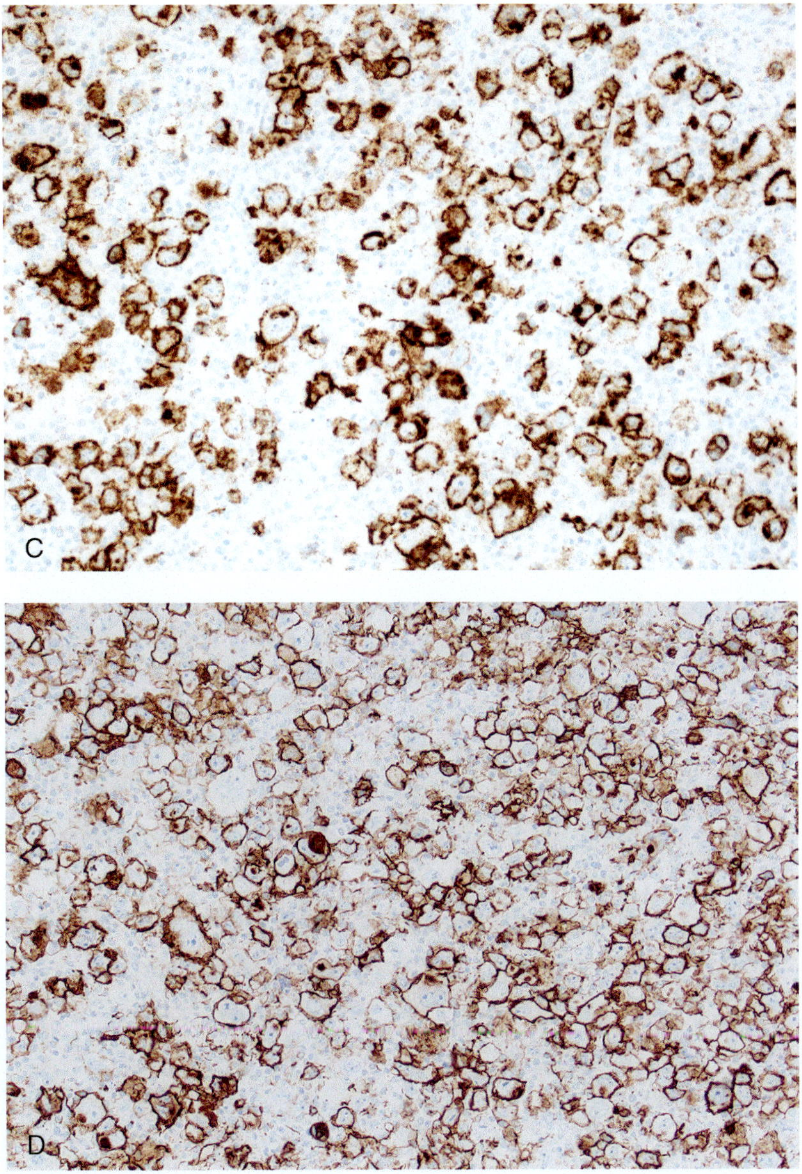

FIGURE 5.54 (*Continued*)

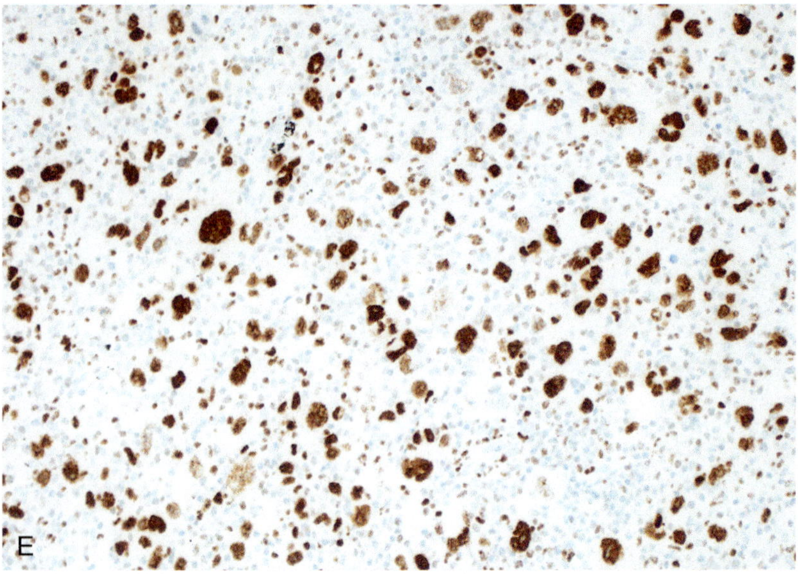

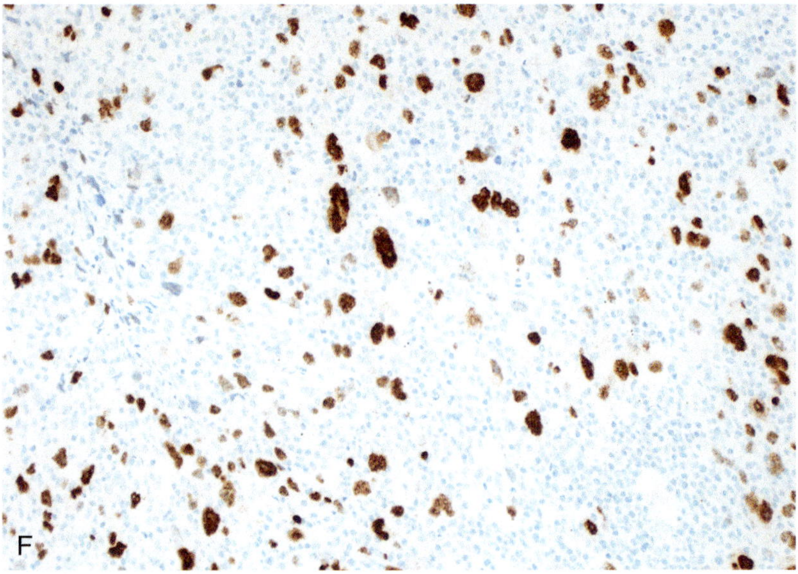

FIGURE 5.54 (*Continued*)

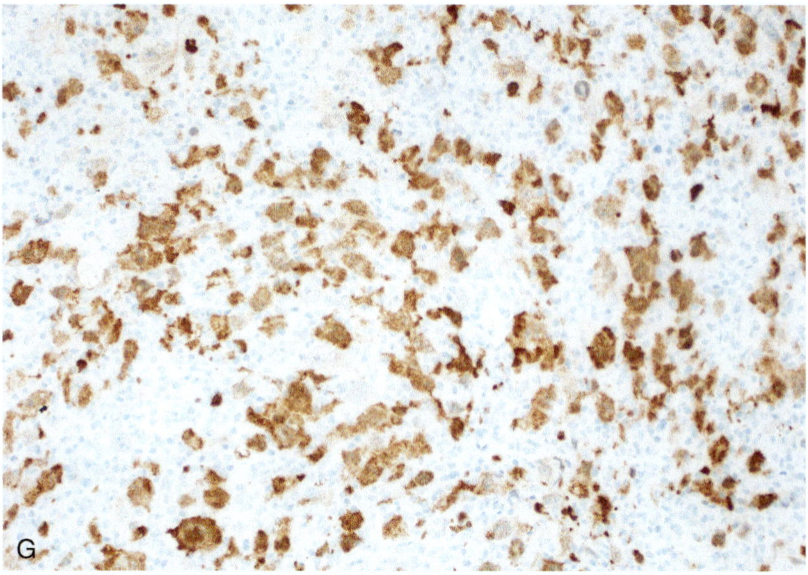

FIGURE 5.54 A, Mediastinal gray zone lymphoma (MGZL) can show a tumor-cell-rich Hodgkin-like pattern. B, On high power cells may be a mixture of large pleomorphic cells and more typical centroblasts or immunoblasts. C, Strong expression of CD30 is typical. D, In cases that otherwise might be diagnosed as Hodgkin lymphoma, strong expression of at least two B-cell markers including CD20, (E) OCT2, (F) PAX5, and (G) BOB.1 support a diagnosis of MGZL.

REFERENCES

1. Campo E, Jaffe ES, Cook JR, et al. The International Consensus Classification of Mature Lymphoid Neoplasms: A Report from the Clinical Advisory Committee. *Blood*. 2022.
2. Swerdlow SH CE, Harris NL, et al. *WHO Classification of Tumors of Haematopoetic and Lymphoid Tissues (Revised 4th Edition)*. IARC; 2017.
3. Link BK, Maurer MJ, Nowakowski GS, et al. Rates and outcomes of follicular lymphoma transformation in the immunochemotherapy era: a report from the University of Iowa/Mayo Clinic Specialized Program of Research Excellence Molecular Epidemiology Resource. *J Clin Oncol*. 2013;31(26):3272-3278.
4. Horn H, Schmelter C, Leich E, et al. Follicular lymphoma grade 3B is a distinct neoplasm according to cytogenetic and immunohistochemical profiles. *Haematologica*. 2011;96(9):1327-1334.
5. Yegappan S, Schnitzer B, Hsi ED. Follicular lymphoma with marginal zone differentiation: microdissection demonstrates the t(14;18) in both the follicular and marginal zone components. *Mod Pathol*. 2001;14(3):191-196.
6. Chapman JR, Alvarez JP, White K, et al. Unusual variants of follicular lymphoma: case-based review. *Am J Surg Pathol*. 2020;44(3):329-339.
7. Lai R, Arber DA, Chang KL, Wilson CS, Weiss LM. Frequency of bcl-2 expression in non-Hodgkin's lymphoma: a study of 778 cases with comparison of marginal zone lymphoma and monocytoid B-cell hyperplasia. *Mod Pathol*. 1998;11(9):864-869.
8. Wang SA, Wang L, Hochberg EP, Muzikansky A, Harris NL, Hasserjian RP. Low histologic grade follicular lymphoma with high proliferation index: morphologic and clinical features. *Am J Surg Pathol*. 2005;29(11):1490-1496.

9. Payne K, Wright P, Grant JW, et al. BIOMED-2 PCR assays for IGK gene rearrangements are essential for B-cell clonality analysis in follicular lymphoma. *Br J Haematol.* 2011;155(1):84-92.
10. Keller CE, Nandula S, Vakiani E, Alobeid B, Murty VV, Bhagat G. Intrachromosomal rearrangement of chromosome 3q27: an under recognized mechanism of BCL6 translocation in B-cell non-Hodgkin lymphoma. *Hum Pathol.* 2006;37(8):1093-1099.
11. Cuneo A, Bigoni R, Roberti MG, et al. Molecular cytogenetic characterization of marginal zone B-cell lymphoma: correlation with clinicopathologic findings in 14 cases. *Haematologica.* 2001;86(1):64-70.
12. Dierlamm J, Pittaluga S, Stul M, et al. BCL6 gene rearrangements also occur in marginal zone B-cell lymphoma. *Br J Haematol.* 1997;98(3):719-725.
13. Siddiqi IN, Friedman J, Barry-Holson KQ, et al. Characterization of a variant of t(14;18) negative nodal diffuse follicular lymphoma with CD23 expression, 1p36/TNFRSF14 abnormalities, and STAT6 mutations. *Mod Pathol.* 2016;29(6):570-581.
14. Ziemba JB, Wolf Z, Weinstock M, Asakrah S. Double-hit and triple-hit follicular lymphoma. *Am J Clin Pathol.* 2020;153(5):672-685.
15. Morschhauser F, Tilly H, Chaidos A, et al. Tazemetostat for patients with relapsed or refractory follicular lymphoma: an open-label, single-arm, multicentre, phase 2 trial. *Lancet Oncol.* 2020;21(11):1433-1442.
16. Louissaint A, Ackerman AM, Dias-Santagata D, et al. Pediatric-type nodal follicular lymphoma: an indolent clonal proliferation in children and adults with high proliferation index and no BCL2 rearrangement. *Blood.* 2012;120(12):2395-2404.
17. Louissaint A, Schafernak KT, Geyer JT, et al. Pediatric-type nodal follicular lymphoma: a biologically distinct lymphoma with frequent MAPK pathway mutations. *Blood.* 2016;128(8):1093-1100.
18. Liu QY, Salaverria I, Pittaluga S, et al. Follicular lymphomas in children and young adults a comparison of the pediatric variant with usual follicular lymphoma. *Am J Surg Pathol.* 2013;37(3):333-343.
19. Cong PJ, Raffeld M, Teruya-Feldstein J, Sorbara L, Pittaluga S, Jaffe ES. In situ localization of follicular lymphoma: description and analysis by laser capture microdissection. *Blood.* 2002;99(9):3376-3382.
20. Jegalian AG, Eberle FC, Pack SD, et al. Follicular lymphoma in situ: clinical implications and comparisons with partial involvement by follicular lymphoma. *Blood.* 2011;118(11):2976-2984.
21. van den Brand M, van der Velden WJ, Diets IJ, et al. Clinical features of patients with nodal marginal zone lymphoma compared to follicular lymphoma: similar presentation, but differences in prognostic factors and rate of transformation. *Leuk Lymphoma.* 2016;57(7):1649-1656.
22. van den Brand M, Mathijssen JJ, Garcia-Garcia M, et al. Immunohistochemical differentiation between follicular lymphoma and nodal marginal zone lymphoma – combined performance of multiple markers. *Haematologica.* 2015;100(9):e358-360.
23. van den Brand M, Balagué O, van Cleef PH, et al. A subset of low-grade B cell lymphomas with a follicular growth pattern but without a BCL2 translocation shows features suggestive of nodal marginal zone lymphoma. *J Hematop.* 2016;9(1):3-8.
24. van den Brand M, van Krieken JH. Recognizing nodal marginal zone lymphoma: recent advances and pitfalls. A systematic review. *Haematologica.* 2013;98(7):1003-1013.
25. Egan C, Laurent C, Alejo JC, et al. Expansion of PD1-positive T cells in nodal marginal zone lymphoma: a potential diagnostic pitfall. *Am J Surg Pathol.* 2020;44(5):657-664.

26. Hamadeh F, MacNamara SP, Aguilera NS, Swerdlow SH, Cook JR. MYD88 L265P mutation analysis helps define nodal lymphoplasmacytic lymphoma. *Mod Pathol.* 2015;28(4):564-574.
27. Martinez-Lopez A, Curiel-Olmo S, Mollejo M, et al. MYD88 (L265P) somatic mutation in marginal zone B-cell lymphoma. *Am J Surg Pathol.* 2015;39(5):644-651.
28. Pillonel V, Juskevicius D, Ng CKY, et al. High-throughput sequencing of nodal marginal zone lymphomas identifies recurrent BRAF mutations. *Leukemia.* 2018;32(11):2412-2426.
29. Spina V, Khiabanian H, Messina M, et al. The genetics of nodal marginal zone lymphoma. *Blood.* 2016;128(10):1362-1373.
30. Taddesse-Heath L, Pittaluga S, Sorbara L, Bussey M, Raffeld M, Jaffe ES. Marginal zone B-cell lymphoma in children and young adults. *Am J Surg Pathol.* 2003;27(4):522-531.
31. Sander B, Quintanilla-Martinez L, Ott G, et al. Mantle cell lymphoma–a spectrum from indolent to aggressive disease. *Virchows Arch.* 2016;468(3):245-257.
32. Ruan J, Martin P. Which patients with mantle cell lymphoma do not need aggressive therapy. *Curr Hematol Malig Rep.* 2016;11(3):234-240.
33. Jares P, Colomer D, Campo E. Molecular pathogenesis of mantle cell lymphoma. *J Clin Investig.* 2012;122(10):3416-3423.
34. Narurkar R, Alkayem M, Liu DL. SOX11 is a biomarker for cyclin D1-negative mantle cell lymphoma. *Biomark Res.* 2016;4:6.
35. Mozos A, Royo C, Hartmann E, et al. SOX11 expression is highly specific for mantle cell lymphoma and identifies the cyclin D1-negative subtype. *Haematologica.* 2009;94(11):1555-1562.
36. Raty R, Franssila K, Joensuu H, Teerenhovi L, Elonen E. Ki-67 expression level, histological subtype, and the International Prognostic Index as outcome predictors in mantle cell lymphoma. *Eur J Haematol.* 2002;69(1):11-20.
37. Tiemann M, Schrader C, Klapper W, et al. Histopathology, cell proliferation indices and clinical outcome in 304 patients with mantle cell lymphoma (MCL): a clinicopathological study from the European MCL Network. *Br J Haematol.* 2005;131(1):29-38.
38. Polonis K, Schultz MJ, Olteanu H, et al. Detection of cryptic CCND1 rearrangements in mantle cell lymphoma by next generation sequencing. *Ann Diagn Pathol.* 2020;46:151533.
39. Shiller SM, Zieske A, Holmes H III, Feldman AL, Law ME, Saad R. CD5-positive, cyclinD1-negative mantle cell lymphoma with a translocation involving the CCND2 gene and the IGL locus. *Cancer Genet.* 2011;204(3):162-164.
40. Eskelund CW, Dahl C, Hansen JW, et al. TP53 mutations identify younger mantle cell lymphoma patients who do not benefit from intensive chemoimmunotherapy. *Blood.* 2017;130(17):1903-1910.
41. Nordström L, Sernbo S, Eden P, et al. SOX11 and TP53 add prognostic information to MIPI in a homogenously treated cohort of mantle cell lymphoma–a Nordic Lymphoma Group study. *Br J Haematol.* 2014;166(1):98-108.
42. King RL, Gonsalves WI, Ansell SM, et al. Lymphoplasmacytic lymphoma with a non-IgM paraprotein shows clinical and pathologic heterogeneity and may harbor MYD88 L265P mutations. *Am J Clin Pathol.* 2016;145(6):843-851.
43. Fang H, Kapoor P, Gonsalves WI, et al. Defining lymphoplasmacytic lymphoma: does MYD88L265P define a pathologically distinct entity among patients with an IgM paraprotein and bone marrow-based low-grade B-cell lymphomas with plasmacytic differentiation? *Am J Clin Pathol.* 2018;150(2):168-176.

44. Treon SP, Tripsas CK, Meid K, et al. Ibrutinib in previously treated Waldenström's macroglobulinemia. *N Engl J Med.* 2015;372(15):1430-1440.
45. Treon SP, Cao Y, Xu L, Yang G, Liu X, Hunter ZR. Somatic mutations in MYD88 and CXCR4 are determinants of clinical presentation and overall survival in Waldenstrom macroglobulinemia. *Blood.* 2014;123(18):2791-2796.
46. Gibson SE, Swerdlow SH, Ferry JA, et al. Reassessment of small lymphocytic lymphoma in the era of monoclonal B-cell lymphocytosis. *Haematologica.* 2011;96(8):1144-1152.
47. Ciccone M, Agostinelli C, Rigolin GM, et al. Proliferation centers in chronic lymphocytic leukemia: correlation with cytogenetic and clinicobiological features in consecutive patients analyzed on tissue microarrays. *Leukemia.* 2012;26(3):499-508.
48. Xiao W, Chen WW, Sorbara L, et al. Hodgkin lymphoma variant of Richter transformation: morphology, Epstein-Barr virus status, clonality, and survival analysis-with comparison to Hodgkin-like lesion. *Hum Pathol.* 2016;55:108-116.
49. King RL, Gupta A, Kurtin PJ, et al. Chronic lymphocytic leukemia (CLL) with Reed-Sternberg-like cells vs Classic Hodgkin lymphoma transformation of CLL: does this distinction matter? *Blood Cancer J.* 2022;12(1):18.
50. Horna P, Pearce KE, Ketterling RP, Peterson J. Recurrent chromosomal abnormalities in tumoral lesions of small lymphocytic lymphoma/chronic lymphocytic leukemia: a large-scale fluorescent in-situ hybridization study on tissue biopsy sections. *Blood.* 2019;134(suppl 1):4282.
51. Hamblin T, Davis Z, Gardiner A. Unmutated Ig V(H) genes are associated with a more aggressive form of chronic lymphocytic leukemia. *Blood.* 1999;94:1848-1854.
52. Oscier D, Gardiner A, Mould S. Multivariate analysis of prognostic factors in CLL: clinical stage, IGVH gene mutational status, and loss or mutation of the p53 gene are independent prognostic factors. *Blood.* 2002;100:1177-1184.
53. Zenz T, Eichhorst B, Busch R. TP53 mutation and survival in chronic lymphocytic leukemia. *J Clin Oncol.* 2010;28:4473-4479.
54. Wierda WG, Byrd JC, Abramson JS, et al. Chronic lymphocytic leukemia/small lymphocytic lymphoma, Version 4.2020, NCCN Clinical Practice Guidelines in Oncology. *J Natl Compr Canc Netw.* 2020;18(2):185-217.
55. Dasari S, Theis JD, Vrana JA, et al. Amyloid typing by mass spectrometry in clinical practice: a comprehensive review of 16,175 samples. *Mayo Clin Proc.* 2020;95(9):1852-1864.
56. D'Souza A, Theis J, Quint P, et al. Exploring the amyloid proteome in immunoglobulin-derived lymph node amyloidosis using laser microdissection/tandem mass spectrometry. *Am J Hematol.* 2013;88(7):577-580.
57. Verstovsek G, Chakraborty S, Ramzy I, Jorgensen JL. Large B-cell lymphomas: Fine-needle aspiration plays an important role in initial diagnosis of cases which are falsely negative by flow cytometry. *Diagn Cytopathol.* 2002;27(5):282-285.
58. Swerdlow SH, Campo E, Harris NL, et al. *WHO Classification of Tumours of Haematopoietic and Lymphoid Tissues.* Revised 4th ed. IARC; 2017.
59. Cucco F, Barrans S, Sha C, et al. Distinct genetic changes reveal evolutionary history and heterogeneous molecular grade of DLBCL with MYC/BCL2 double-hit. *Leukemia.* 2020;34(5):1329-1341.
60. A clinical evaluation of the International Lymphoma Study Group classification of non-Hodgkin's lymphoma. The Non-Hodgkin's Lymphoma Classification Project. *Blood.* 1997;89(11):3909-3918.
61. Anderson JR, Armitage JO, Weisenburger DD. Epidemiology of the non-Hodgkin's lymphomas: distributions of the major subtypes differ by geographic locations. *Ann Oncol.* 1998;9(7):717-720.

62. Arber DA, George TI. Bone marrow biopsy involvement by non-Hodgkin's lymphoma: frequency of lymphoma types, patterns, blood involvement, and discordance with other sites in 450 specimens. *Am J Surg Pathol.* 2005;29(12):1549-1557.
63. Campbell J, Seymour JF, Matthews J, Wolf M, Stone J, Juneja S. The prognostic impact of bone marrow involvement in patients with diffuse large cell lymphoma varies according to the degree of infiltration and presence of discordant marrow involvement. *Eur J Haematol.* 2006;76(6):473-480.
64. Hernandez-Ilizaliturri FJ, Deeb G, Zinzani PL, et al. Higher response to lenalidomide in relapsed/refractory diffuse large B-cell lymphoma in nongerminal center B-cell-like than in germinal center B-cell-like phenotype. *Cancer.* 2011;117(22):5058-5066.
65. Dunleavy K, Pittaluga S, Czuczman MS, et al. Differential efficacy of bortezomib plus chemotherapy within molecular subtypes of diffuse large B-cell lymphoma. *Blood.* 2009;113(24):6069-6076.
66. Hans CP, Weisenburger DD, Greiner TC, Gascoyne RD. Confirmation of the molecular classification of diffuse large B-cell lymphoma by immunohistochemistry using a tissue microarray. *Blood.* 2004;103(1):275-282.
67. Coutinho R, Clear AJ, Owen A, et al. Poor concordance among nine immunohistochemistry classifiers of cell-of-origin for diffuse large B-cell lymphoma: implications for therapeutic strategies. *Clin Cancer Res.* 2013;19(24):6686-6695.
68. Bobée V, Ruminy P, Marchand V, et al. Determination of molecular subtypes of diffuse large B-cell lymphoma using a reverse transcriptase multiplex ligation-dependent probe amplification classifier. *J Mol Diagn.* 2017;19(6):892-904.
69. Clipson A, Wang M, de Leval L, et al. KLF2 mutation is the most frequent somatic change in splenic marginal zone lymphoma and identifies a subset with distinct genotype. *Leukemia.* 2015;29(5):1177-1185.
70. Iqbal S, DePew ZS, Kurtin PJ, et al. Endobronchial ultrasound and lymphoproliferative disorders: a retrospective study. *Ann Thorac Surg.* 2012;94(6):1830-1834.
71. Scott DW, King RL, Staiger AM, et al. High-grade B-cell lymphoma with MYC and BCL2 and/or BCL6 rearrangements with diffuse large B-cell lymphoma morphology. *Blood.* 2018;131(18):2060-2064.
72. Meriranta L, Pasanen A, Alkodsi A, Haukka J, Karjalainen-Lindsberg ML, Leppa S. Molecular background delineates outcome of double protein expressor diffuse large B-cell lymphoma. *Blood Adv.* 2020;4(15):3742-3753.
73. Chapuy B, Stewart C, Dunford AJ, et al. Molecular subtypes of diffuse large B cell lymphoma are associated with distinct pathogenic mechanisms and outcomes. *Nat Med.* 2018;24(5):679-690.
74. Bea S, Valdes-Mas R, Navarro A, et al. Landscape of somatic mutations and clonal evolution in mantle cell lymphoma. *Proc Natl Acad Sci USA.* 2013;110(45):18250-18255.
75. Pittaluga S, Nicolae A, Wright GW, et al. Gene expression profiling of mediastinal gray zone lymphoma and its relationship to primary mediastinal B-cell lymphoma and classical hodgkin lymphoma. *Blood Cancer Discov.* 2020;1(2):155-161.
76. Alaggio R, Amador C, Anagnostopoulos I, et al. The 5th edition of the World Health Organization Classification of Haematolymphoid Tumours: lymphoid neoplasms. *Leukemia.* 2022;36(7):1720-1748.
77. Greer JP, Macon WR, Lamar RE, et al. T-cell-rich B-cell lymphomas: diagnosis and response to therapy of 44 patients. *J Clin Oncol.* 1995;13(7):1742-1750.
78. Ramsay AD, Smith WJ, Isaacson PG. T-cell-rich B-cell lymphoma. *Am J Surg Pathol.* 1988;12(6):433-443.
79. Achten R, Verhoef G, Vanuytsel L, De Wolf-Peeters C. Histiocyte-rich, T-cell-rich B-cell lymphoma: a distinct diffuse large B-cell lymphoma subtype showing characteristic morphologic and immunophenotypic features. *Histopathology.* 2002;40(1):31-45.

80. Kunder C, Cascio MJ, Bakke A, Venkataraman G, O'Malley DP, Ohgami RS. Predominance of CD4+ T cells in T-cell/histiocyte-rich large B-cell lymphoma and identification of a subset of patients with peripheral B-cell lymphopenia. *Am J Clin Pathol.* 2017;147(6):596-603.

81. Beltran BE, Morales D, Quinones P, Medeiros LJ, Miranda RN, Castillo JJ. EBV-positive diffuse large B-cell lymphoma in young immunocompetent individuals. *Clin Lymphoma Myeloma Leuk.* 2011;11(6):512-516.

82. Cohen M, Narbaitz M, Metrebian F, De Matteo E, Preciado MV, Chabay PA. Epstein-Barr virus-positive diffuse large B-cell lymphoma association is not only restricted to elderly patients. *Int J Cancer.* 2014;135(12):2816-2824.

83. Hu S, Xu-Monette ZY, Tzankov A, et al. MYC/BCL2 protein coexpression contributes to the inferior survival of activated B-cell subtype of diffuse large B-cell lymphoma and demonstrates high-risk gene expression signatures: a report from The International DLBCL Rituximab-CHOP Consortium Program. *Blood.* 2013;121(20):4021-4031. quiz 4250.

84. Dojcinov SD, Venkataraman G, Pittaluga S, et al. Age-related EBV-associated lymphoproliferative disorders in the Western population: a spectrum of reactive lymphoid hyperplasia and lymphoma. *Blood.* 2011;117(18):4726-4735.

85. Brudno J, Tadmor T, Pittaluga S, Nicolae A, Polliack A, Dunleavy K. Discordant bone marrow involvement in non-Hodgkin lymphoma. *Blood.* 2016;127(8):965-970.

86. Oyama T, Yamamoto K, Asano N, et al. Age-related EBV-associated B-cell lymphoproliferative disorders constitute a distinct clinicopathologic group: a study of 96 patients. *Clin Cancer Res.* 2007;13(17):5124-5132.

87. Starr A, Kwon DH, Kallakury B. Epstein-Barr Virus–positive CD20- and CD45-negative diffuse large B-cell lymphoma: a diagnostic challenge. *Int J Surg Pathol.* 2019;27(1):98-101.

88. Zinzani PL, Martelli M, Poletti V, et al. Practice guidelines for the management of extranodal non-Hodgkin's lymphomas of adult non-immunodeficient patients. Part I: primary lung and mediastinal lymphomas. A project of the Italian Society of Hematology, the Italian Society of Experimental Hematology and the Italian Group for Bone Marrow Transplantation. *Haematologica.* 2008;93(9):1364-1371.

89. Cazals-Hatem D, Lepage E, Brice P, et al. Primary mediastinal large B-cell lymphoma. A clinicopathologic study of 141 cases compared with 916 nonmediastinal large B-cell lymphomas, a GELA ("Groupe d'Etude des Lymphomes de l'Adulte") study. *Am J Surg Pathol.* 1996;20(7):877-888.

90. Lazzarino M, Orlandi E, Paulli M, et al. Treatment outcome and prognostic factors for primary mediastinal (thymic) B-cell lymphoma: a multicenter study of 106 patients. *J Clin Oncol.* 1997;15(4):1646-1653.

91. Falini B, Pileri S, Zinzani PL, et al. ALK+ lymphoma: clinico-pathological findings and outcome. *Blood.* 1999;93(8):2697-2706.

92. Pileri SA, Gaidano G, Zinzani PL, et al. Primary mediastinal B-cell lymphoma: high frequency of BCL-6 mutations and consistent expression of the transcription factors OCT-2, BOB.1, and PU.1 in the absence of immunoglobulins. *Am J Pathol.* 2003;162(1):243-253.

93. Higgins JP, Warnke RA. CD30 expression is common in mediastinal large B-cell lymphoma. *Am J Clin Pathol.* 1999;112(2):241-247.

94. Feuerhake F, Kutok JL, Monti S, et al. NFkappaB activity, function, and target-gene signatures in primary mediastinal large B-cell lymphoma and diffuse large B-cell lymphoma subtypes. *Blood.* 2005;106(4):1392-1399.

95. Twa DD, Chan FC, Ben-Neriah S, et al. Genomic rearrangements involving programmed death ligands are recurrent in primary mediastinal large B-cell lymphoma. *Blood.* 2014;123(13):2062-2065.

96. Gentry M, Bodo J, Durkin L, Hsi ED. Performance of a commercially available MAL antibody in the diagnosis of primary mediastinal large B-cell lymphoma. *Am J Surg Pathol.* 2017;41(2):189-194.

97. Copie-Bergman C, Plonquet A, Alonso MA, et al. MAL expression in lymphoid cells: further evidence for MAL as a distinct molecular marker of primary mediastinal large B-cell lymphomas. *Mod Pathol.* 2002;15(11):1172-1180.

98. Mottok A, Wright G, Rosenwald A, et al. Molecular classification of primary mediastinal large B-cell lymphoma using routinely available tissue specimens. *Blood.* 2018;132(22):2401-2405.

99. Scarpa A, Moore PS, Rigaud G, et al. Molecular features of primary mediastinal B-cell lymphoma: involvement of p16INK4A, p53 and c-myc. *Br J Haematol.* 1999;107(1):106-113.

100. Laurent C, Do C, Gascoyne RD, et al. Anaplastic lymphoma kinase-positive diffuse large B-cell lymphoma: a rare clinicopathologic entity with poor prognosis. *J Clin Oncol.* 2009;27(25):4211-4216.

101. Gascoyne RD, Lamant L, Martin-Subero JI, et al. ALK-positive diffuse large B-cell lymphoma is associated with Clathrin-ALK rearrangements: report of 6 cases. *Blood.* 2003;102(7):2568-2573.

102. Onciu M, Behm FG, Downing JR, et al. ALK-positive plasmablastic B-cell lymphoma with expression of the NPM-ALK fusion transcript: report of 2 cases. *Blood.* 2003;102(7):2642-2644.

103. Colomo L, Loong F, Rives S, et al. Diffuse large B-cell lymphomas with plasmablastic differentiation represent a heterogeneous group of disease entities. *Am J Surg Pathol.* 2004;28(6):736-747.

104. Hertel N, Merz H, Bernd HW, et al. Performance of international prognostic indices in plasmablastic lymphoma: a comparative evaluation. *J Cancer Res Clin Oncol.* 2021;147(10):3043-3050.

105. Delecluse HJ, Anagnostopoulos I, Dallenbach F, et al. Plasmablastic lymphomas of the oral cavity: a new entity associated with the human immunodeficiency virus infection. *Blood.* 1997;89(4):1413-1420.

106. Borenstein J, Pezzella F, Gatter KC. Plasmablastic lymphomas may occur as post-transplant lymphoproliferative disorders. *Histopathology.* 2007;51(6):774-777.

107. Castillo JJ, Bibas M, Miranda RN. The biology and treatment of plasmablastic lymphoma. *Blood.* 2015;125(15):2323-2330.

108. Valera A, Balague O, Colomo L, et al. IG/MYC rearrangements are the main cytogenetic alteration in plasmablastic lymphomas. *Am J Surg Pathol.* 2010;34(11):1686-1694.

109. Lebbe C, Porcher R, Marcelin AG, et al. Human herpesvirus 8 (HHV8) transmission and related morbidity in organ recipients. *Am J Transplant.* 2013;13(1):207-213.

110. Oksenhendler E, Boulanger E, Galicier L, et al. High incidence of Kaposi sarcoma-associated herpesvirus-related non-Hodgkin lymphoma in patients with HIV infection and multicentric Castleman disease. *Blood.* 2002;99(7):2331-2336.

111. Dupin N, Diss TL, Kellam P, et al. HHV-8 is associated with a plasmablastic variant of Castleman disease that is linked to HHV-8–positive plasmablastic lymphoma. *Blood.* 2000;95(4):1406-1412.

112. Gonzalez-Farre B, Martinez D, Lopez-Guerra M, et al. HHV8-related lymphoid proliferations: a broad spectrum of lesions from reactive lymphoid hyperplasia to overt lymphoma. *Mod Pathol.* 2017;30(5):745-760.

113. Roithmann S, Toledano M, Tourani JM, et al. HIV-associated non-Hodgkin's lymphomas: clinical characteristics and outcome. The experience of the French Registry of HIV-associated tumors. *Ann Oncol.* 1991;2(4):289-295.

114. Diehl V, Klimm B, Re D. Hodgkin lymphoma: a curable disease–what comes next? *Eur J Haematol Suppl.* 2005(66):6-13.
115. Gibson TM, Morton LM, Shiels MS, Clarke CA, Engels EA. Risk of non-Hodgkin lymphoma subtypes in HIV-infected people during the HAART era: a population-based study. *AIDS.* 2014;28(15):2313-2318.
116. Burkitt D. A sarcoma involving the jaws in African children. *Br J Surg.* 1958;46(197):218-223.
117. Schrager JA, Pittaluga S, Raffeld M, Jaffe ES. Granulomatous reaction in Burkitt lymphoma: correlation with EBV positivity and clinical outcome. *Am J Surg Pathol.* 2005;29(8):1115-1116.
118. Gualco G, Queiroga EM, Weiss LM, Klumb CE, Harrington WJ Jr, Bacchi CE. Frequent expression of multiple myeloma 1/interferon regulatory factor 4 in Burkitt lymphoma. *Hum Pathol.* 2009;40(4):565-571.
119. Haralambieva E, Boerma EJ, van Imhoff GW, et al. Clinical, immunophenotypic, and genetic analysis of adult lymphomas with morphologic features of Burkitt lymphoma. *Am J Surg Pathol.* 2005;29(8):1086-1094.
120. Chamberlain WD, Falta MT, Kotzin BL. Functional subsets within clonally expanded CD8(+) memory T cells in elderly humans. *Clin Immunol.* 2000;94(3):160-172.
121. Gonzalez-Farre B, Ramis-Zaldivar JE, Salmeron-Villalobos J, et al. Burkitt-like lymphoma with 11q aberration: a germinal center derived lymphoma genetically unrelated to Burkitt lymphoma. *Haematologica.* 2019;104(9):1822-1829.
122. Salaverria I, Martin-Guerrero I, Wagener R, et al. A recurrent 11q aberration pattern characterizes a subset of MYC-negative high-grade B-cell lymphomas resembling Burkitt lymphoma. *Blood.* 2014;123(8):1187-1198.
123. Sarkozy C, Traverse-Glehen A, Coiffier B. Double-hit and double-protein-expression lymphomas: aggressive and refractory lymphomas. *Lancet Oncol.* 2015;16(15):e555-e567.
124. Gebauer N, Witte HM, Merz H, et al. Aggressive B-cell lymphoma cases with 11q aberration patterns indicate a spectrum beyond Burkitt-like lymphoma. *Blood Adv.* 2021;5(23):5220-5225.
125. Kanagal-Shamanna R, Medeiros LJ, Lu G, et al. High-grade B cell lymphoma, unclassifiable, with blastoid features: an unusual morphological subgroup associated frequently with BCL2 and/or MYC gene rearrangements and a poor prognosis. *Histopathology.* 2012;61(5):945-954.
126. Johnson NA, Savage KJ, Ludkovski O, et al. Lymphomas with concurrent BCL2 and MYC translocations: the critical factors associated with survival. *Blood.* 2009;114(11):2273-2279.
127. Bhavsar S, Liu YC, Gibson SE, Moore EM, Swerdlow SH. Mutational landscape of TdT+ large B-cell lymphomas supports their distinction from B-lymphoblastic neoplasms: a multiparameter study of a rare and aggressive entity. *Am J Surg Pathol.* 2022;46(1):71-82.
128. Rosenwald A, Bens S, Advani R, et al. Prognostic significance of MYC rearrangement and translocation partner in diffuse large B-cell lymphoma: a study by the Lunenburg Lymphoma Biomarker Consortium. *J Clin Oncol.* 2019;37.
129. Larson DP, Peterson JF, Nowakowski GS, McPhail ED. A practical approach to FISH testing for MYC rearrangements and brief review of MYC in aggressive B-cell lymphomas. *J Hematopathol.* 2020;13(3):127-135.
130. Ennishi D, Jiang A, Boyle M, et al. Double-hit gene expression signature defines a distinct subgroup of germinal center B-cell-like diffuse large B-cell lymphoma. *J Clin Oncol.* 2019;37(3):190-201.

131. Hilton LK, Tang J, Ben-Neriah S, et al. The double-hit signature identifies double-hit diffuse large B-cell lymphoma with genetic events cryptic to FISH. *Blood*. 2019;134(18):1528-1532.
132. Traverse-Glehen A, Felman P, Callet-Bauchu E, et al. A clinicopathological study of nodal marginal zone B-cell lymphoma. A report on 21 cases. *Histopathology*. 2006;48(2):162-173.
133. Pilichowska M, Pittaluga S, Ferry JA, et al. Clinicopathologic consensus study of gray zone lymphoma with features intermediate between DLBCL and classical HL. *Blood Adv*. 2017;1(26):2600-2609.
134. Sarkozy C, Copie-Bergman C, Damotte D, et al. Gray-zone lymphoma between cHL and large B-cell lymphoma: a histopathologic series from the LYSA. *Am J Surg Pathol*. 2019;43(3):341-351.
135. Sarkozy C, Chong L, Takata K, et al. Gene expression profiling of gray zone lymphoma. *Blood Adv*. 2020;4(11):2523-2535.

6

MATURE T-CELL NEOPLASMS

ANAMARIJA M. PERRY

Mature T/natural killer (NK)-cell neoplasms are relatively rare and comprise fewer than 15% of non-Hodgkin lymphomas (NHLs) in the Western world (ie, North America and Europe), while the relative frequency is somewhat higher in Asian countries.[1] T/NK-cell NHLs can occur as primary nodal or as primary extranodal lymphomas with secondary involvement of lymph nodes. This chapter will focus on primary nodal T-cell lymphomas including peripheral T-cell lymphoma, not otherwise specified (PTCL, NOS), follicular helper T-cell lymphomas (including angioimmunoblastic T-cell lymphoma [AITL], follicular helper T-cell lymphoma, follicular type, and follicular helper T-cell lymphoma, NOS), and anaplastic large cell lymphoma (ALCL), ALK-positive and ALK-negative.[2] Furthermore, several primary extranodal lymphomas that frequently involve lymph nodes (T-cell prolymphocytic leukemia [T-PLL], adult T-cell leukemia/lymphoma [ATLL], and mycosis fungoides [MF]) will also be covered.

The general "consensus" among pathologists who deal with lymph node pathology is that T-cell lymphomas are challenging. There are several reasons for this, one of the most important being the relative rarity of these cases, even in practices with large volume of specimens. Increasing practice of performing needle core, rather than larger incisional or excisional, biopsies has further complicated this issue, since T-cell lymphomas can show overlapping features with other lymphomas, as well as benign conditions. Proper assessment of lymph node architecture is critically important in these cases, and this is not always possible on a small/needle core biopsy. Some of the common pitfalls in evaluation of potential T-cell lymphoma in a needle core biopsy (and in a larger biopsy too) include the following:

- *Relatively bland looking infiltrate*–some T-cell lymphomas, such as AITL or PTCL, NOS, show a polymorphous infiltrate with relatively bland-appearing lymphoma cells intermixed with abundant inflammatory cells. These cases that do not appear overtly malignant can be easily mistaken for a benign condition.

- *Reactive conditions that mimic T-cell lymphoma*–some benign conditions such as Kikuchi lymphadenitis, and drug-induced lymphadenopathy, are characterized by expanded T-cell compartments and may show cytologic atypia.
- *Presence of Hodgkin-like and Reed-Sternberg-like (HRS-like) cells*–T-cell lymphomas may show HRS-like cells in a polymorphous background, which can be mistaken for classic Hodgkin lymphoma (CHL).
- *Presence of hyperplastic B-cell follicles or an increased number of B-cells*–these features can be seen in AITL, for example, and diagnosis can be extremely challenging on a needle core biopsy.
- *Partial/low-level involvement*–ALCL, for example, can show subtle sinusoidal involvement; similarly, early involvement of lymph node by MF can be very difficult to appreciate even on a large biopsy.

In addition to the above-mentioned pitfalls, interpretation of immunohistochemical stains and demonstration of aberrant phenotype can be challenging on a small biopsy. Flow cytometry and molecular studies for T-cell gene rearrangement can be very helpful in establishing a diagnosis. However, it is important to remember that clonal T-cell gene rearrangement supports the diagnosis of T-cell lymphoma but is not synonymous with malignancy as it can be seen in some reactive conditions too.

When evaluating nodal T-cell lymphoma, the goal is to try to classify it into one of the defined subtypes. PTCL, NOS, should be used as a diagnosis of exclusion; however, if there is insufficient material or clinical history a diagnosis of "T-cell lymphoma," with a note stating that additional tissue and/or clinical history is needed for complete subclassification, is preferred. Knowledge of clinical history is very important for proper classification; for example, a previous history of MF will change one's approach to a lymph node showing dermatopathic change. For T-cell lymphoma the differential diagnosis is sometimes broad, and an algorithmic approach, as outlined in Figure 6.1, is recommended by the 2022 International Consensus Classification (ICC).[2,3] An initial immunohistochemical panel that should be done includes CD20, CD3, CD4, CD8, CD2, CD5, CD7, and CD30. Epstein-Barr virus (EBV)-encoded RNA in situ hybridization (EBER-ISH) can also be included in the upfront panel or performed in subsequent steps. The results of this panel will help guide further workup, which may include ALK, TCR-BetaF1, TCR-delta, TIA1, granzyme B, and markers of T-follicular helper phenotype (discussed below). It is important to emphasize that, in addition to CD30, EBER-ISH is very helpful when entertaining the diagnosis of T-cell lymphoma, as these markers are defining for some entities or at least diagnostically useful.[4] Moreover, expression of CD30 is important for therapeutic purposes, since patients can be potentially treated with anti-CD30 antibody brentuximab vedotin.[5]

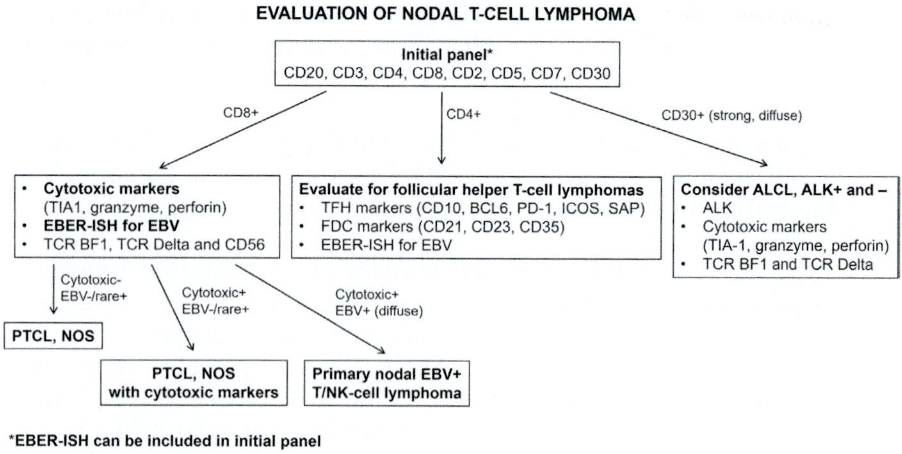

FIGURE 6.1 Algorithm for immunohistochemical evaluation and classification of nodal T-cell lymphomas.

PERIPHERAL T-CELL LYMPHOMA, NOT OTHERWISE SPECIFIED

PTCL, NOS is a name for a heterogeneous group of mature T-cell lymphomas that cannot be classified into any other defined T-cell lymphoma category. In other words, PTCL, NOS is a diagnosis of exclusion. Currently, PTCL, NOS comprises around 30% of T-cell lymphomas and is one of the most commonly diagnosed nodal T-cell lymphomas in the Western world.[6,7] Patients are usually older with a median age of presentation in the sixth to seventh decade, and men are more commonly affected. Most patients present with lymphadenopathy; however, involvement of extranodal sites (eg, liver, spleen, bone marrow) is common, and most patients are in advanced clinical stage. PTCL, NOS is typically an aggressive disease with frequent relapses and relatively low survival rates.[1,4]

Morphology

Lymph nodes with PTCL, NOS can show either partial involvement, typically with paracortical expansion, or complete diffuse effacement of the architecture. This group of lymphomas is very morphologically heterogeneous, with lymphoma cells ranging from small to large and showing variable degree of pleomorphism and nuclear atypia. Frequently, there is a mixture of cell sizes (Figure 6.2). Cases that show predominantly small cells can be very challenging on a needle core biopsy where the lymph node architecture cannot be properly assessed (Figure 6.3). Frequently, there is an inflammatory background composed of small lymphocytes, plasma cells, eosinophils, and epithelioid histiocytes (occasionally with sarcoid-like granulomas) (Figure 6.4). A subset of cases show HRS-like cells, and in these cases the differential diagnosis includes CHL (Figure 6.5).

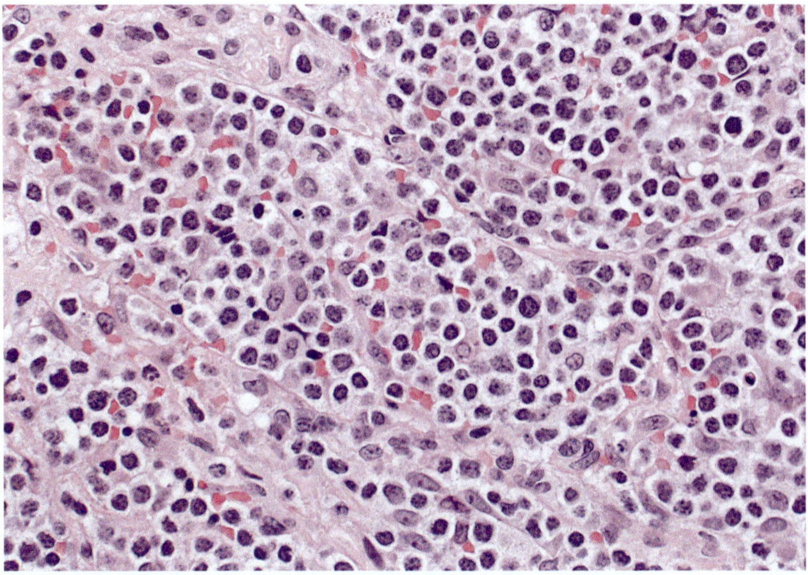

FIGURE 6.2 **Peripheral T-cell lymphoma, not otherwise specified.** The lymphoma cells are medium sized with round to irregular nuclei and moderately abundant pale cytoplasm.

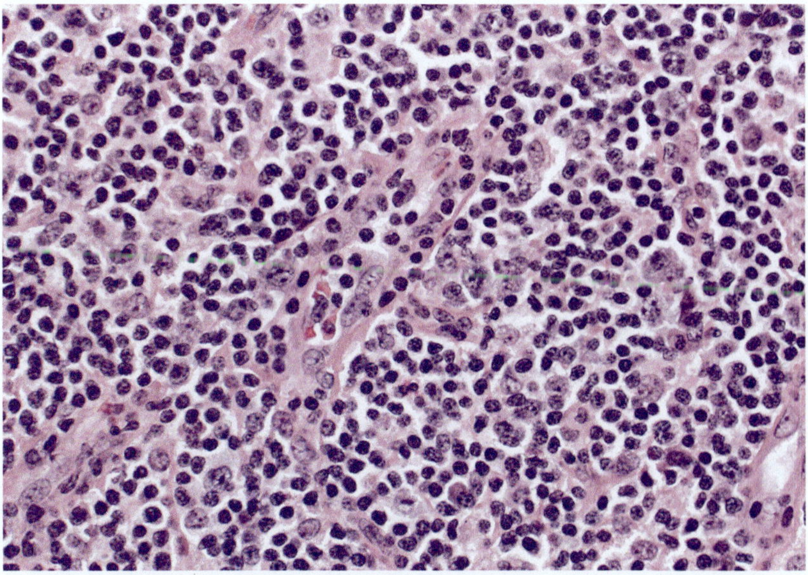

FIGURE 6.3 **Peripheral T-cell lymphoma, not otherwise specified.** The lymphoma cells are small in size and relatively bland appearing.

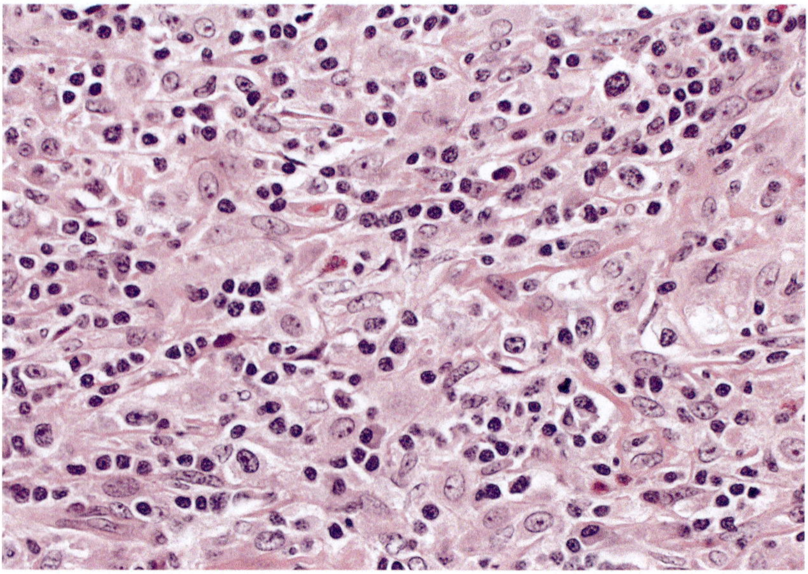

FIGURE 6.4 Case of PTCL, NOS showing lymphoma cells in an inflammatory background composed of histiocytes, small lymphocytes, plasma cells, and eosinophils.

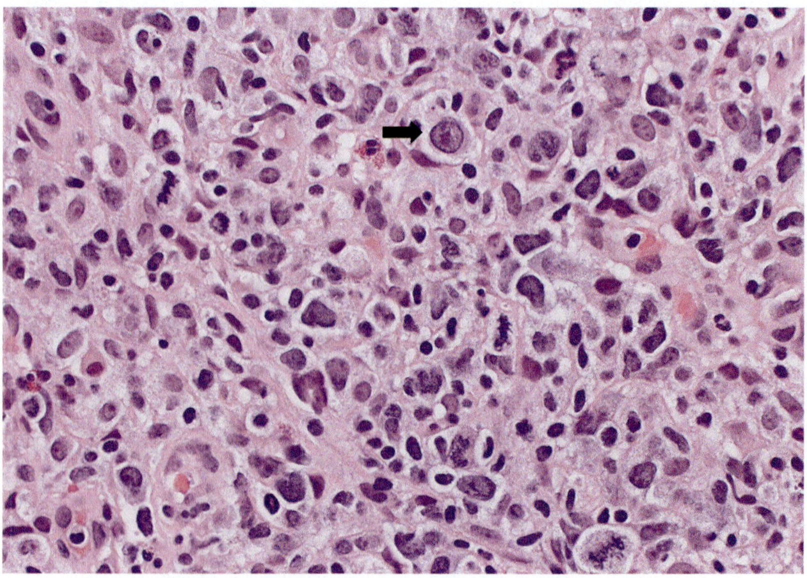

FIGURE 6.5 Hodgkin-like cells (arrow) in a case of PTCL, NOS.

Furthermore, prominent sclerosis can be occasionally seen (Figure 6.6).[1,4] One common morphologic variant is the lymphoepithelioid variant (Lennert lymphoma). This variant is characterized by prominent infiltrate of epithelioid histiocytes, typically in small clusters. The lymphoma cells are typically small with slightly irregular nuclei, admixed with some larger

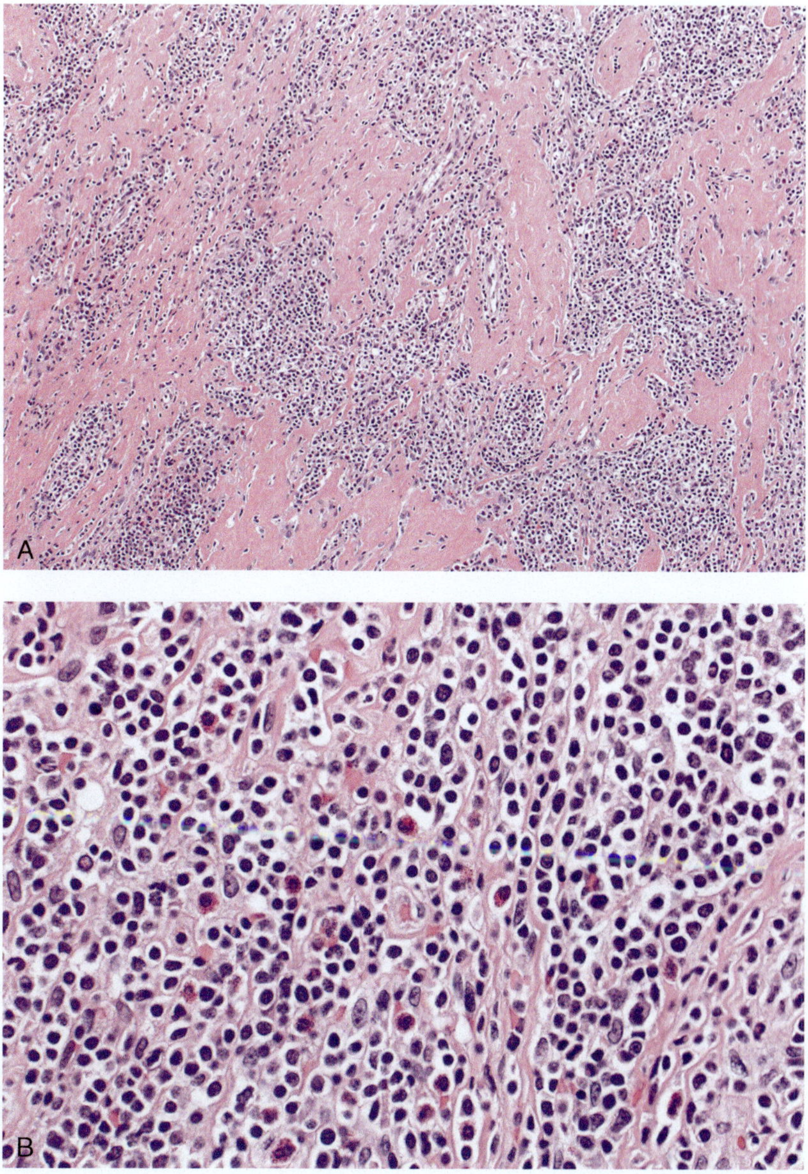

FIGURE 6.6 Case of PTCL, NOS showing prominent sclerotic bands (A). On higher magnification, the lymphoma cells are small and monotonous appearing, admixed with scattered eosinophils (B).

cells and occasional HRS-like cells (Figure 6.7). Based on the limited data in the literature, cases of Lennert lymphoma appear to have a more favorable clinical course. Moreover, they appear to have different molecular signature from other PTCL, NOS cases[8,9]; however, they are currently still diagnosed as PTCL, NOS.

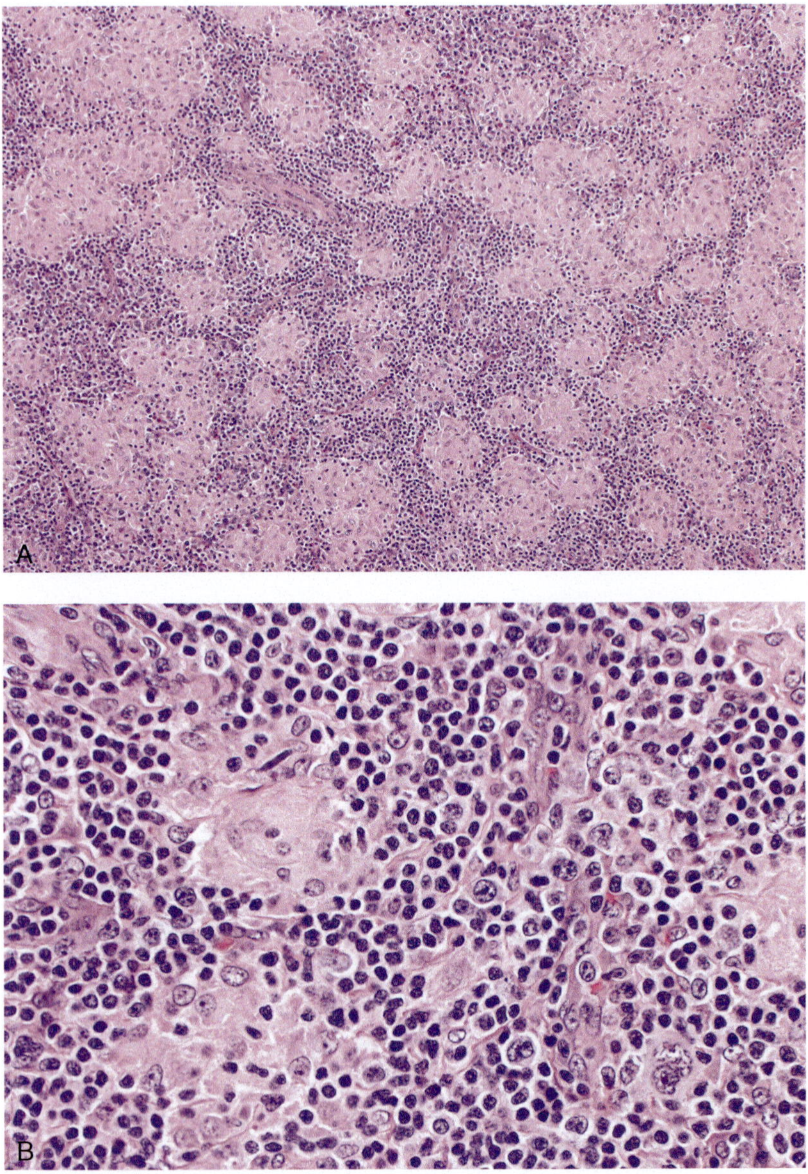

FIGURE 6.7 Lymphoepithelioid variant or PTCL, NOS (Lennert lymphoma) characterized by clusters of epithelioid histiocytes (A). On higher magnification, the lymphoma cells are small with slightly irregular nuclei and scattered larger cells admixed (B).

Phenotype

The lymphoma cells express pan-T-cell markers including CD2, CD3, CD5, CD7, and CD43. Many cases show aberrant loss of one or more markers, which is a very helpful diagnostic feature, especially in a limited biopsy. The majority are CD4-positive, while CD8-positive cases are much less common. Some cases are double negative or rarely double positive for CD4/CD8. TCR alpha/beta is seen in majority of cases, while small subset shows TCR gamma/delta positivity. When dealing with limited biopsies, submission of additional tissue (or fine needle aspirate) for flow cytometric evaluation can be very useful, since flow cytometry can provide information about aberrant phenotype and robustly assess for T-cell clonality with a TRBC1 antibody.[10] Importantly, markers of immaturity including CD1a and TdT are negative in PTCL, NOS. Other markers that should be performed, particularly when dealing with CD8-positive case, are cytotoxic molecules including TIA-1, granzyme, and/or perforin, which will be positive in 15% to 30% of cases. The cases that express cytotoxic molecules may be clinically more aggressive.[11-13] CD30 is expressed in the majority of cases, usually only in subset of cells and with variable intensity. Strong and diffuse staining should raise a differential diagnosis of ALCL. Up to 50% of cases will show some positivity for EBV in background B cells, with only small subset of cells staining.[14] The tumor cells are EBV-negative. Diffuse EBER staining in T/NK cells should prompt consideration of a primary nodal EBV-positive T/NK-cell lymphoma, an aggressive lymphoma that is a provisional entity in 2022 ICC, or extranodal NK/T-cell lymphoma, nasal type in extranodal sites.[2,15]

The differential diagnosis of PTCL, NOS primarily includes other defined subtypes of mature T-cell lymphomas, including the ones discussed in this chapter. An algorithmic approach to ruling out other entities (Figure 6.1), as well as correlation with clinical history, is needed in every case before this diagnosis can be made.

Genetics

The majority of PTCL, NOS cases have a clonal T-cell receptor gene rearrangement, which can be very helpful in supporting malignancy (with the caveats discussed previously). By conventional cytogenetic analysis, cases of PTCL, NOS typically have a complex karyotype.[16] Gene expression profiling (GEP) studies have identified two prognostically important groups–PTCL-TBX21 (resembling Th1 cells) with better prognosis, and PTCL-GATA3 (resembling Th2 cells) having worse prognosis.[12] Moreover, an immunohistochemical algorithm has been proposed to reproduce GEP findings that uses four antibodies including TBX21, CXCR3, GATA3, and CCR4 (Figure 6.8).[17] This algorithm is not currently used in clinical risk stratification but may represent a future direction.

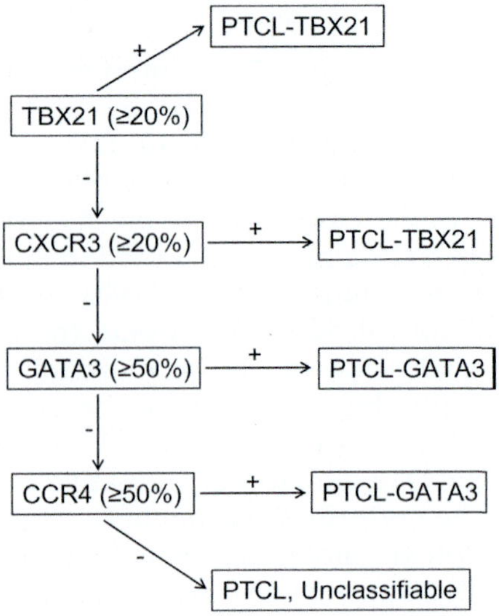

FIGURE 6.8 Immunohistochemical algorithm for determination of prognostically important groups (TBX21 vs GATA3) of PTCL, NOS.

FOLLICULAR HELPER T-CELL LYMPHOMAS

Lymphomas of T-follicular helper (TFH) cells were first grouped into a separate category in the 2017 Revision of World Health Organization Classification. The 2022 ICC further reinforced this and created a unified entity of follicular helper T-cell lymphoma encompassing three subtypes–AITL, follicular helper T-cell lymphoma, follicular type, and follicular helper T-cell lymphoma, NOS.[2,4] These lymphomas are characterized by TFH phenotype and have common genetic features, as outlined below.[18,19]

Angioimmunoblastic T-cell Lymphoma

AITL is the most common defined subtype of TFH lymphomas. This lymphoma shows some geographic variability and is more common in the Western world than in Asian countries.[4,20,21] The median age of patients is 60 years, and it more commonly occurs in males. Clinically, the patients usually present in advanced stage with generalized lymphadenopathy. Extranodal sites of involvement include skin, liver, spleen, and bone marrow. B-symptoms (fever, night sweats, and weight loss) are common, as well as body cavity effusions (eg, pleural, peritoneal), autoimmune phenomena including hemolytic anemia, skin rash, and polyclonal hypergammaglobulinemia. AITL is an aggressive lymphoma with a median survival of less than 3 years.[4,22,23]

Morphology

Lymph nodes involved by AITL show variable effacement of nodal architecture by a polymorphous infiltrate composed of small to medium-sized lymphoma cells with variably irregular nuclei and pale cytoplasm, admixed with reactive small lymphocytes, plasma cells, histiocytes, and eosinophils (Figure 6.9). Some cases are "tumor cell rich" and more monotonous in appearance. A helpful histologic feature is involvement of perinodal tissue by lymphoma with sparing of the subcapsular sinus, which is patent (Figure 6.10). Increased vascularity due to proliferation of high endothelial venules (HEVs) is seen in the paracortex (Figure 6.11). Clusters of tumor cells with pale cytoplasm can be seen associated with HEVs. There is a proliferation of follicular dendritic cells (FDCs), characteristically around small vessels, best seen by immunohistochemistry for CD21 and/or CD23. Some cases have an abundance of plasma cells, which are usually polyclonal, but rarely can be monoclonal.[1,11] Three histologic patterns have been described, which are thought to represent histologic evolution of AITL. In pattern 1, which is the least common, there are hyperplastic B-cell follicles with poorly formed mantle zones, with clusters of lymphoma cells in the perifollicular distribution and polymorphous infiltrate in the paracortex (Figure 6.12). Pattern 2 is characterized by the presence of regressed follicles, while in pattern 3 the architecture is diffusely effaced.[24] Another characteristic morphologic feature of AITL is the presence of B immunoblasts, scattered in the polymorphous infiltrate, as well as occasional HRS-like cells in some cases. A subset of the B immunoblasts are EBV-positive in the majority of cases (over 80%), another diagnostically helpful feature.[25,26] Occasionally, the EBV-positive immunoblastic proliferation will progress into diffuse large B-cell lymphoma (DLBCL) (Figure 6.13).[1,27]

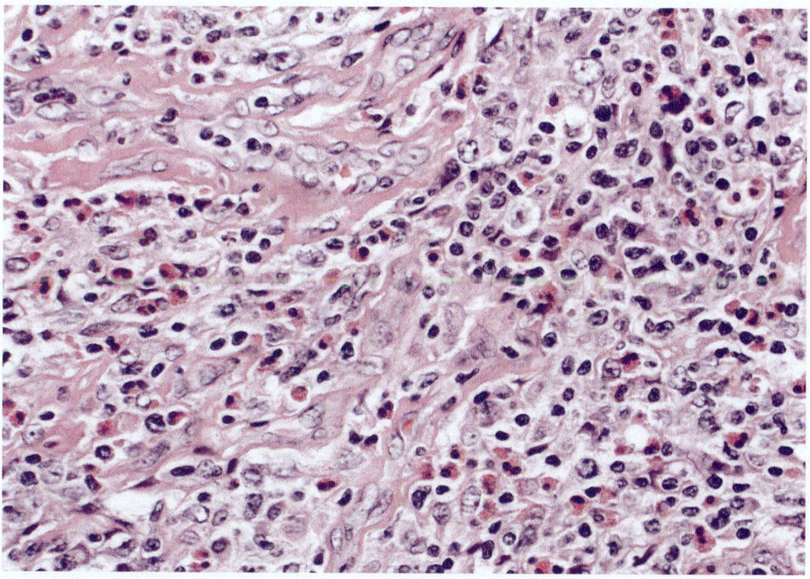

FIGURE 6.9 **Angioimmunoblastic T-cell lymphoma.** Polymorphous infiltrate with medium-sized lymphoma cells, admixed with histiocytes, small lymphocytes, and eosinophils.

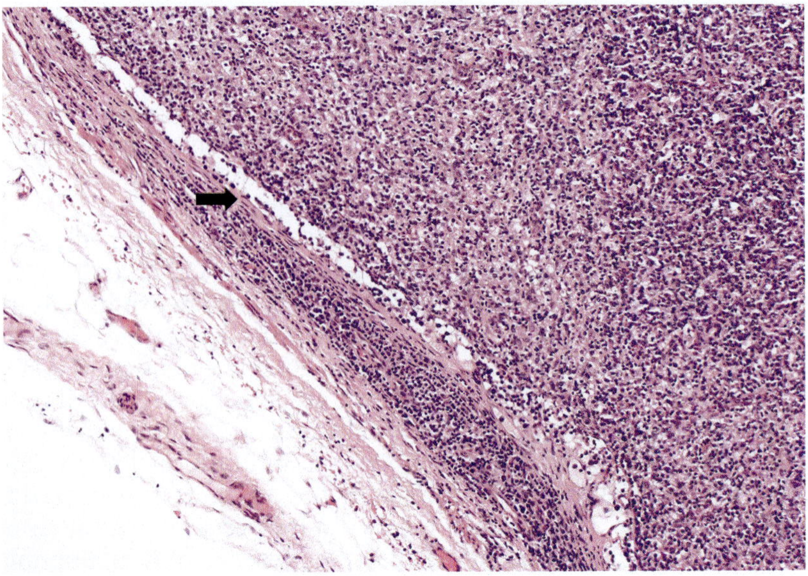

FIGURE 6.10 AITL showing involvement of perinodal soft tissue and patent subcapsular sinus (arrow), a helpful morphologic clue.

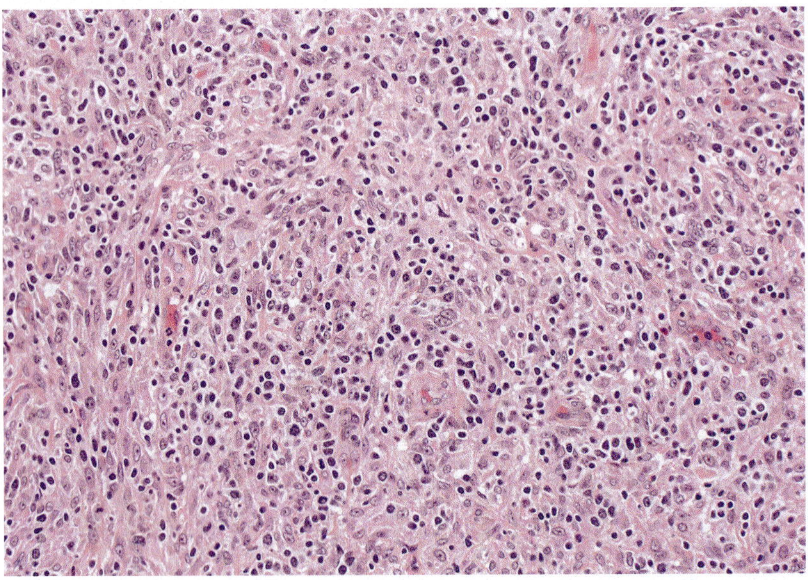

FIGURE 6.11 Prominent vascularity/proliferation of high endothelial venules in a case of AITL.

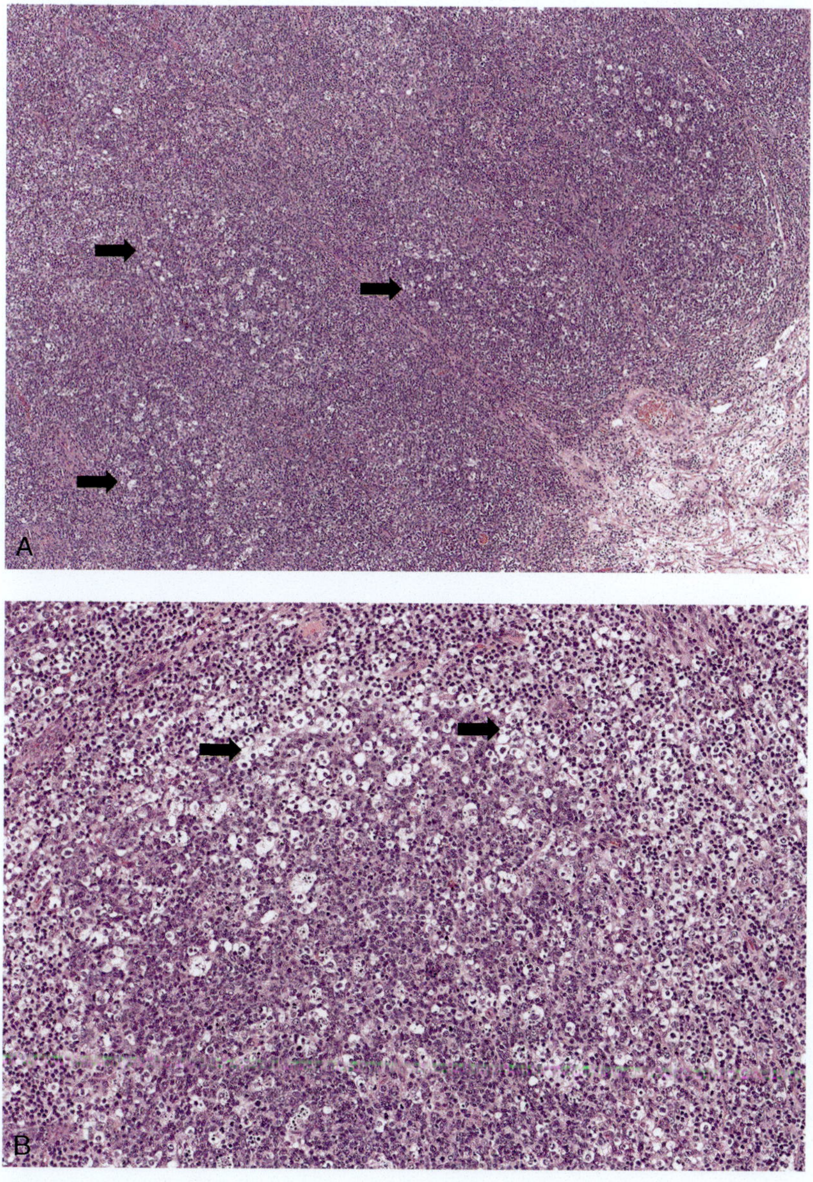

FIGURE 6.12 (*Continued*)

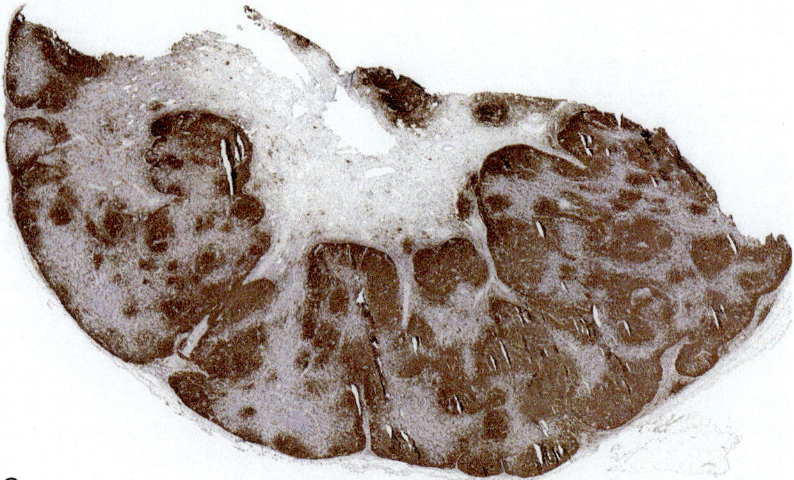

C

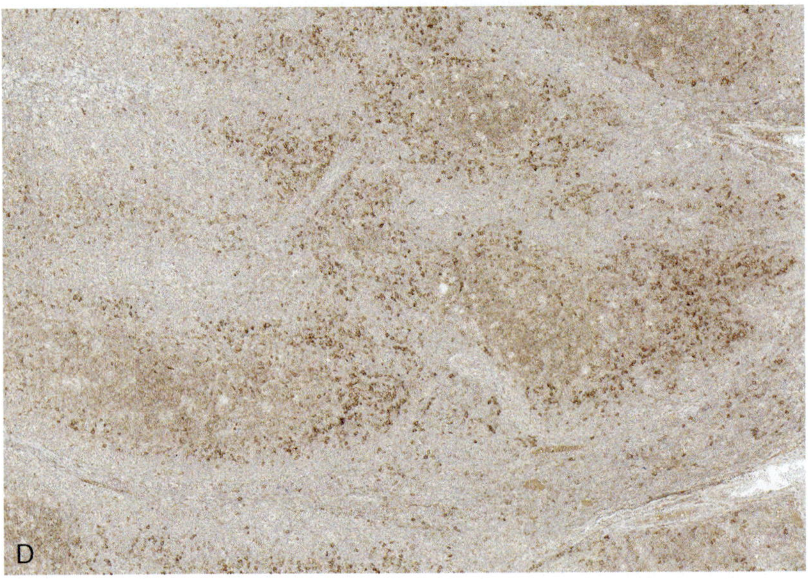

D

FIGURE 6.12 *(Continued)*

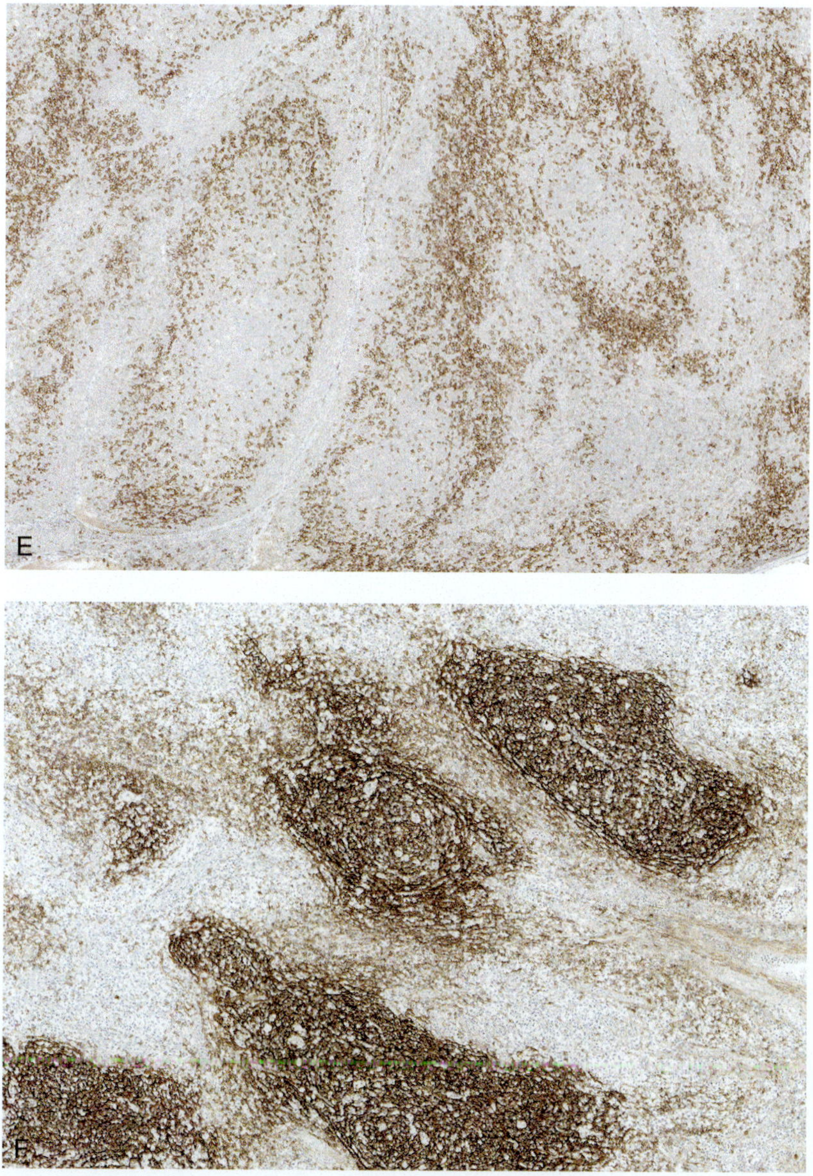

FIGURE 6.12 **Angioimmunoblastic T-cell lymphoma, histologic pattern 1.** A, Hyperplastic B-cell follicles with absence of mantle zones (arrows); (B) clusters of lymphoma cells with abundant pale cytoplasm at the periphery of the hyperplastic follicle (arrows). Immunohistochemical stain for CD20 (C) shows B-cell follicles; perifollicular distribution of lymphoma cells is highlighted by CD10 (bright compared with follicular B cells) (D) and PD-1 (E). CD21 (F) highlights slightly expanded follicular dendritic cell meshworks in the interfollicular areas.

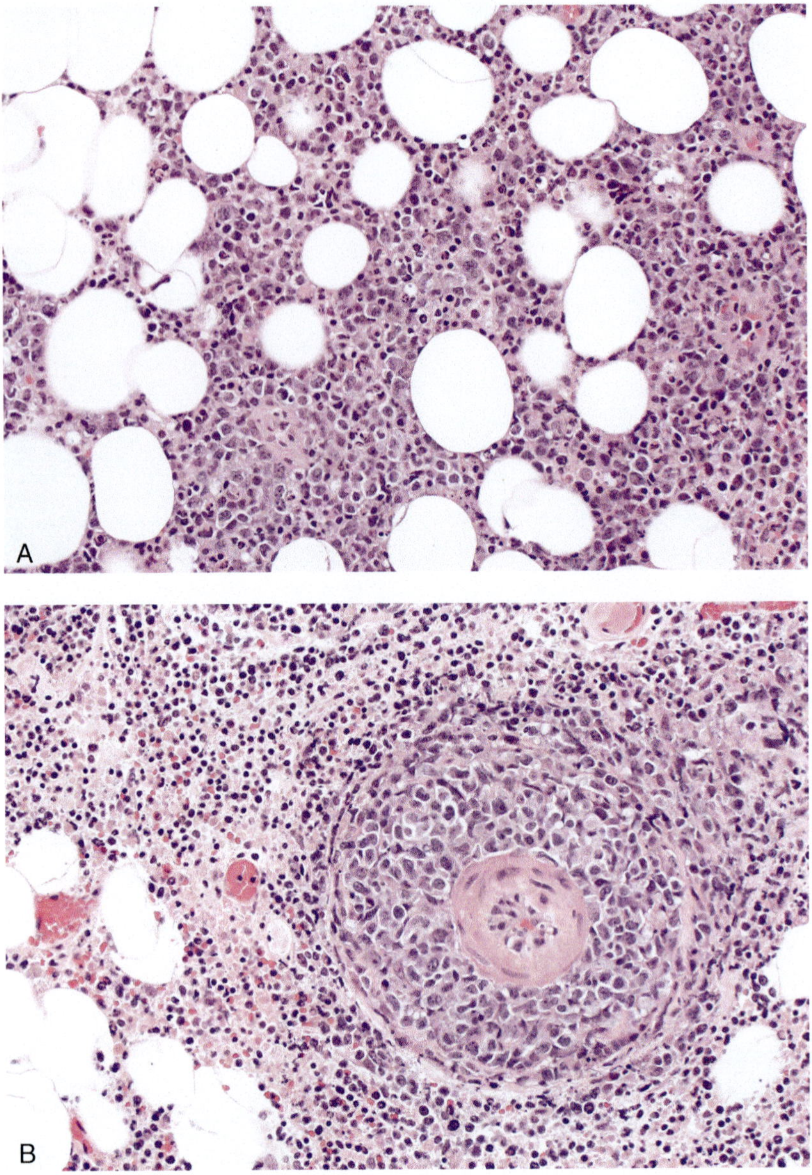

FIGURE 6.13 (*Continued*)

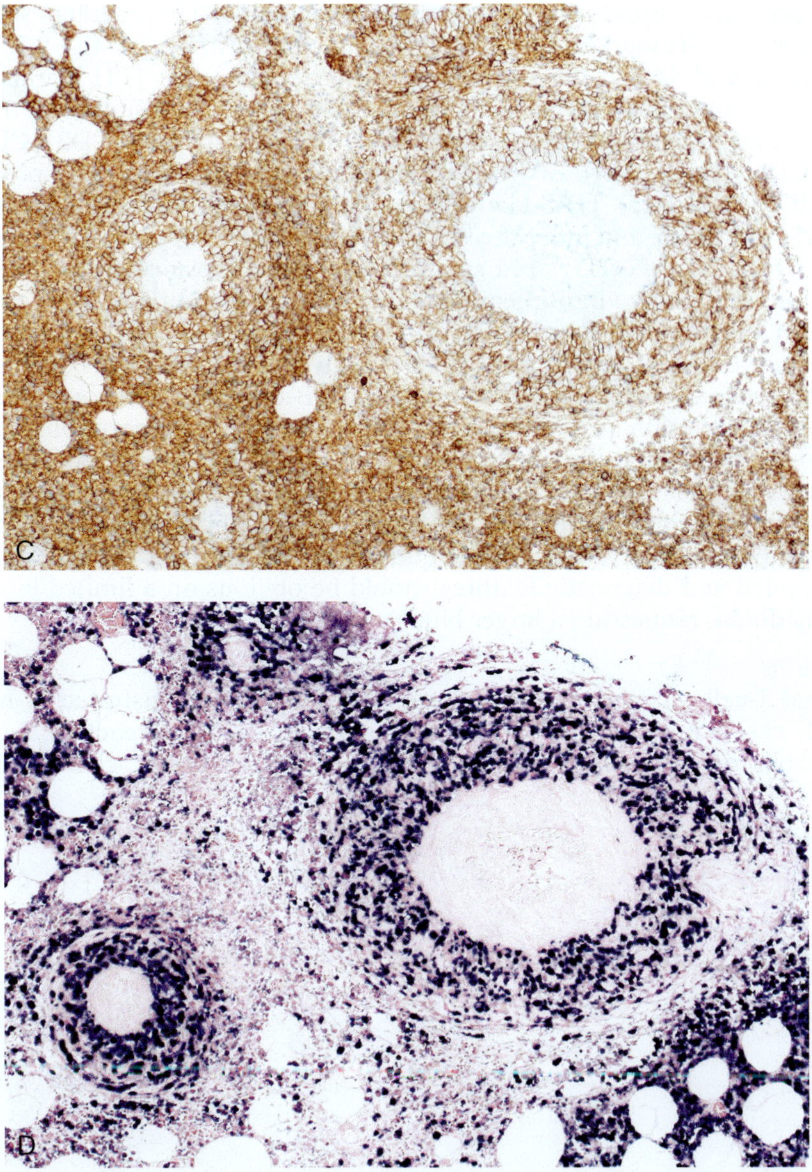

FIGURE 6.13 **Diffuse large B-cell lymphoma that arose in a patient with AITL.** Sheets of large lymphoma cells infiltrate adipose tissue (A); angioinvasion and prominent necrosis is seen (B). CD20 stain (C); EBER (D).

Phenotype

The lymphoma cells express pan-T-cell markers CD2, CD3, and CD5. Surface CD3 can be absent in flow cytometric analysis, but immunohistochemistry will be positive due to expression of cytoplasmic CD3. CD7, and occasionally CD5, can be reduced or absent. Consistent with TFH cell origin, lymphoma cells are CD4-positive, and two (and preferably three) TFH markers should be positive. TFH markers include (among others) CD10, BCL6, PD-1, ICOS, CXCL13, and SAP. It is recommended to use four to five TFH markers in routine immunophenotypic analysis of these cases. Proliferation of FDC meshworks is demonstrated by immunohistochemical stains for CD21, CD23, and CD35 (Figure 6.14). EBER-ISH will demonstrate scattered EBV-positive B cells (Figure 6.15). HRS-like cells are variably positive for CD20, CD30, CD15, and PAX5, and in most cases EBER-positive.[1,4,19,26]

Diagnosis of AITL on a small/needle core biopsy requires extreme caution, as there are multiple pitfalls that one can encounter. Diagnosis of pattern 1 is particularly problematic, since hyperplastic B-cell follicles can be very prominent and clusters of perifollicular lymphoma cells quite subtle. Moreover, B-cell-rich cases can resemble B-cell lymphoma on a limited biopsy. Cases with prominent HRS-like cells in a polymorphous background can be very difficult to distinguish from CHL. Furthermore, even in cases with complete architectural effacement, the polymorphous nature of the infiltrate frequently does not look overtly malignant especially on a limited biopsy. Strict morphologic and immunophenotypic criteria should be applied and diagnostic features should be obvious on a limited biopsy. If any doubt, requesting a larger biopsy is prudent.

Genetics

Clonal T-cell receptor gene rearrangement can be demonstrated in most AITL cases; however, the large number of background reactive T cells may obscure the clone. Clonal immunoglobulin heavy chain (IGH)

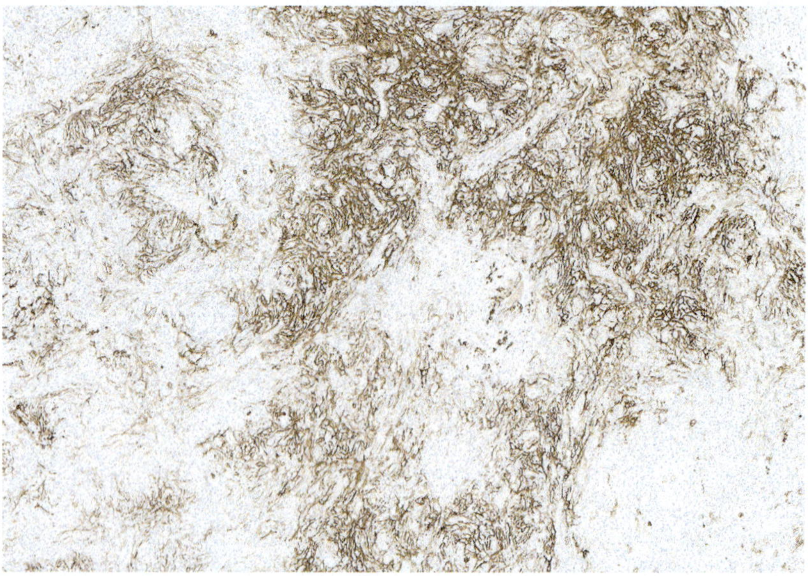

FIGURE 6.14 Markedly expanded follicular dendritic cell meshworks in AITL, highlighted by CD23 immunohistochemical stain.

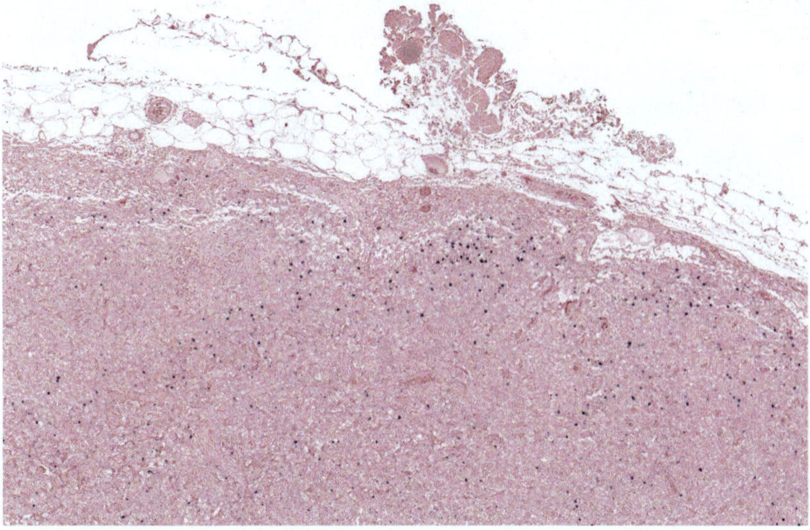

FIGURE 6.15 Scattered EBV-positive cells, a typical finding in AITL.

rearrangement is seen in approximately one-third of cases and is not synonymous with concurrent B-cell lymphoma.[1,28] Mutational analyses showed frequent mutations of *TET2*, *DNMT3A*, *IDH2* R172, and *RHOA* G17V, as well as other mutations of the T-cell receptor signaling pathway.[12,29-32]

Follicular Helper T-cell Lymphoma, Follicular Type

This rare lymphoma shows a nodular/follicular growth pattern and lacks extrafollicular proliferation of high endothelial venules or FDC meshwork. Clinical features overlap with those of AITL.

Morphologically, three growth patterns are recognized–follicular lymphoma–like, progressive transformation of germinal center (PTGC)-like, and marginal zone–like. In the follicular lymphoma–like pattern, lymphoma cells form nodules. Neoplastic T cells are admixed with remnants of germinal center B cells. Lymphoma cells are usually medium sized, irregular, and with abundant pale cytoplasm (Figure 6.16). In the PTGC-like variant, macronodules are seen resembling PTGC (Figure 6.17). Lymphoma cells are arranged in clusters and surrounded by numerous small mantle zone B cells, which can be highlighted with IgD immunostain. A subset of cases show scattered HRS-like cells and can mimic CHL (lymphocyte-rich subtype), especially in the PTGC-like variant.[1,22,26,33-35] This rare T-cell lymphoma is extremely challenging to diagnose on a needle core biopsy and can be easily mistaken for a B-cell lymphoma (eg, follicular lymphoma, marginal zone lymphoma, or nodular lymphocyte predominant B-cell lymphoma) or a benign condition, such as PTGC.

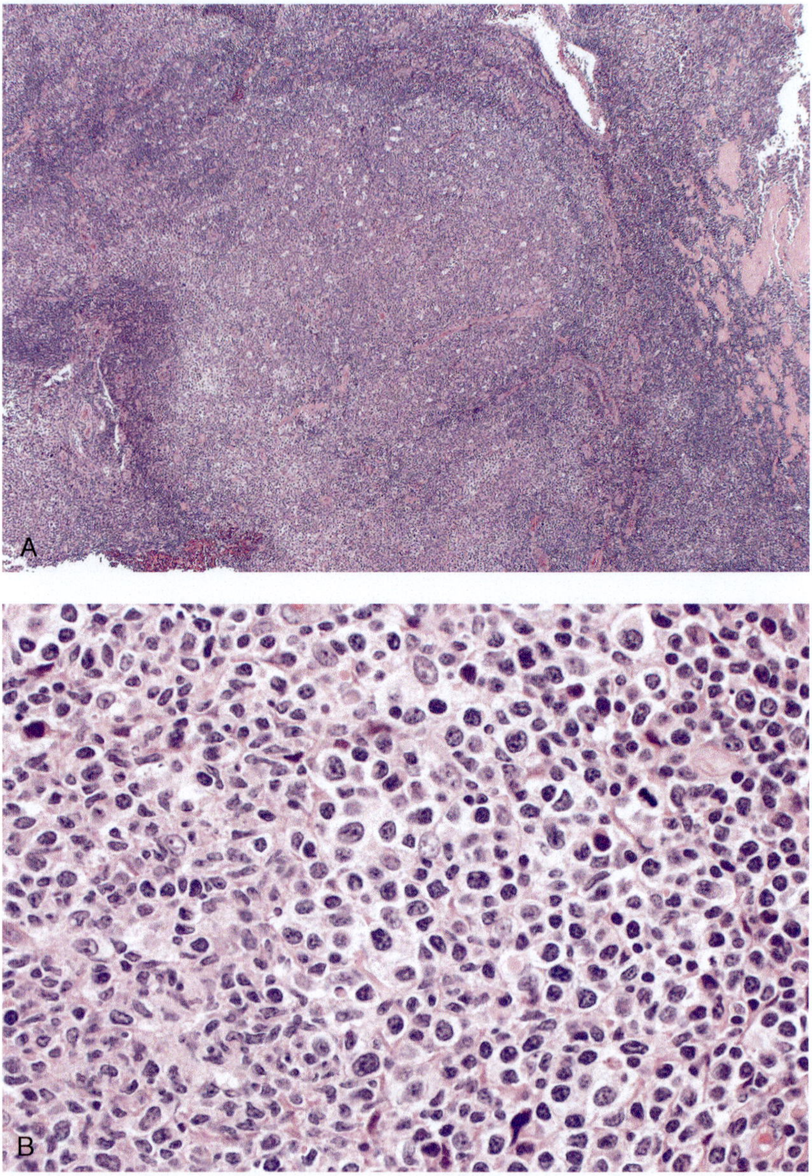

FIGURE 6.16 **Follicular helper T-cell lymphoma, follicular type.** A, The lymphoma forms neoplastic nodules. B, On high magnification, the lymphoma cells show some pleomorphism with round to irregular nuclei and abundant pale cytoplasm.

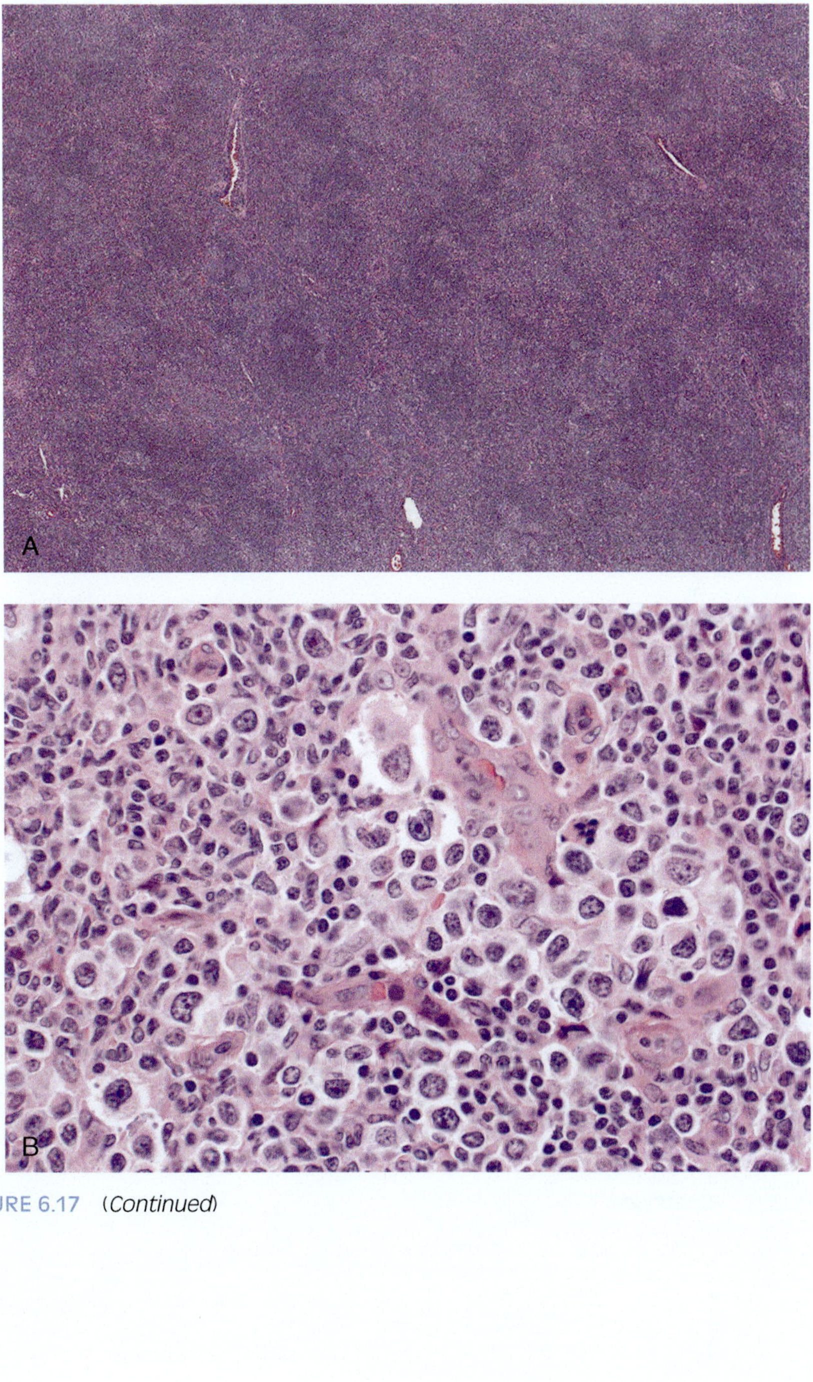

FIGURE 6.17 (*Continued*)

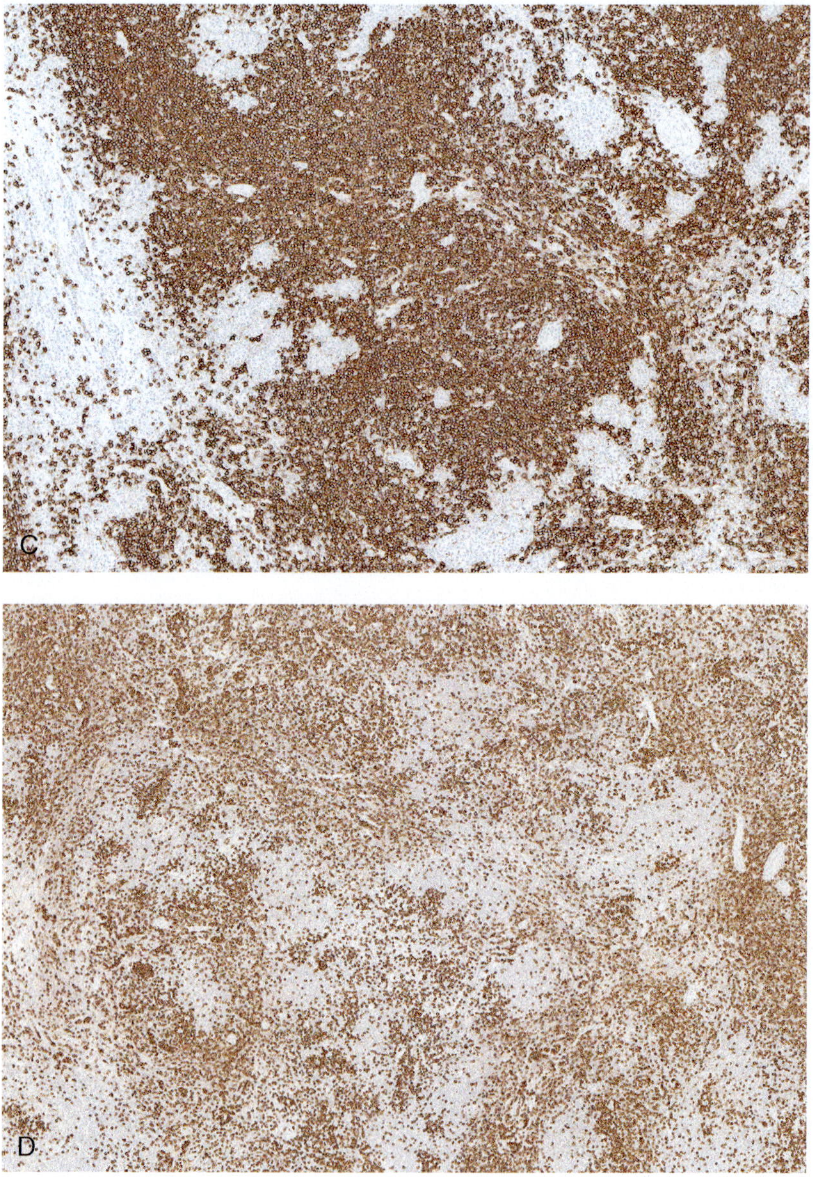

FIGURE 6.17 (*Continued*)

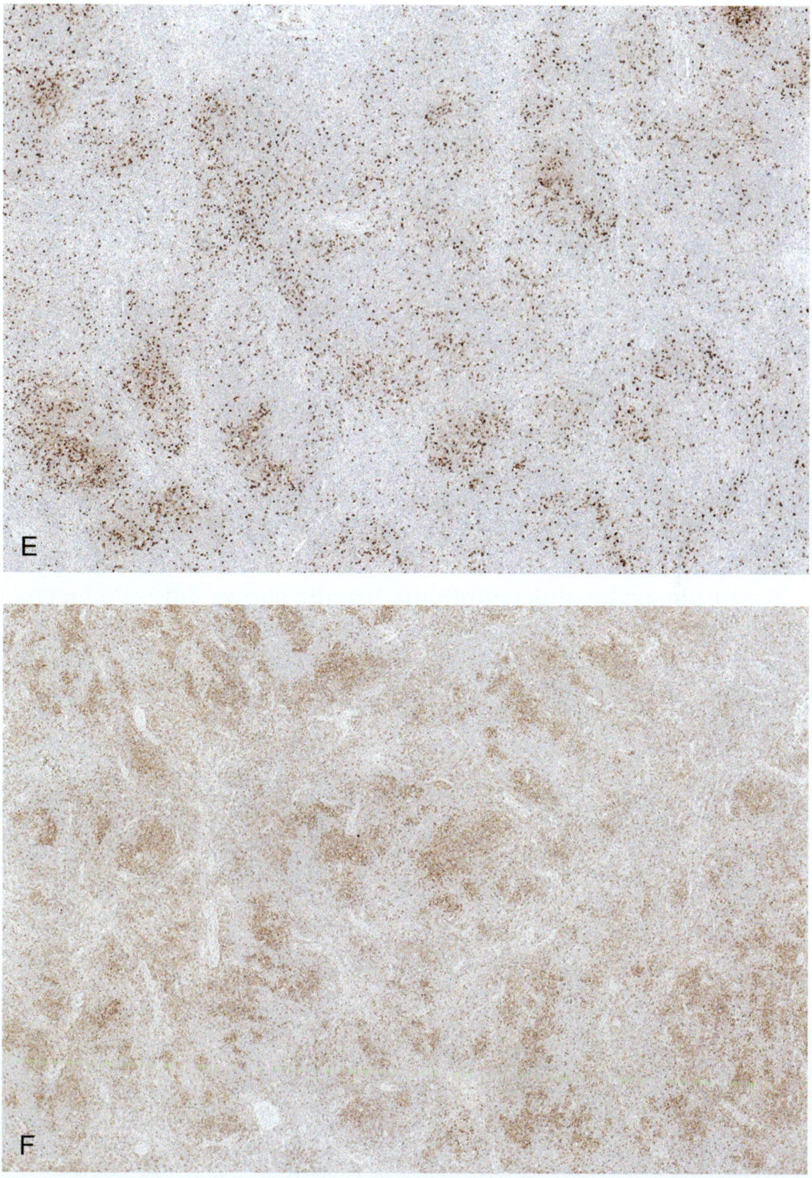

FIGURE 6.17 **Follicular helper T-cell lymphoma, follicular type.** This case shows progressive transformation of germinal center (PTGC)-like growth pattern (A). Clusters of markedly atypical lymphoma cells (B). Immunohistochemical stain for CD20 (C) highlights expanded B-cell nodules, while CD3 (D), CD10 (E), and PD-1 (F) demonstrate clusters of lymphoma cells.

In addition to T-cell markers (CD3, CD5, CD4), these lymphomas by definition express several TFH markers. HRS-like cells are consistently positive for CD30 and PAX5 and frequently positive for EBV.

Translocation t(5;9)(q33;q22) leading to *ITK-SYK* fusion can be seen in this lymphoma, and it has also been reported in rare cases of AITL.[36,37]

Follicular Helper T-cell Lymphoma, NOS

This lymphoma is characterized by expression of CD4 and at least two (preferably three) TFH markers (as outlined above) and can show some morphologic features of AITL (eg, proliferation of high endothelial venules or FDC meshwork), but these are insufficient for definitive diagnosis of AITL. It most commonly occurs in adults (median fifth to seventh decade) with slight male predominance. Patients usually present with generalized lymphadenopathy, and in about half of patients there is extranodal involvement with liver, spleen, and bone marrow being most commonly involved. Some patients have polyclonal hypergammaglobulinema, Coombs-positive hemolytic anemia, and leukocytosis, findings that are commonly seen in AITL.[1,4,22]

Morphologically, this lymphoma usually shows diffuse effacement of lymph node architecture by sheets of small to medium-sized cells with irregular nuclei and pale cytoplasm (Figures 6.18 and 6.19). Some inflammatory cells can be seen in the background, but these are not prominent

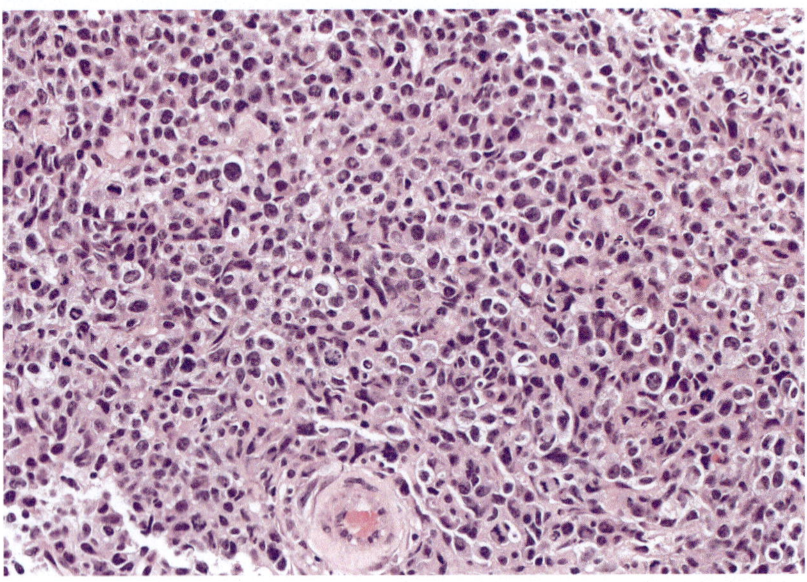

FIGURE 6.18 **Follicular helper T-cell lymphoma, NOS.** Sheets of lymphoma cells ranging in size from small to medium sized with no significant inflammatory background.

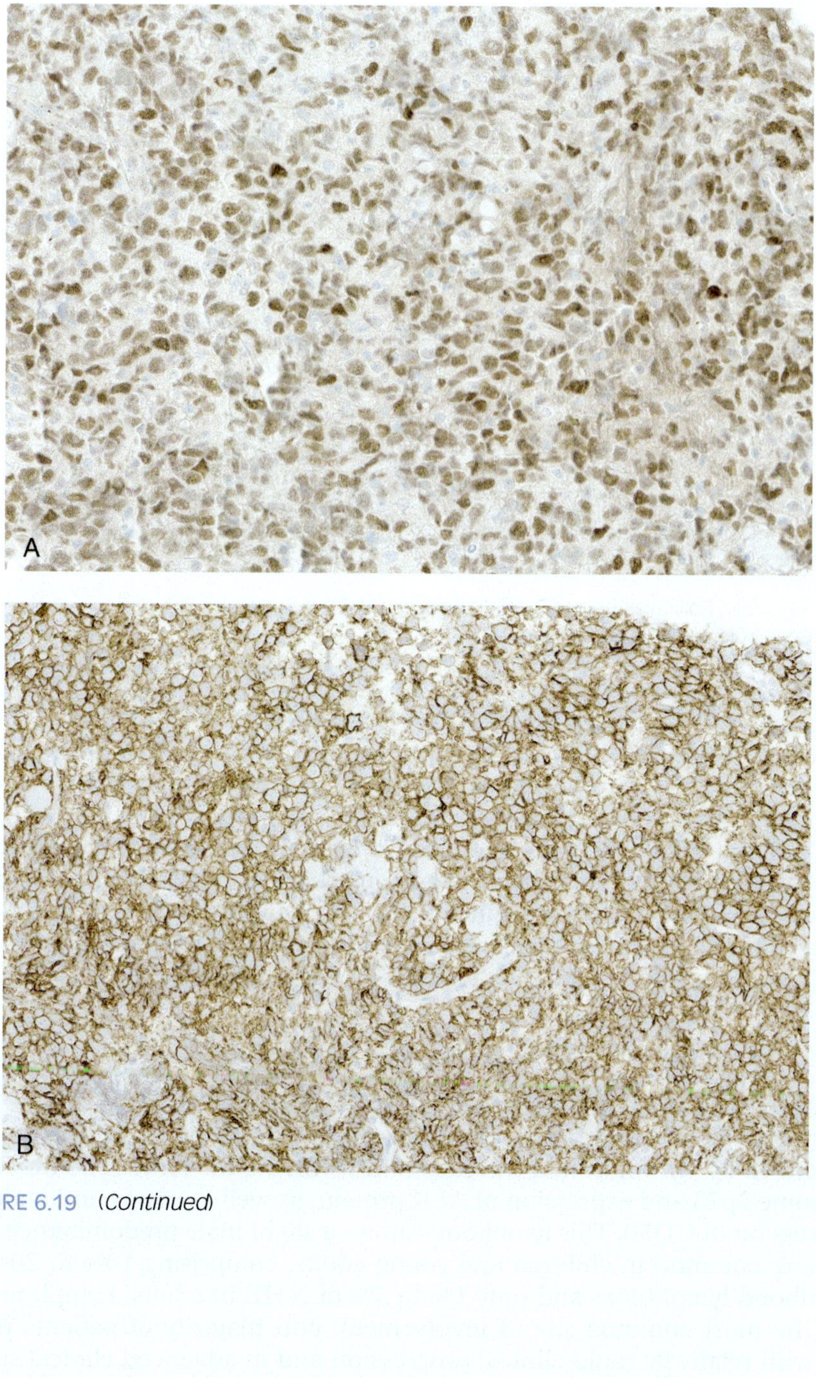

FIGURE 6.19 (*Continued*)

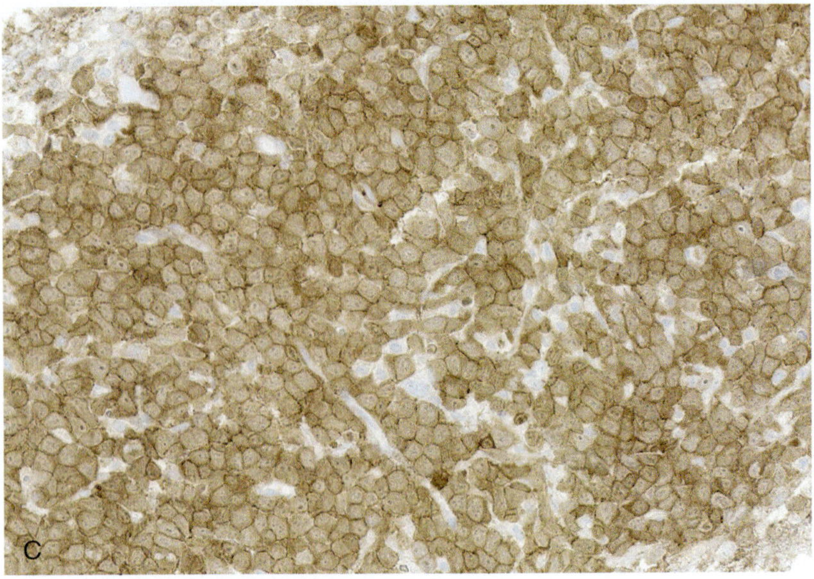

FIGURE 6.19 Follicular helper T-cell lymphoma, NOS-positive for 3 T follicular helper cell markers—BCL6 (A), ICOS (B), and SAP (C).

and, in contrast to AITL, they are typically rich in neoplastic T cells. Scattered HRS-like cells are frequently seen. As mentioned above, some proliferation of high endothelial venules and/or FDC meshwork can be seen, but not as robust as seen in AITL.[1,22]

Clonal T-cell receptor gene rearrangements are seen in most cases and are a useful tool to support the diagnosis in morphologically challenging cases. Next-generation sequencing of this lymphoma, as well as follicular type for TFH lymphoma, showed a mutational profile similar to that of AITL with mutations of *TET2, DNMT3A*, and *RHOA*.[18]

ANAPLASTIC LARGE-CELL LYMPHOMA, ALK-POSITIVE

ALCL is divided into four distinct entities–ALK+ ALCL, ALK– ALCL, primary cutaneous ALCL, and breast implant–associated ALCL.[2] ALK+ ALCL is defined by chromosomal translocation involving the *ALK* gene on chromosome 2p23 and expression of ALK protein, as well as strong and uniform expression of CD30. This lymphoma shows a slight male predominance and is more common in children and young adults, comprising 10% to 20% of childhood lymphomas and only 1% to 3% of NHL in adults. Lymph nodes are the most common site of involvement, and majority of patients present with relatively rapid clinical progression and in advanced clinical stage. Extranodal sites (such as spleen, skin, bones, lungs) are involved in approximately half of patients. The disease is curable in majority of patients with a 5-year overall survival of 70% to 80%.[1,4,38-40]

Morphology

ALK+ ALCL most commonly involves lymph node in a diffuse pattern and completely obliterates the architecture. In some cases, the lymph node is involved in a sinusoidal pattern, that is, lymphoma cells fill and distend the sinuses (especially the subcapsular sinus) (Figures 6.20 and 6.21). In cases with relatively subtle sinusoidal involvement, it can be very difficult to appreciate lymphoma cells since the lymph node architecture is essentially preserved. Moreover, when needle core biopsies are performed in these cases only small number of lymphoma cells can be present in the section, or the lymphoma cells can be absent in a limited sample. The lymphoma cells show a broad morphologic spectrum, and four histologic variants are recognized–common (70% of cases), lymphohistiocytic, small cell, and Hodgkin-like. Some cases show a composite pattern (usually two different patterns). Also, very rare morphologic variants such as sarcomatoid, giant cell–rich, and neutrophil and eosinophil rich have been described. Although the morphologic appearance can vary considerably, all cases have variable number of "hallmark" cells, that is, lymphoma cells with eccentric horseshoe-shaped nuclei, with eosinophilic paranuclear region, consistent with Golgi region (Figure 6.22). Sometimes, the lymphoma cells appear to have intranuclear inclusions, the so-called donut cells. In the common pattern, the lymphoma cells are large, pleomorphic with round to variably irregular, and occasionally anaplastic nuclei. Giant and multinucleated lymphoma cells are seen in some cases. The chromatin is finely clumped,

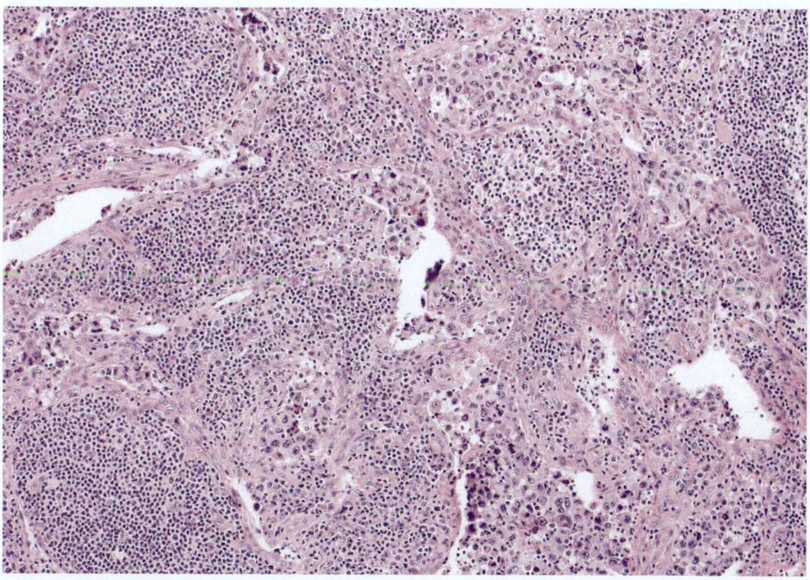

FIGURE 6.20 Anaplastic large cell lymphoma, ALK-positive (ALCL, ALK+) showing sinusoidal pattern of involvement with large lymphoma cells filling and distending the cortical sinuses.

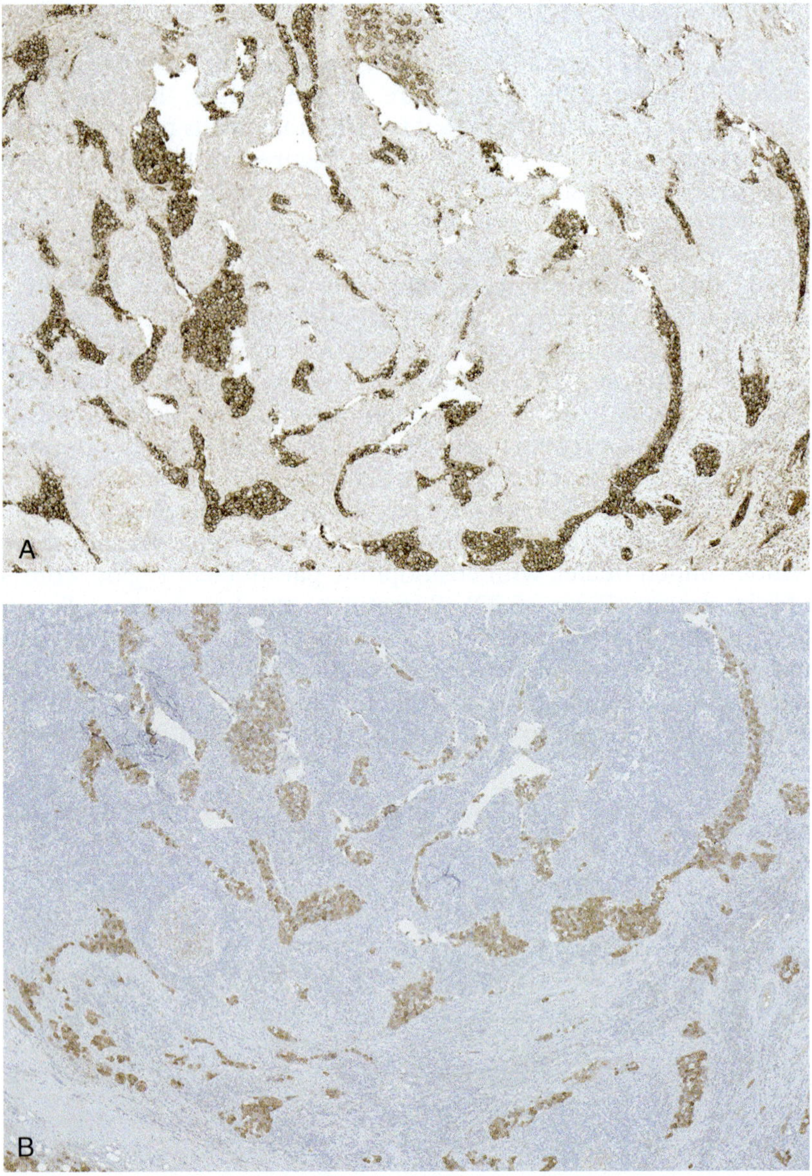

FIGURE 6.21 Immunohistochemical stains for CD30 (A) and ALK (B) highlight the sinusoidal pattern of involvement in anaplastic large cell lymphoma, ALK-positive.

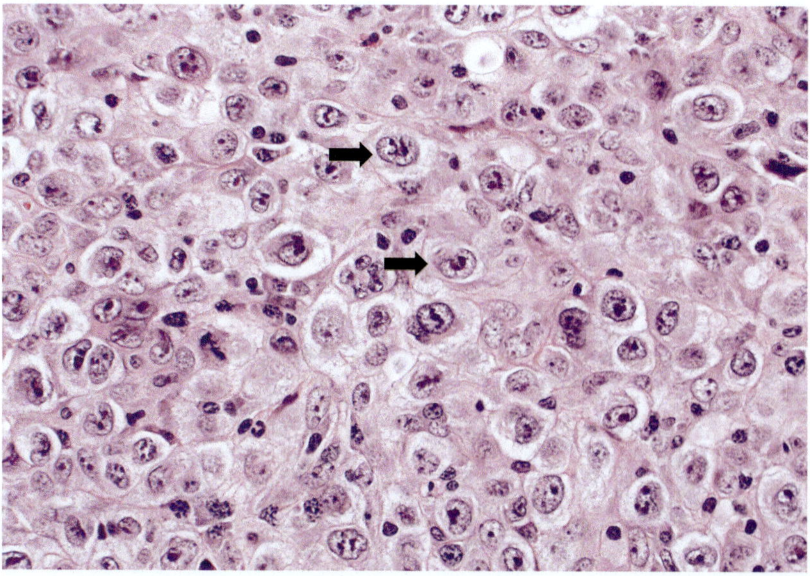

FIGURE 6.22 **ALCL, ALK+. Sheets of large pleomorphic lymphoma cells with prominent nucleoli and abundant eosinophilic cytoplasm.** Scattered "hallmark" cells are seen (arrows).

nucleoli are usually conspicuous, and cells have abundant eosinophilic or basophilic cytoplasm. In the relatively rare lymphohistiocytic variant, lymphoma cells are scattered among the abundant small lymphocytes and histiocytes. Frequently, the lymphoma cells will cluster around blood vessels. These cases can be very challenging and mistaken for nonneoplastic/reactive conditions. CD30 and ALK will highlight neoplastic cells in the reactive background. The small cell variant is characterized by predominantly small to medium-sized lymphoma cells with occasional large cells admixed. The cells have abundant pale cytoplasm, imparting a fried egg appearance, and tend to cluster around blood vessels (Figure 6.23A). This variant too can be very challenging to diagnose, especially on a limited biopsy, since typically only a subset of cells (usually larger ones) are CD30-positive (Figure 6.23B). The Hodgkin-like variant of ALK+ ALCL is for all practical purposes morphologically indistinguishable from CHL, most frequently the nodular sclerosis subtype. It is prudent to perform PAX5 immunohistochemical stain on cases that morphologically look like CHL, and if negative or equivocal, perform ALK stain.[1,11,41-44]

Phenotype

ALK+ ALCL is positive for the ALK protein, with several patterns of expression in lymphoma cells, corresponding to different translocation partners of the *ALK* gene. In approximately 80% of cases, the most common translocation t(2;5)(p23;q25) leads to nuclear and cytoplasmic ALK staining (Figure 6.24). Most other translocations lead to cytoplasmic pattern[4,43] (Figure 6.25). Expression of CD30 is strong and uniform showing

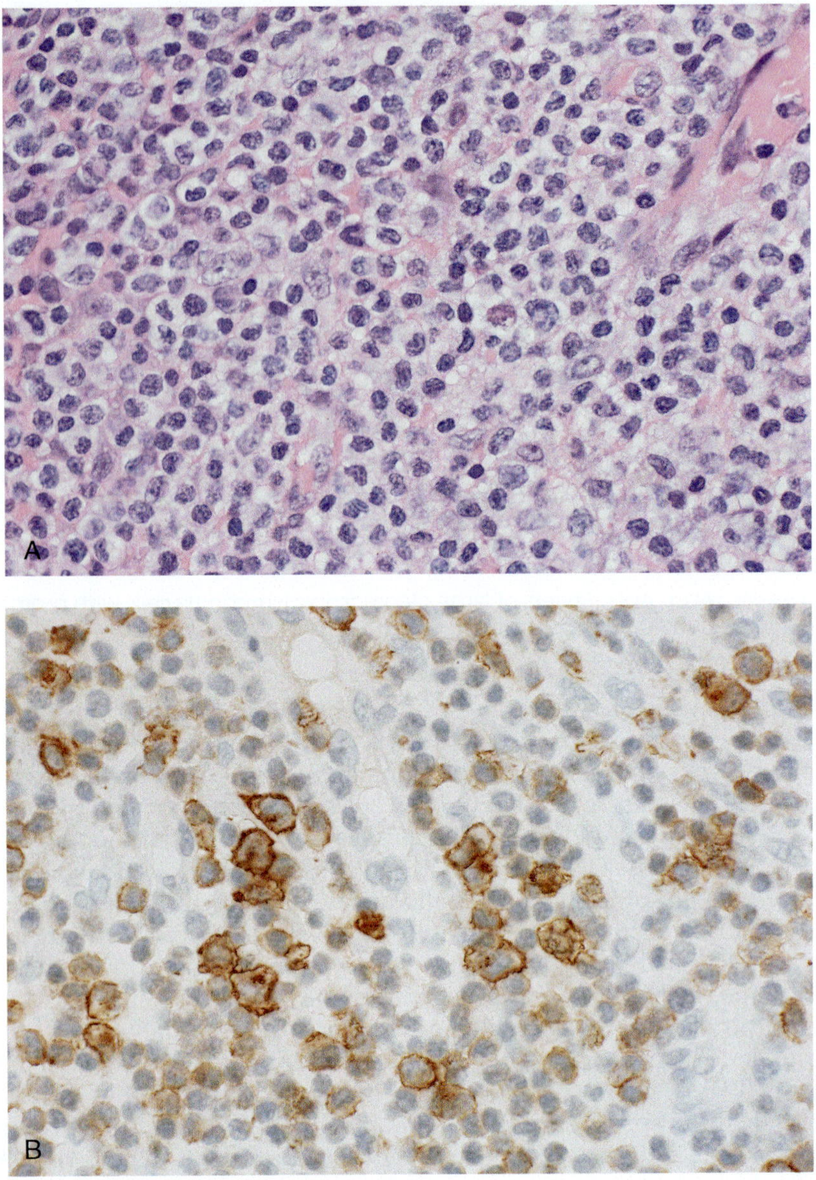

FIGURE 6.23 **ALCL, ALK+, small cell variant.** The lymphoma cells are predominantly small to medium sized and have abundant pale cytoplasm, imparting a fried egg appearance (A). Lymphoma cells show variable staining for CD30 with only larger cells showing strong staining (B).

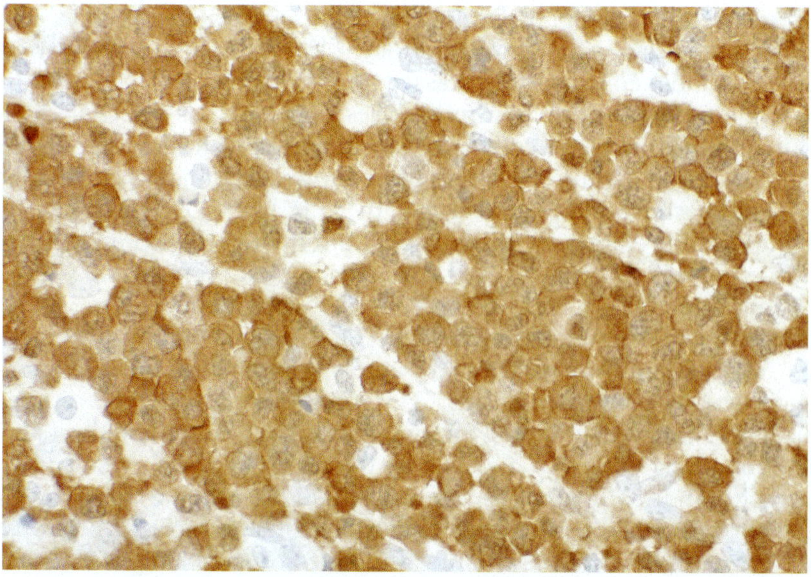

FIGURE 6.24 ALK immunohistochemical stain shows nuclear and cytoplasmic staining of lymphoma cells, indicating the presence of the most common translocation t(2;5)(p23q25) *NPM1-ALK* in ALCL, ALK+.

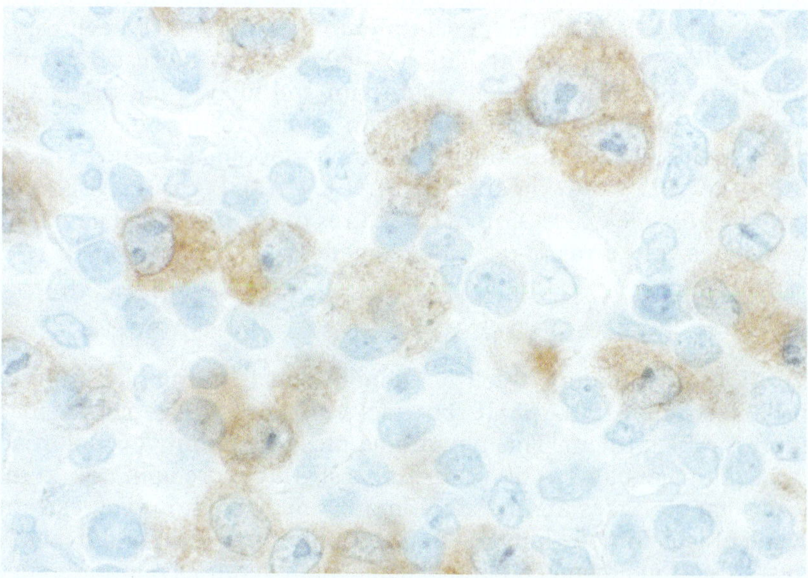

FIGURE 6.25 ALK immunohistochemical stain shows granular cytoplasmic staining of lymphoma cells, indicating the presence of variant translocation of *ALK* gene (ie, other than *NPM1-ALK*).

membranous and Golgi pattern. The exceptions are the small cell variant (as described above) and the lymphohistiocytic variant where some variability is seen. The most commonly expressed T-cell markers are CD2, CD4, and CD5, while CD3 is negative in most cases. Rarely, cases are CD8-positive. In some cases, lymphoma cells have so-called null-cell phenotype with no expression of T-cell markers. These cases, however, typically have a clonal T-cell gene rearrangement, although with ALK and CD30 positivity this is rarely needed for diagnosis. Other useful and frequently expressed markers include cytotoxic molecules (TIA-1, granzyme, and perforin) CD43, EMA, CD25, and clusterin. CD45 is expressed in more than half of cases, frequently with variable intensity. EBER-ISH for EBV is negative. Even though ALK+ ALCL can morphologically resemble a number of other lymphomas and nonhematopoietic neoplasms, ALK positivity narrows the differential diagnosis to a limited number of entities. ALK+ large B-cell lymphoma is one hematopoietic neoplasm to consider in the differential diagnosis; however, this lymphoma usually shows plasmablastic differentiation and is negative for CD30. Nonhematopoietic entities, such as inflammatory myofibroblastic tumor, breast cancer, neural tumors, and alveolar rhabdomyosarcoma, can show ALK positivity, but they are usually morphologically distinct and negative for other markers associated with ALCL.[45-47]

Genetics

Most cases (90%) show clonal T-cell receptor gene rearrangement. All cases of ALK+ ALCL have a fusion gene involving *ALK* (2p23), with different partners. The most common translocation (>80% of cases) is t(2;5)(p23;q35) with *NPM1*, but over 10 different partners have been reported so far.[1,4] *ALK* rearrangement can be detected by fluorescence in situ hybridization (FISH); however, this is not routinely done or needed as positive ALK immunohistochemical stain is diagnostic. Gene expression profiling studies showed distinct and also overlapping signatures of ALK+ and ALK– ALCL.[48,49] Compared with ALK– ALCL cases, ALK+ ALCL was enriched for the expression of signatures of HIF1-α target genes, IL10-induced genes, and h-ras/k-ras-induced genes.[49]

ANAPLASTIC LARGE-CELL LYMPHOMA, ALK-NEGATIVE

ALCL, ALK– is a mature T-cell lymphoma that is morphologically indistinguishable from ALK+ ALCL but lacks *ALK* rearrangement and does not express ALK protein. This lymphoma most commonly occurs in adults with a median age of 40 to 60 years and is slightly more common in males. Clinically, lymph nodes are most commonly involved; however, extranodal involvement is common (lungs, skin, gastrointestinal tract, and liver). Most patients present in advanced clinical stage and overall have poorer survival than patients with ALK+ ALCL, with a 5-year overall survival of 40% to 50%. However, ALK– ALCL is a genetically heterogeneous lymphoma with prognostically important genetic abnormalities, as discussed below.[1,4,50-52]

Morphology

ALK– ALCL morphologically resembles the common variant of ALK+ ALCL with cohesive sheets of large lymphoma cells that frequently involve the sinuses. Paracortical involvement with sparing of lymphoid follicles is also commonly seen. Similar to ALK+ ALCL, cases with partial or sinusoidal involvement can be challenging on a needle core biopsy since the pattern of growth can be difficult to appreciate. The lymphoma cells are pleomorphic with round to irregular and sometimes anaplastic nuclei, occasional multinucleated cells, conspicuous nucleoli, and abundant eosinophilic or basophilic cytoplasm. Horseshoe-shaped hallmark cells are usually easy to find, and "donut" cells with nuclear pseudoinclusions are commonly seen (Figure 6.26). Some cases have scattered neutrophils or eosinophils in the background, which is a helpful morphologic clue for diagnosing this entity (Figure 6.27). In contrast to ALK+ ALCL, morphologic variants are generally not recognized in the ALK– ALCL category.[1]

Phenotype

All cases are strongly and uniformly positive for CD30 in a membranous and Golgi pattern (Figure 6.28). This is a very important feature as other T-cell lymphomas, such as PTCL, NOS frequently show CD30 expression, most commonly in only a subset of cells or with variable intensity. However, some cases of PTCL, NOS have strong and diffuse CD30 expression. In these cases, as outlined above, cohesive sheets of large pleomorphic cells with scattered hallmark cells favor the diagnosis of ALK– ALCL. The most

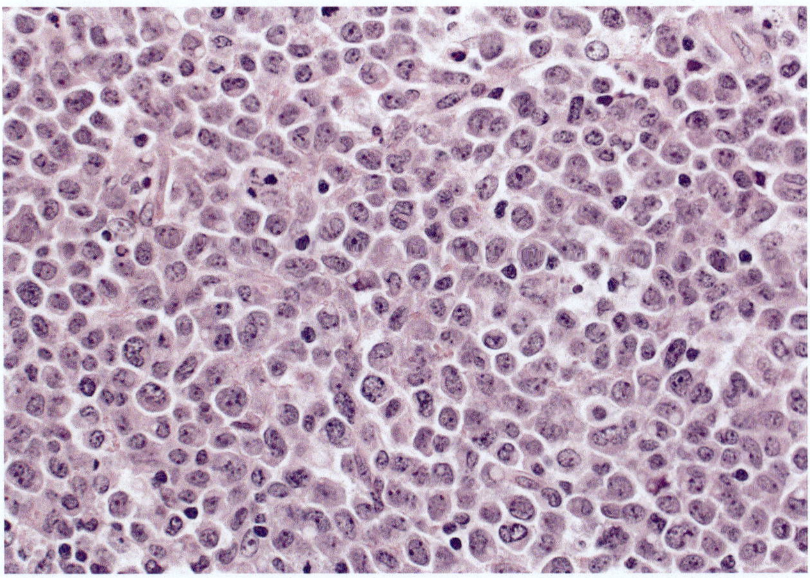

FIGURE 6.26 Anaplastic large cell lymphoma, ALK-negative, showing sheets of large pleomorphic lymphoma cells, morphologically indistinguishable from ALCL, ALK+.

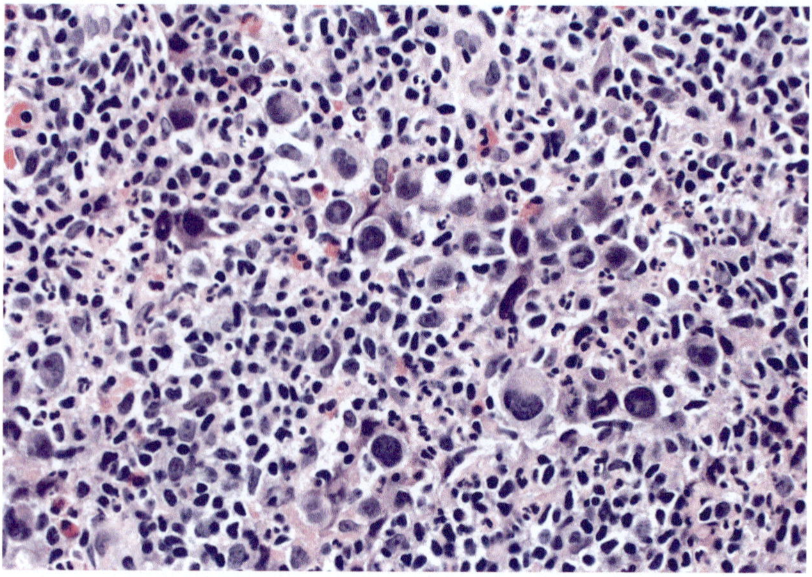

FIGURE 6.27 ALCL, ALK−. Scattered large lymphoma cells in an inflammatory background with neutrophils and eosinophils.

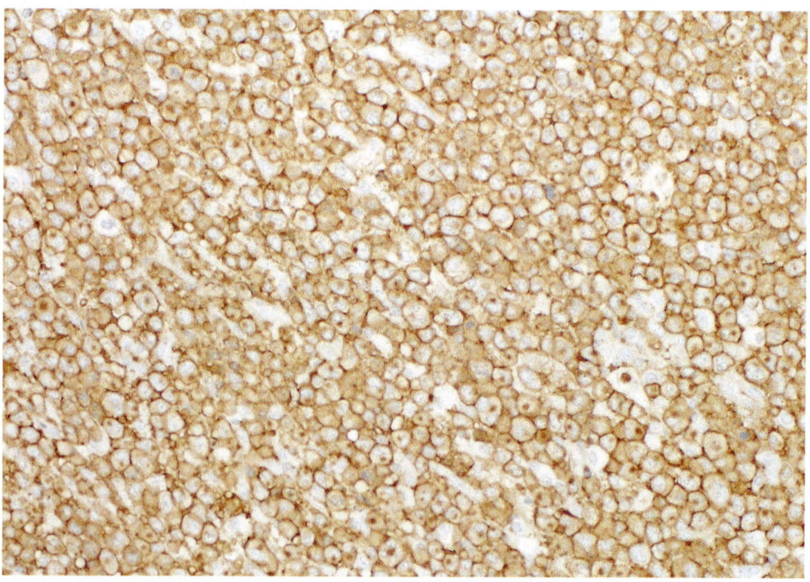

FIGURE 6.28 ALCL, ALK− showing strong and uniform staining for CD30 in membranous and Golgi pattern.

commonly expressed T-cell markers are CD2, CD3, CD4, CD5, and CD43, while CD7 is negative in most cases. However, loss of several or even all T-cell markers is not uncommon. Rarely, cases can be CD8-positive or double negative for CD4/CD8. Other frequently positive markers include CD45, cytotoxic molecules (TIA-1, granzyme, and perforin), MUM1, EMA, and clusterin. EBER-ISH is negative. A few other markers are worth mentioning as they can lead to diagnostic errors. Rare cases are positive for keratins (such as AE1/AE3 and OSCAR), which coupled with cohesive growth of lymphoma cells can be interpreted as carcinoma. The most difficult differential diagnosis is with CHL, especially in rare cases of ALK– ALCL that show fibrous bands and background rich in eosinophils.[1,53] In an overwhelming majority of cases, this differential diagnosis can be resolved with immunohistochemistry. ALK– ALCL will usually be positive for at least some T-cell markers, EMA, and CD45 and negative for PAX5. Of note, CD15 can be rarely seen in ALK– ALCL, and very rarely PAX5 can be expressed too.[54]

Genetics

Most cases show a clonal T-cell receptor gene rearrangement. Two prognostically important abnormalities in ALK– ALCL are *DUSP22* (6p25.3) rearrangement detected in up to 30% of cases and *TP63* (3q28) rearrangement found in <10% of cases. FISH for these rearrangements should be routinely done in all cases of ALK– ALCL. Patients with *TP63* rearrangement have poor prognosis. As for *DUSP22* rearrangement, survival data in the literature are somewhat controversial with some studies reporting excellent and some intermediate survival.[50,55] Cases with *DUSP22* rearrangement are defined as a distinct genetic subtype of systemic ALK– ALCL in 2022 ICC.[2] They have somewhat characteristic morphology with medium-sized monomorphic cells with abundant hallmark cells and frequent doughnut cells (Figure 6.29). Moreover, they lack expression of cytotoxic molecules.[56,57] Next-generation sequencing data showed that ALK– ALCL cases have frequent activation of the JAK-STAT pathway similar to ALK+ ALCL, albeit through different mechanisms.[58]

OTHER T-CELL LYMPHOMAS THAT CAN INVOLVE LYMPH NODES

T-cell Prolymphocytic Leukemia

T-PLL is a rare aggressive neoplasm of mature postthymic T cells. The median age at diagnosis is 65 years with a male to female ratio of 2:1. Patients with ataxia telangiectasia (mutation of *ATM* gene) have an increased risk of T-PLL compared with the general population, and in these patients T-PLL occurs earlier (third to fifth decade of life). Clinically, patients usually present with prominent lymphocytosis, frequently $>100 \times 10^9$/L, with accompanying anemia and/or thrombocytopenia. Other typical presenting signs include hepatosplenomegaly, lymphadenopathy, and in subset of patients skin lesions. Median survival is 1 to 2 years.[4,11,59-61]

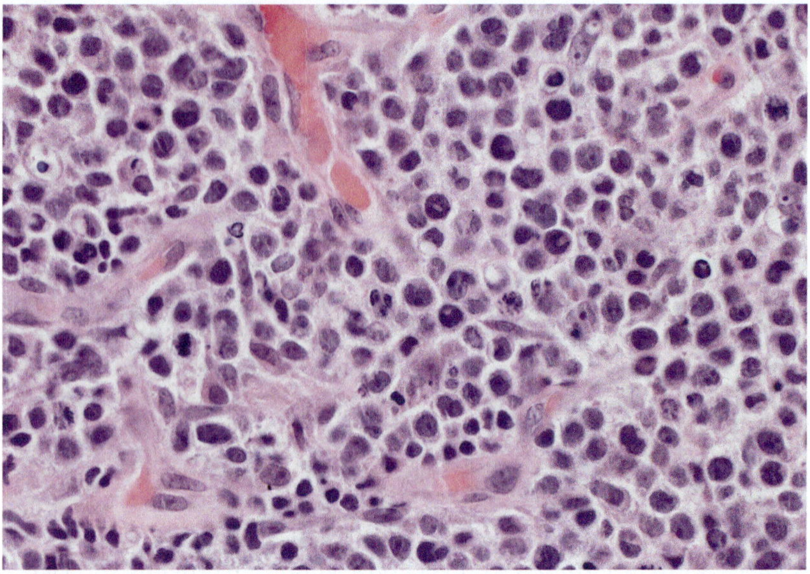

FIGURE 6.29 **ALCL, ALK–, *DUSP22* rearranged.** There are numerous uniformly sized hallmark cells with deeply indented nuclei and occasional "donut" cells.

Morphology

The morphologic features of T-PLL are best appreciated on peripheral blood and bone marrow smears. The lymphoma cells are small to medium-sized prolymphocytes with round to irregular nuclei, conspicuous nucleoli, and scant deeply basophilic cytoplasm that frequently shows blebs (Figure 6.30). However, in a subset of cases nuclei are small and nucleoli are not seen; the morphology here resembles CLL/SLL. Lymph nodes are uncommonly biopsied in T-PLL since the diagnosis is usually made by examination of bone marrow and peripheral blood. In lymph nodes, lymphoma cells diffusely involve paracortical areas and sometimes completely replace lymph node architecture (Figure 6.31). Reactive residual germinal centers can be seen.

Phenotype

T-PLL is positive for pan-T-cell markers CD2, CD3, CD5, and CD7. The majority of cases are CD4+/CD8–, with the CD4+/CD8+ phenotype seen in 25% of cases. In cases that are double positive for CD4/CD8, a differential diagnosis of T-lymphoblastic lymphoma should be excluded by performing TdT, CD1a, CD10, and CD34, all of which are negative in T-PLL. On the other hand, the CD4+/CD8+ phenotype is very helpful in the context of differential diagnosis with other mature T-cell lymphomas, as this phenotype is extremely uncommon in other T-cell lymphomas. Another helpful marker is TCL1, which is expressed in the majority of cases (Figure 6.32). CD52 is expressed at a higher density compared with normal T and B cells.

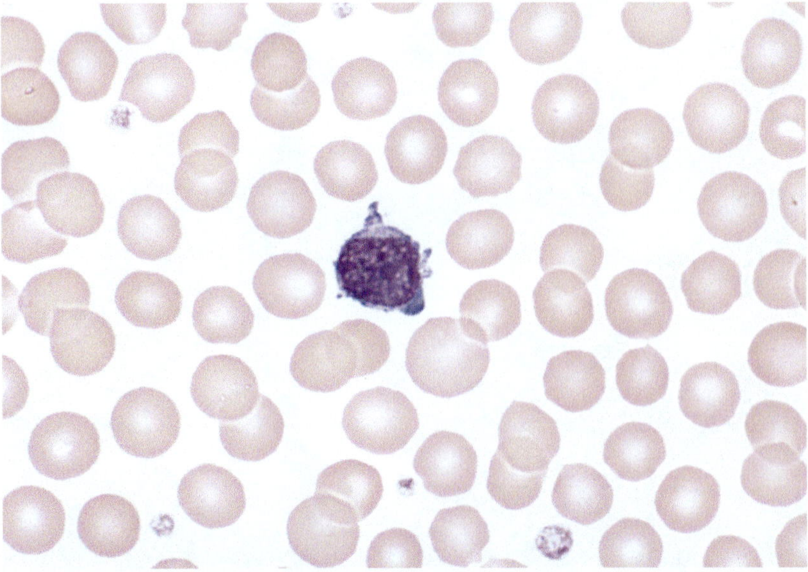

FIGURE 6.30 **T-cell prolymphocytic leukemia in the peripheral blood.** A neoplastic cell with slightly irregular nucleus, small nucleolus, and deeply basophilic cytoplasm with blebs.

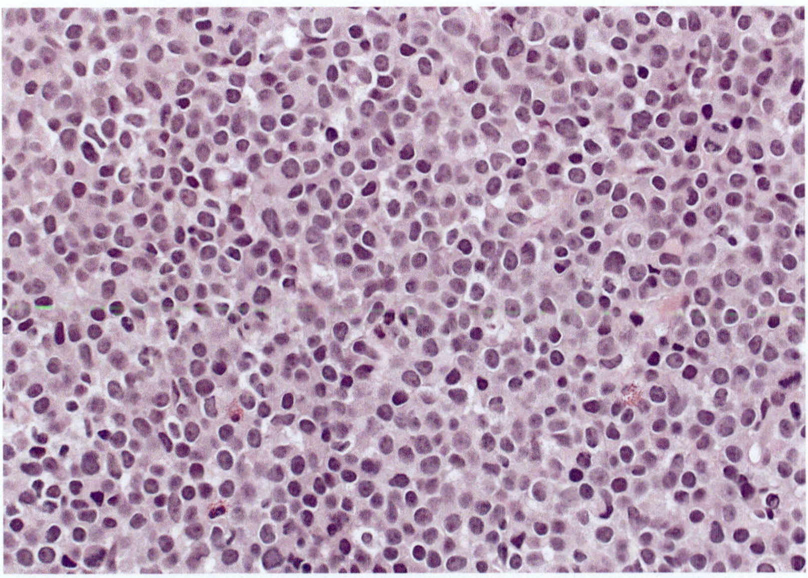

FIGURE 6.31 **T-cell prolymphocytic leukemia involving the lymph node.** Sheets of T-prolymphocytes with round to slightly irregular nuclei and small central nucleoli.

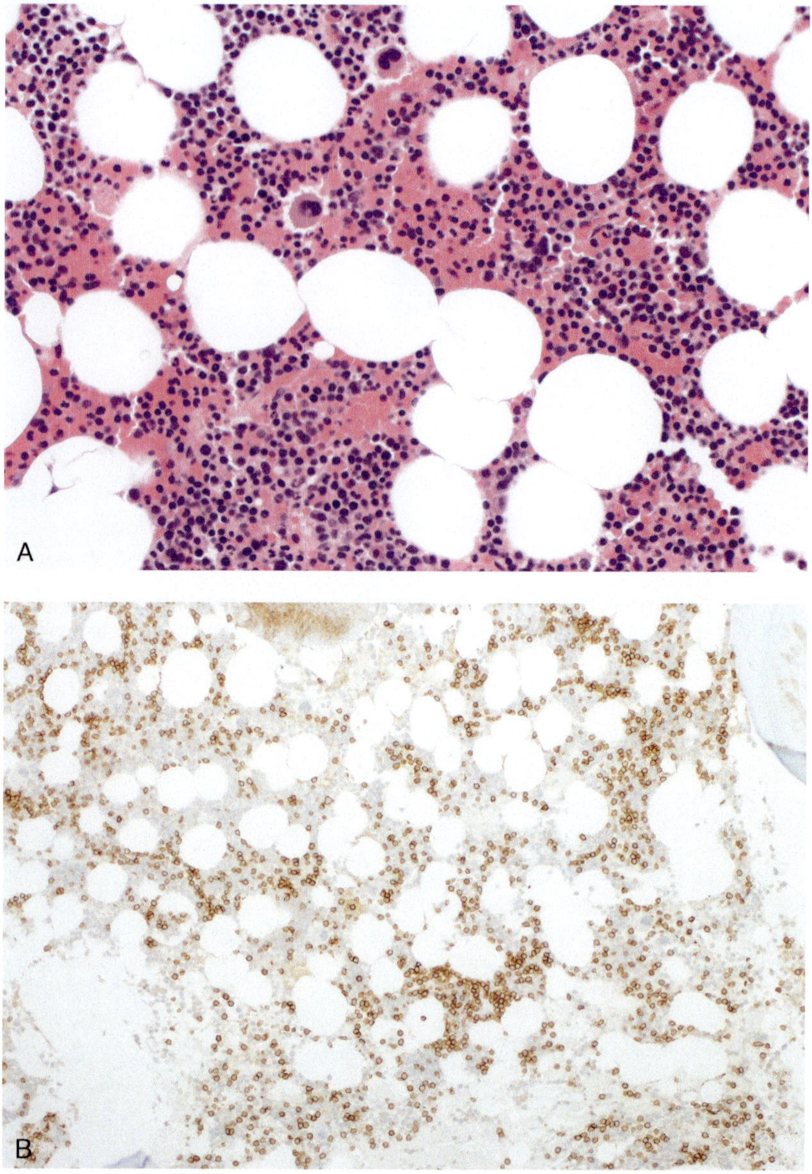

FIGURE 6.32 (*Continued*)

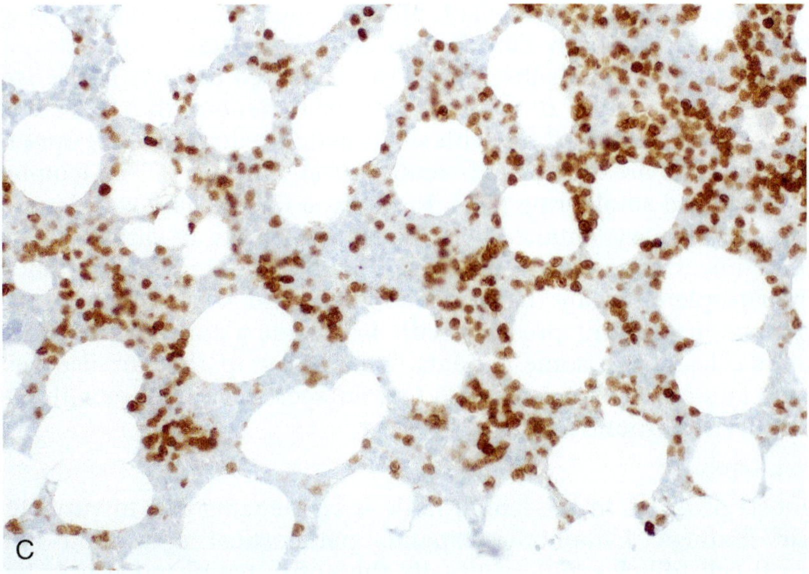

FIGURE 6.32 T-PLL showing diffuse interstitial infiltrate in the bone marrow (A). The neoplastic cells are positive for CD3 (B) and TCL-1 (C).

The differential diagnosis of T-PLL includes other mature T-cell lymphomas that show peripheral blood involvement such as adult T-cell leukemia lymphoma, mycosis fungoides, and T-cell large granular lymphocytic leukemia. A combination of clinical, morphologic, and phenotypic findings usually successfully resolves the differential diagnosis.[4,62,63]

Genetics

T-PLL cases show clonal T-cell receptor gene rearrangements. The most common genetic abnormalities (around 90% of cases) include inv(14)(q11q32) or t(14;14)(q11;q32), which juxtapose the TCRA/D locus on chromosome 14q11 with *TCL1A* and *TCLB1* oncogenes at 14q32.1. Occasionally, t(X;14)(q28;q11) is seen, which involves *MTCP1* gene. FISH for these abnormalities can help confirm the diagnosis, especially in cases in which immunohistochemistry for TCL1 is negative. Other common abnormalities are unbalanced rearrangements of chromosome 8, most commonly trisomy 8, as well as deletions at 11q23 (*ATM* locus) and mutations at the *ATM* locus. Sequencing studies show frequent mutations in the JAK/STAT pathway.[11,64-66]

Adult T-cell Leukemia/Lymphoma

ATLL is a mature T-cell lymphoma that occurs in people infected with human T-lymphotropic virus type 1 (HTLV-1), a virus that is endemic in Japan, parts of South America, the Caribbean, and parts of Africa. However, due to travel and migration, ATLL incidence has increased in parts of the United States (eg, south Florida and New York state) and Europe.[4,67,68] ATLL occurs in a small subset of HTLV-1 infected patients (<5% overall) after a latency period of 20 to 30 years. Most patients with ATLL are in the fifth to seventh decade of life with slight male predominance. Four classic clinical variants are recognized–acute (60%), chronic (15%), lymphomatous (20%), and smoldering (5%). Recently, a fifth variant was described–extranodal primary cutaneous. Clinical presentation varies depending on the clinical variant, and the most common findings are lymphocytosis, hepatosplenomegaly, lymphadenopathy, and skin involvement. The lymphomatous variant presents with lymphadenopathy with associated extranodal lesions in some patients. Lymphadenopathy can also be seen in acute and chronic variants. ATLL is an aggressive disease with overall 5-year survival around 25%.[1,69,70]

Morphology

Diagnosis of ATLL in the lymph node is challenging due to variable histologic findings. Lymphoma expands paracortical areas and initially spares B-cell follicles, but eventually the entire lymph node may be diffusely replaced. The T cells vary in size from small to large, with irregular nuclear contours. The infiltrate can be pleomorphic with a mixture of cell sizes or be more uniform in appearance (Figure 6.33). The cells can be immunoblastic or centroblastic and morphologically resemble DLBCL (Figure 6.34). Furthermore, HRS-like cells can be occasionally seen.

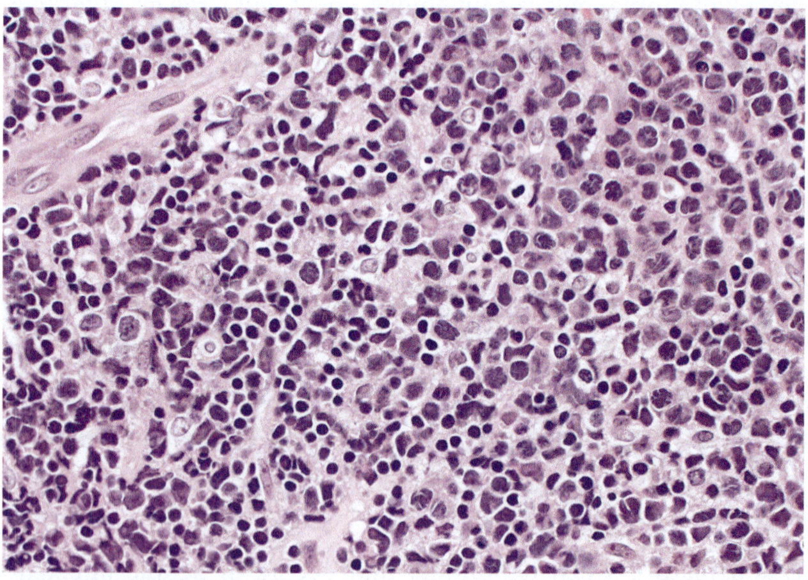

FIGURE 6.33 **Adult T-cell leukemia/lymphoma.** The lymphoma cells are medium sized to large and have markedly irregular nuclei.

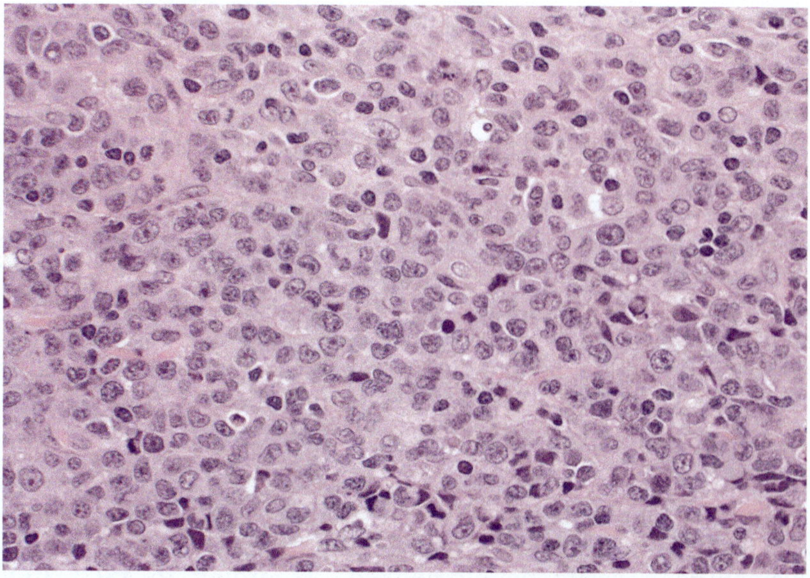

FIGURE 6.34 A case of ATLL with predominantly large cells.

Multiple morphologic patterns have been described and include pleomorphic small-cell, pleomorphic medium- and large-cell, ALCL-like, AITL-like, and Hodgkin lymphoma–like pattern.[1,69-71] In other words, ATLL can mimic a number of other mature T-cell lymphomas and diagnosis requires a high level of suspicion in people with appropriate demographic background. Since definitive diagnosis requires knowledge of patient's HTLV-1 status, it is best to sign these cases out as "Peripheral T-cell lymphoma" and recommend testing for HTLV-1.

Phenotype

The lymphoma cells are positive for pan-T-cell markers including CD2, CD3, and CD5, with loss of CD7. In over 90% of cases, lymphoma cells are CD4+/CD8−; however, rarely other phenotypes (CD4−/CD8+, CD4+/CD8+, or CD4−/CD8−) can be seen. CD25 is also expressed in a majority of cases, while CD30 is typically positive in cases with large cells, which can be particularly challenging in ATLL cases with ALCL-like morphology.[69]

Genetics

Clonal T-cell receptor rearrangement can be detected in virtually all cases, and HTLV-1 provirus is inserted clonally within lymphoma cells.[4]

Mycosis Fungoides and Sézary Syndrome

Mycosis fungoides (MF) is primary cutaneous epidermotropic T-cell lymphoma, composed of markedly irregular/convoluted lymphoma cells. MF is the most common primary cutaneous lymphoma.[72] It usually occurs in older adults, but it can occur in younger people, including children. The male to female ratio is 2:1. Clinically, MF is characterized by skin patches, plaques, and tumors, typically in sun protected areas. It is an indolent disease, usually with slow clinical evolution over years to decades. Peripheral blood, lymph nodes, and extranodal/visceral sites are usually involved later in the disease course. The most important prognostic factor is clinical stage according to International Society for Cutaneous Lymphomas/European Organization of Research and Treatment of Cancer (ISCL/EORTC).[73] Sézary syndrome (SS) is defined as a triad of erythroderma, generalized lymphadenopathy, and the presence of clonally related neoplastic T cells with cerebriform nuclei in skin, lymph nodes, and peripheral blood. Some patients have a clinical history of MF, while in others SS arises de novo (ie, primary SS).[1,4]

Morphology

The lymph nodes from patients with MF are uncommonly biopsied. Knowledge of clinical history of MF is essential; otherwise, lymph node involvement can easily be overlooked. According to ISCL/EORTC guidelines, the lymph node has to be at least 1.5 cm in diameter to be considered "abnormal"; moreover, any lymph node that is firm, irregular, or fixed is also abnormal.[73] Histologic changes in the lymph node show a spectrum, and the ISCL/EORTC group has integrated two grading systems (Dutch System and National Cancer Institute Classification) into four categories–N0-N3 (Table 6.1).[73-75] In the early stage (N1) the lymph node shows dermatopathic change with expanded paracortex, containing small lymphocytes, histiocytes with focal pigment, interdigitating dendritic cells, and Langerhans cells. Lymphoma cells are not morphologically apparent. However, studies have shown that, in subset of cases with only dermatopathic change, molecular analysis detects clonal T-cell gene rearrangement.[76] Stage N2 is morphologically the most challenging to diagnose. Lymph nodes show prominent dermatopathic change with lymphoma cells in the paracortex, distributed singly or in small clusters. The lymphoma cells are medium sized and have markedly irregular (cerebriform) nuclei, but they are hard to appreciate on lower magnifications and are best seen on high magnification or even using the oil objective. As lymphoma cells proliferate, clusters become larger and eventually the entire architecture is diffusely replaced by MF cells (stage N3) (Figure 6.35). In lymph nodes that are diffusely replaced, there are usually increased number of large cells, similar to large cell transformation observed in the skin.[1,73] Evaluation of lymph node involvement on a needle core biopsy can be extremely challenging, particularly in early stages (N1 and N2), where lymphoma cells are not numerous. In SS, lymph nodes usually do not show dermatopathic change and lymphoma cells expand the paracortex.[1,74,75]

TABLE 6.1 Histologic Staging of Lymph Nodes in Mycosis Fungoides and Sézary Syndrome

Updated ISCL/EORTC Classification[73]	Dutch System[74]	NCI-VA Classification[75]
N1	Grade 1: Dermatopathic lymphadenopathy (DL)	LN0: No atypical lymphocytes LN1: Occasional and isolated atypical lymphocytes (not in clusters) LN2: Many atypical lymphocytes or in 3-6 cell clusters
N2	Grade 2: DL; early involvement by MF (presence of cerebriform nuclei >7.5 μm)	LN3: Aggregates of atypical lymphocytes; nodal architecture preserved
N3	Grade 3: Partial effacement of lymph node architecture Grade 4: Complete effacement	LN4: Partial/complete effacement of nodal architecture by atypical lymphocytes or frankly neoplastic cells

NCI-VA, National Cancer Institute-Veterans Administration.

Phenotype

The lymphoma cells in MF express pan-T-cell antigens CD2, CD3, CD5, and CD45RO and are usually CD4-positive, with rare cases being CD4−/CD8+. Most cases are positive for TCR alpha/beta, but rare CD8+ cases can be positive for TCR gamma/delta. CD7 and CD26 are usually absent. CD30 is usually expressed in large cells, and in some cases of large cell transformation there is also expression of cytotoxic molecules (TIA-1, granzyme, and perforin).[4] The differential diagnosis in those cases includes ALCL and can be very challenging as phenotypes overlap. Knowledge of clinical history of MF is needed to correctly diagnose transformed cases. SS shows an immunophenotype similar to that of MF.

Genetics

Clonal T-cell receptor rearrangement can be detected in most MF cases.[77] In lymph nodes (regardless of biopsy size), T-cell clonality studies should be done on all cases where the histologic involvement is not clearly seen on hematoxylin & eosin stain or by immunohistochemistry.

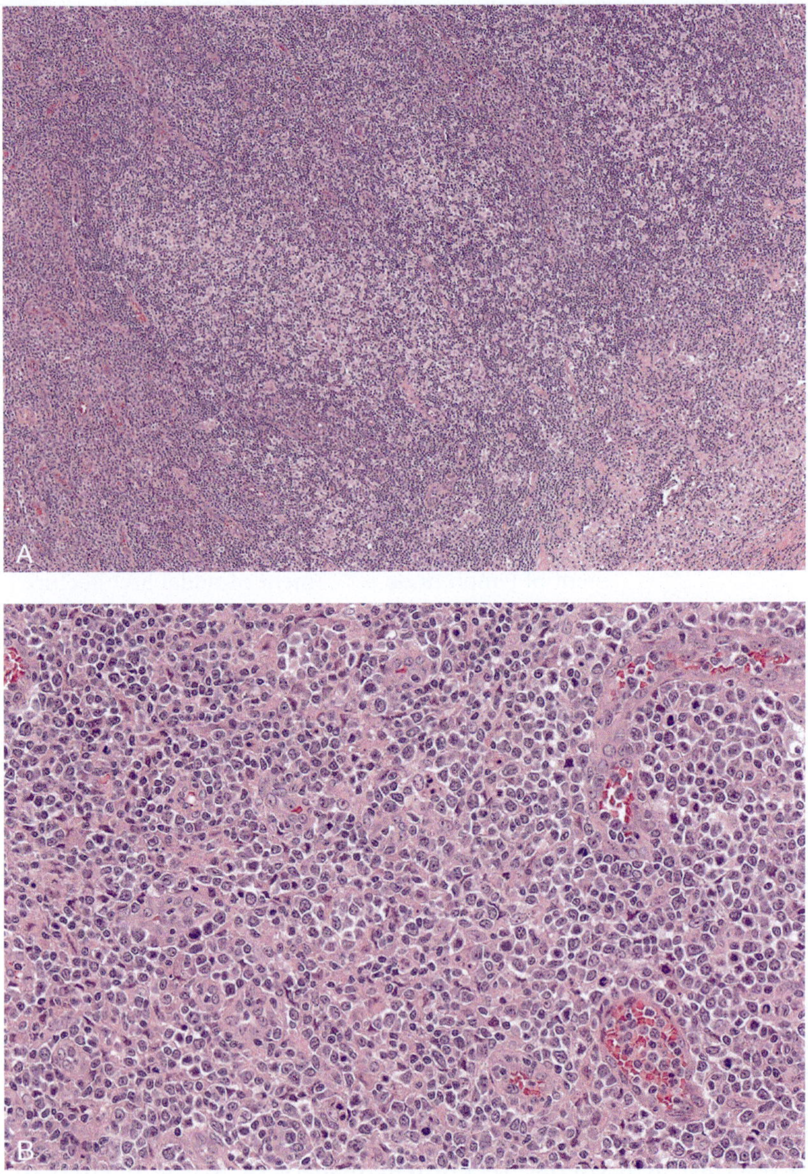

FIGURE 6.35 **Lymph node involved by mycosis fungoides.** Prominent dermatopathic change is seen in some areas (A), while the others show sheets of lymphoma cells (B).

REFERENCES

1. Medeiros LJ. *Ioachim's Lymph Node Pathology*. 5th ed. Wolters Kluwer; 2021.
2. Campo E, Jaffe ES, Cook JR, et al. The International Consensus Classification of Mature Lymphoid Neoplasms: a report from the Clinical Advisory Committee. *Blood.* 2022;140(11):1229-1253.
3. Vega F, Medeiros LJ. A suggested immunohistochemical algorithm for the classification of T-cell lymphomas involving lymph nodes. *Hum Pathol.* 2020;102:104-116.
4. Swerdlow SH, Campo E, Harris NL, et al. *WHO Classification of Tumours of Haematopoietic and Lymphoid Tissues*. IARC; 2017.
5. Shea L, Mehta-Shah N. Brentuximab vedotin in the treatment of peripheral T cell lymphoma and cutaneous T cell lymphoma. *Curr Hematol Malig Rep*. 2020;15(1):9-19.
6. Morton LM, Wang SS, Devesa SS, Hartge P, Weisenburger DD, Linet MS. Lymphoma incidence patterns by WHO subtype in the United States, 1992-2001. *Blood.* 2006;107(1):265-276.
7. Weisenburger DD, Savage KJ, Harris NL, et al. Peripheral T-cell lymphoma, not otherwise specified: a report of 340 cases from the International Peripheral T-cell Lymphoma Project. *Blood*. 2011;117(12):3402-3408.
8. Kurita D, Miyoshi H, Yoshida N, et al. A clinicopathologic study of Lennert lymphoma and possible prognostic factors: the importance of follicular helper T-cell markers and the association with angioimmunoblastic T-cell lymphoma. *Am J Surg Pathol.* 2016;40(9):1249-1260.
9. Etebari M, Navari M, Agostinelli C, et al. Transcriptional analysis of Lennert lymphoma reveals a unique profile and identifies novel therapeutic targets. *Front Genet.* 2019;10:780.
10. Berg H, Otteson GE, Corley H, et al. Flow cytometric evaluation of TRBC1 expression in tissue specimens and body fluids is a novel and specific method for assessment of T-cell clonality and diagnosis of T-cell neoplasms. *Cytometry B Clin Cytom.* 2021;100(3):361-369.
11. Jaffe ESAD, Campo E, Harris NL, Quintanilla-Martinez L. *Hematopathology*. 2nd ed. Elsevier; 2017.
12. Heavican TB, Bouska A, Yu J, et al. Genetic drivers of oncogenic pathways in molecular subgroups of peripheral T-cell lymphoma. *Blood*. 2019;133(15):1664-1676.
13. Nicolae A, Bouilly J, Lara D, et al. Nodal cytotoxic peripheral T-cell lymphoma occurs frequently in the clinical setting of immunodysregulation and is associated with recurrent epigenetic alterations. *Mod Pathol*. 2022;35(8):1126-1136.
14. Dupuis J, Emile JF, Mounier N, et al. Prognostic significance of Epstein-Barr virus in nodal peripheral T-cell lymphoma, unspecified: a Groupe d'Etude des Lymphomes de l'Adulte (GELA) study. *Blood*. 2006;108(13):4163-4169.
15. Kato S, Yamashita D, Nakamura S. Nodal EBV+ cytotoxic T-cell lymphoma: a literature review based on the 2017 WHO classification. *J Clin Exp Hematop*. 2020;60(2):30-36.
16. Nelson M, Horsman DE, Weisenburger DD, et al. Cytogenetic abnormalities and clinical correlations in peripheral T-cell lymphoma. *Br J Haematol*. 2008;141(4):461-469.
17. Amador C, Greiner TC, Heavican TB, et al. Reproducing the molecular subclassification of peripheral T-cell lymphoma-NOS by immunohistochemistry. *Blood*. 2019;134(24):2159-2170.
18. Dobay MP, Lemonnier F, Missiaglia E, et al. Integrative clinicopathological and molecular analyses of angioimmunoblastic T-cell lymphoma and other nodal lymphomas of follicular helper T-cell origin. *Haematologica*. 2017;102(4):e148-e151.
19. Basha BM, Bryant SC, Rech KL, et al. Application of a 5 marker panel to the routine diagnosis of peripheral T-cell lymphoma with T-follicular helper phenotype. *Am J Surg Pathol*. 2019;43(9):1282-1290.

20. Rudiger T, Weisenburger DD, Anderson JR, et al. Peripheral T-cell lymphoma (excluding anaplastic large-cell lymphoma): results from the Non-Hodgkin's Lymphoma Classification Project. *Ann Oncol.* 2002;13(1):140-149.
21. de Leval L, Parrens M, Le Bras F, et al. Angioimmunoblastic T-cell lymphoma is the most common T-cell lymphoma in two distinct French information data sets. *Haematologica.* 2015;100(9):e361-e364.
22. de Leval L. Approach to nodal-based T-cell lymphomas. *Pathology.* 2020;52(1):78-99.
23. Federico M, Rudiger T, Bellei M, et al. Clinicopathologic characteristics of angioimmunoblastic T-cell lymphoma: analysis of the international peripheral T-cell lymphoma project. *J Clin Oncol.* 2013;31(2):240-246.
24. Tan LH, Tan SY, Tang T, et al. Angioimmunoblastic T-cell lymphoma with hyperplastic germinal centres (pattern 1) shows superior survival to patterns 2 and 3: a meta-analysis of 56 cases. *Histopathology.* 2012;60(4):570-585.
25. Merchant SH, Amin MB, Viswanatha DS. Morphologic and immunophenotypic analysis of angioimmunoblastic T-cell lymphoma: emphasis on phenotypic aberrancies for early diagnosis. *Am J Clin Pathol.* 2006;126(1):29-38.
26. Nicolae A, Pittaluga S, Venkataraman G, et al. Peripheral T-cell lymphomas of follicular T-helper cell derivation with Hodgkin/Reed-Sternberg cells of B-cell lineage: both EBV-positive and EBV-negative variants exist. *Am J Surg Pathol.* 2013;37(6):816-826.
27. Willenbrock K, Brauninger A, Hansmann ML. Frequent occurrence of B-cell lymphomas in angioimmunoblastic T-cell lymphoma and proliferation of Epstein-Barr virus-infected cells in early cases. *Br J Haematol.* 2007;138(6):733-739.
28. Shah ZH, Harris S, Smith JL, Hodges E. Monoclonality and oligoclonality of T cell receptor beta gene in angioimmunoblastic T cell lymphoma. *J Clin Pathol.* 2009;62(2):177-181.
29. Vallois D, Dobay MP, Morin RD, et al. Activating mutations in genes related to TCR signaling in angioimmunoblastic and other follicular helper T-cell-derived lymphomas. *Blood.* 2016;128(11):1490-1502.
30. Sakata-Yanagimoto M, Enami T, Yoshida K, et al. Somatic RHOA mutation in angioimmunoblastic T cell lymphoma. *Nat Genet.* 2014;46(2):171-175.
31. Wang C, McKeithan TW, Gong Q, et al. IDH2R172 mutations define a unique subgroup of patients with angioimmunoblastic T-cell lymphoma. *Blood.* 2015;126(15):1741-1752.
32. Fujisawa M, Sakata-Yanagimoto M, Nishizawa S, et al. Activation of RHOA-VAV1 signaling in angioimmunoblastic T-cell lymphoma. *Leukemia.* 2018;32(3):694-702.
33. Hu S, Young KH, Konoplev SN, Medeiros LJ. Follicular T-cell lymphoma: a member of an emerging family of follicular helper T-cell derived T-cell lymphomas. *Hum Pathol.* 2012;43(11):1789-1798.
34. Moroch J, Copie-Bergman C, de Leval L, et al. Follicular peripheral T-cell lymphoma expands the spectrum of classical Hodgkin lymphoma mimics. *Am J Surg Pathol.* 2012;36(11):1636-1646.
35. Ikonomou IM, Tierens A, Troen G, et al. Peripheral T-cell lymphoma with involvement of the expanded mantle zone. *Virchows Arch.* 2006;449(1):78-87.
36. Streubel B, Vinatzer U, Willheim M, Raderer M, Chott A. Novel t(5;9)(q33;q22) fuses ITK to SYK in unspecified peripheral T-cell lymphoma. *Leukemia.* 2006;20(2):313-318.
37. Attygalle AD, Feldman AL, Dogan A. ITK/SYK translocation in angioimmunoblastic T-cell lymphoma. *Am J Surg Pathol.* 2013;37(9):1456-1457.
38. Hapgood G, Savage KJ. The biology and management of systemic anaplastic large cell lymphoma. *Blood.* 2015;126(1):17-25.
39. Sibon D, Nguyen DP, Schmitz N, et al. ALK-positive anaplastic large-cell lymphoma in adults: an individual patient data pooled analysis of 263 patients. *Haematologica.* 2019;104(12):e562-e565.

40. d'Amore ES, Menin A, Bonoldi E, et al. Anaplastic large cell lymphomas: a study of 75 pediatric patients. *Pediatr Dev Pathol*. 2007;10(3):181-191.
41. Montes-Mojarro IA, Steinhilber J, Bonzheim I, Quintanilla-Martinez L, Fend F. The pathological spectrum of systemic anaplastic large cell lymphoma (ALCL). *Cancers (Basel)*. 2018;10(4):107.
42. Vassallo J, Lamant L, Brugieres L, et al. ALK-positive anaplastic large cell lymphoma mimicking nodular sclerosis Hodgkin's lymphoma: report of 10 cases. *Am J Surg Pathol*. 2006;30(2):223-229.
43. Falini B, Bigerna B, Fizzotti M, et al. ALK expression defines a distinct group of T/null lymphomas ("ALK lymphomas") with a wide morphological spectrum. *Am J Pathol*. 1998;153(3):875-886.
44. Klapper W, Bohm M, Siebert R, Lennert K. Morphological variability of lymphohistiocytic variant of anaplastic large cell lymphoma (former lymphohistiocytic lymphoma according to the Kiel classification). *Virchows Arch*. 2008;452(6):599-605.
45. Pulford K, Lamant L, Espinos E, et al. The emerging normal and disease-related roles of anaplastic lymphoma kinase. *Cell Mol Life Sci*. 2004;61(23):2939-2953.
46. Casanova M, Brennan B, Alaggio R, et al. Inflammatory myofibroblastic tumor: the experience of the European pediatric Soft Tissue Sarcoma Study Group (EpSSG). *Eur J Cancer*. 2020;127:123-129.
47. Perez-Pinera P, Chang Y, Astudillo A, Mortimer J, Deuel TF. Anaplastic lymphoma kinase is expressed in different subtypes of human breast cancer. *Biochem Biophys Res Commun*. 2007;358(2):399-403.
48. Lamant L, de Reynies A, Duplantier MM, et al. Gene-expression profiling of systemic anaplastic large-cell lymphoma reveals differences based on ALK status and two distinct morphologic ALK+ subtypes. *Blood*. 2007;109(5):2156-2164.
49. Iqbal J, Wright G, Wang C, et al. Gene expression signatures delineate biological and prognostic subgroups in peripheral T-cell lymphoma. *Blood*. 2014;123(19):2915-2923.
50. Parrilla Castellar ER, Jaffe ES, Said JW, et al. ALK-negative anaplastic large cell lymphoma is a genetically heterogeneous disease with widely disparate clinical outcomes. *Blood*. 2014;124(9):1473-1480.
51. Shustov A, Cabrera ME, Civallero M, et al. ALK-negative anaplastic large cell lymphoma: features and outcomes of 235 patients from the International T-Cell Project. *Blood Adv*. 2021;5(3):640-648.
52. Savage KJ, Harris NL, Vose JM, et al. ALK- anaplastic large-cell lymphoma is clinically and immunophenotypically different from both ALK+ ALCL and peripheral T-cell lymphoma, not otherwise specified: report from the International Peripheral T-Cell Lymphoma Project. *Blood*. 2008;111(12):5496-5504.
53. Fratoni S, Niscola P, Zhao XF, et al. ALK-negative anaplastic large cell lymphoma with "Hodgkin-like" cytomorphology and nuclear expression of PAX5. *Pathol Res Pract*. 2020;216(2):152724.
54. Feldman AL, Law ME, Inwards DJ, Dogan A, McClure RF, Macon WR. PAX5-positive T-cell anaplastic large cell lymphomas associated with extra copies of the PAX5 gene locus. *Mod Pathol*. 2010;23(4):593-602.
55. Hapgood G, Ben-Neriah S, Mottok A, et al. Identification of high-risk DUSP22-rearranged ALK-negative anaplastic large cell lymphoma. *Br J Haematol*. 2019;186(3):e28-e31.
56. King RL, Dao LN, McPhail ED, et al. Morphologic features of ALK-negative anaplastic large cell lymphomas with DUSP22 rearrangements. *Am J Surg Pathol*. 2016;40(1):36-43.
57. Onaindia A, de Villambrosia SG, Prieto-Torres L, et al. DUSP22-rearranged anaplastic lymphomas are characterized by specific morphological features and a lack of cytotoxic and JAK/STAT surrogate markers. *Haematologica*. 2019;104(4):e158-e162.
58. Crescenzo R, Abate F, Lasorsa E, et al. Convergent mutations and kinase fusions lead to oncogenic STAT3 activation in anaplastic large cell lymphoma. *Cancer Cell*. 2015;27(4):516-532.

59. Taylor AM, Metcalfe JA, Thick J, Mak YF. Leukemia and lymphoma in ataxia telangiectasia. *Blood.* 1996;87(2):423-438.
60. Matutes E, Brito-Babapulle V, Swansbury J, et al. Clinical and laboratory features of 78 cases of T-prolymphocytic leukemia. *Blood.* 1991;78(12):3269-3274.
61. Dearden C. How I treat prolymphocytic leukemia. *Blood.* 2012;120(3):538-551.
62. Hoyer JD, Ross CW, Li CY, et al. True T-cell chronic lymphocytic leukemia: a morphologic and immunophenotypic study of 25 cases. *Blood.* 1995;86(3):1163-1169.
63. Valbuena JR, Herling M, Admirand JH, Padula A, Jones D, Medeiros LJ. T-cell prolymphocytic leukemia involving extramedullary sites. *Am J Clin Pathol.* 2005;123(3):456-464.
64. Maljaei SH, Brito-Babapulle V, Hiorns LR, Catovsky D. Abnormalities of chromosomes 8, 11, 14, and X in T-prolymphocytic leukemia studied by fluorescence in situ hybridization. *Cancer Genet Cytogenet.* 1998;103(2):110-116.
65. Delgado P, Starshak P, Rao N, Tirado CA. A comprehensive update on molecular and cytogenetic abnormalities in T-cell prolymphocytic leukemia (T-pll). *J Assoc Genet Technol.* 2012;38(4):193-198.
66. Kiel MJ, Velusamy T, Rolland D, et al. Integrated genomic sequencing reveals mutational landscape of T-cell prolymphocytic leukemia. *Blood.* 2014;124(9):1460-1472.
67. Shah UA, Shah N, Qiao B, et al. Epidemiology and survival trend of adult T-cell leukemia/lymphoma in the United States. *Cancer.* 2020;126(3):567-574.
68. Malpica L, Pimentel A, Reis IM, et al. Epidemiology, clinical features, and outcome of HTLV-1-related ATLL in an area of prevalence in the United States. *Blood Adv.* 2018;2(6):607-620.
69. Adkins BD, Ramos JC, Bliss-Moreau M, Gru AA. Updates in lymph node and skin pathology of adult T-cell leukemia/lymphoma, biomarkers, and beyond. *Semin Diagn Pathol.* 2020;37(1):1-10.
70. Khanlari M, Ramos JC, Sanchez SP, et al. Adult T-cell leukemia/lymphoma can be indistinguishable from other more common T-cell lymphomas. The University of Miami experience with a large cohort of cases. *Mod Pathol.* 2018;31(7):1046-1063.
71. Ohshima K, Kikuchi M, Yoshida T, Masuda Y, Kimura N. Lymph nodes in incipient adult T-cell leukemia-lymphoma with Hodgkin's disease-like histologic features. *Cancer.* 1991;67(6):1622-1628.
72. Korgavkar K, Xiong M, Weinstock M. Changing incidence trends of cutaneous T-cell lymphoma. *JAMA Dermatol.* 2013;149(11):1295-1299.
73. Olsen E, Vonderheid E, Pimpinelli N, et al. Revisions to the staging and classification of mycosis fungoides and Sezary syndrome: a proposal of the International Society for Cutaneous Lymphomas (ISCL) and the cutaneous lymphoma task force of the European Organization of Research and Treatment of Cancer (EORTC). *Blood.* 2007;110(6):1713-1722.
74. Scheffer E, Meijer CJ, van Vloten WA, Willemze R. A histologic study of lymph nodes from patients with the Sezary syndrome. *Cancer.* 1986;57(12):2375-2380.
75. Sausville EA, Worsham GF, Matthews MJ, et al. Histologic assessment of lymph nodes in mycosis fungoides/Sezary syndrome (cutaneous T-cell lymphoma): clinical correlations and prognostic import of a new classification system. *Hum Pathol.* 1985;16(11):1098-1109.
76. Assaf C, Hummel M, Steinhoff M, et al. Early TCR-beta and TCR-gamma PCR detection of T-cell clonality indicates minimal tumor disease in lymph nodes of cutaneous T-cell lymphoma: diagnostic and prognostic implications. *Blood.* 2005;105(2):503-510.
77. Juarez T, Isenhath SN, Polissar NL, et al. Analysis of T-cell receptor gene rearrangement for predicting clinical outcome in patients with cutaneous T-cell lymphoma: a comparison of Southern blot and polymerase chain reaction methods. *Arch Dermatol.* 2005;141(9):1107-1113.

7

CLASSIC HODGKIN LYMPHOMA AND NODULAR LYMPHOCYTE PREDOMINANT B-CELL LYMPHOMA

LAUREN B. SMITH

Hodgkin lymphoma has historically been separated into classic Hodgkin lymphoma (CHL), which accounts for the vast majority of cases, and nodular lymphocyte predominant Hodgkin lymphoma (NLPHL), which comprises 5% of cases. NLPHL was recently removed from the Hodgkin category by the 2022 International Consensus Classification (ICC) but still remains in the Hodgkin category in the World Health Organization Classification.[1] The ICC 2022 now refers to it as nodular lymphocyte predominant B-cell lymphoma (NLPBL).[2] Regardless of the name, this entity differs from CHL in terms of biology and clinical behavior. Both entities will be discussed in this chapter.

Both CHL and NLPBL share some morphologic features including a paucity of neoplastic cells in an inflammatory background. In CHL, this background may consist of eosinophils, neutrophils, plasma cells, and histiocytes (in variable proportions depending on the subtype), while NLPBL contains a background rich in small lymphocytes and epithelioid histiocytes. The inflammatory background is of paramount importance and is required for appropriate subclassification. For this reason, small biopsies pose a challenge in both conditions, as there are a number of neoplastic and non-neoplastic mimickers, which contain Hodgkin/Reed-Sternberg (HRS)-like cells. Immunohistochemistry is essential for resolving the differential diagnosis, and in some cases a larger biopsy may be needed.

CLASSIC HODGKIN LYMPHOMA

CHL represents around 10% of all lymphoma cases in the United States.[3] Overall, it is more common in males than females, but females can outnumber males in late adolescence. It has a bimodal age of onset, with a first peak occurring in adolescents and young adults between 15 and 35 years of age and the second peak occurring after 50 years of age. The age of onset and clinical presentation of CHL depend on the morphologic subtype. Nodular sclerosis Hodgkin lymphoma (NSHL) comprises approximately 70% of CHL cases in Western countries and is more common in late adolescence and early adulthood. It often presents with a mediastinal mass with contiguous spread to other lymph node groups (eg, mediastinal to cervical), although in the elderly it may have an unusual presentation including retroperitoneal involvement (with or without disease above the diaphragm) and/or bone marrow involvement.[4] Mixed-cellularity Hodgkin lymphoma (MCHL) comprises 20% to 25% of CHL, has a median age of presentation in the fourth decade, and is the most common CHL subtype associated with human immunodeficiency virus (HIV) infection. This subtype also occurs in elderly individuals. Lymphocyte-rich Hodgkin lymphoma (LRHL) is uncommon (5% of all CHL cases) and typically occurs in middle-aged patients. Lymphocyte-depleted CHL (LDHL) is rarely seen (fewer than 1% of cases), and is often diagnosed in the setting of HIV infection with widespread disease. Patients with all types of CHL may present with B-symptoms including fever and night sweats. Pruritus is also common.[5] CHL is primarily a nodal disease that may spread to extranodal sites including spleen, liver, and bone marrow in advanced disease. Involvement of Waldeyer ring, skin, and the tubular gastrointestinal tract is extremely rare, and other differential diagnoses should strongly be considered in these sites.

Morphology

There are four morphologic subtypes of CHL (NSHL, MCHL, LRHL, LDHL) as detailed above. It may be very challenging to subtype CHL on a small core biopsy; however, this is not critically important, since the morphologic subtype does not affect treatment or prognosis significantly with modern therapy.[6]

NSHL typically shows a thickened lymph node capsule and large nodules surrounded by collagen bands (Figure 7.1). The nodules contain a mixed inflammatory infiltrate including variable numbers of lymphocytes, plasma cells, histiocytes, eosinophils, and neutrophils. In addition to the inflammatory cells, there are variable numbers of large, atypical, HRS cells. In NSHL, the HRS cells are often lacunar cells, characterized by retraction of the cytoplasm, which makes a space or lacunae around the cell with wisps of cytoplasm spanning the space (Figure 7.2A and B). The lacunar cells have either single or multiple nuclei, often with prominent nucleoli. "Lacunae" are an artifact of formalin fixation. Other HRS cells that can be seen in NSHL include mummified cells, in which the nuclei are eosinophilic and pyknotic with limited nuclear detail and irregular nuclear outlines (Figure 7.3). Hodgkin cells are uninucleate HRS cells that have a prominent cherry-red nucleolus (Figure 7.4). Occasionally, true Reed-Sternberg cells can be seen in NSHL. These are binucleated with

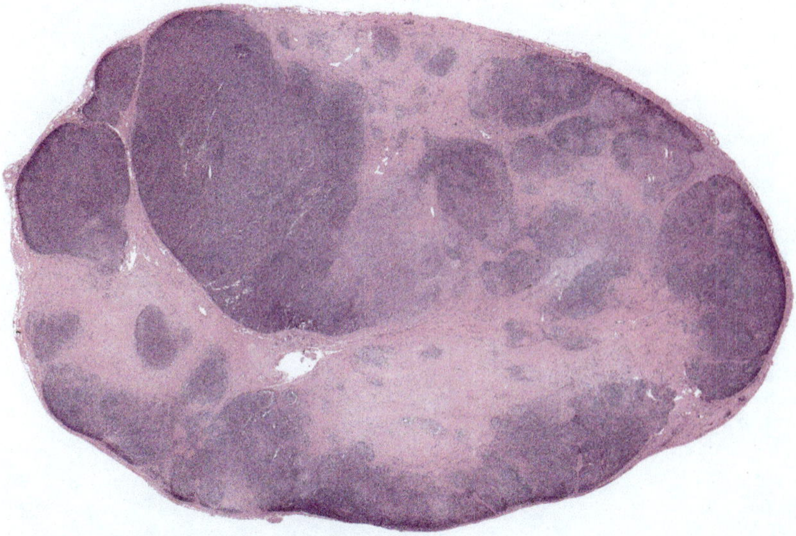

FIGURE 7.1 **Nodular sclerosis Hodgkin lymphoma.** Lymph node with thickened capsule and large nodules surrounded by collagen bands.

prominent nucleoli (Figure 7.5). Multinucleated HRS cells can frequently be seen too (Figure 7.6). Occasional cases of NSHL show cohesive sheets of neoplastic cells, frequently associated with necrosis, the so-called syncytial variant (Figures 7.7 and 7.8). In early NSHL (the so-called cellular phase), the nodules may be less apparent and only early or focal sclerosis is seen. These cases may resemble LRHL.

MCHL shows scattered HRS cells (usually Hodgkin and Reed-Sternberg type) in a mixed inflammatory background, the composition of which varies on a case-by-case basis. Some biopsies may have more small lymphocytes and sheets of histiocytes, whereas others have numerous admixed eosinophils and plasma cells (Figure 7.9). It may be difficult to differentiate NSHL and MCHL on a small core biopsy.

LRHL represents a minority of CHL cases and is uncommonly encountered in routine clinical practice. Morphologically, diffuse and nodular variants exist. In the nodular variant, nodules/follicles with regressed germinal centers and expanded mantle zones are seen, which may sometimes be a clue in helping to distinguish it from NLPBL (Figure 7.10). The HRS cells are often seen within the prominent mantle zones (Figure 7.11) and sometimes may resemble the lymphocyte-predominant (LP) cells seen in NLPBL (Figure 7.12). Other HRS variants, including Hodgkin cells, true Reed-Sternberg cells, and mummified cells, can also be seen. The diffuse variant typically has a background of small lymphocytes and histiocytes and can resemble MCHL.

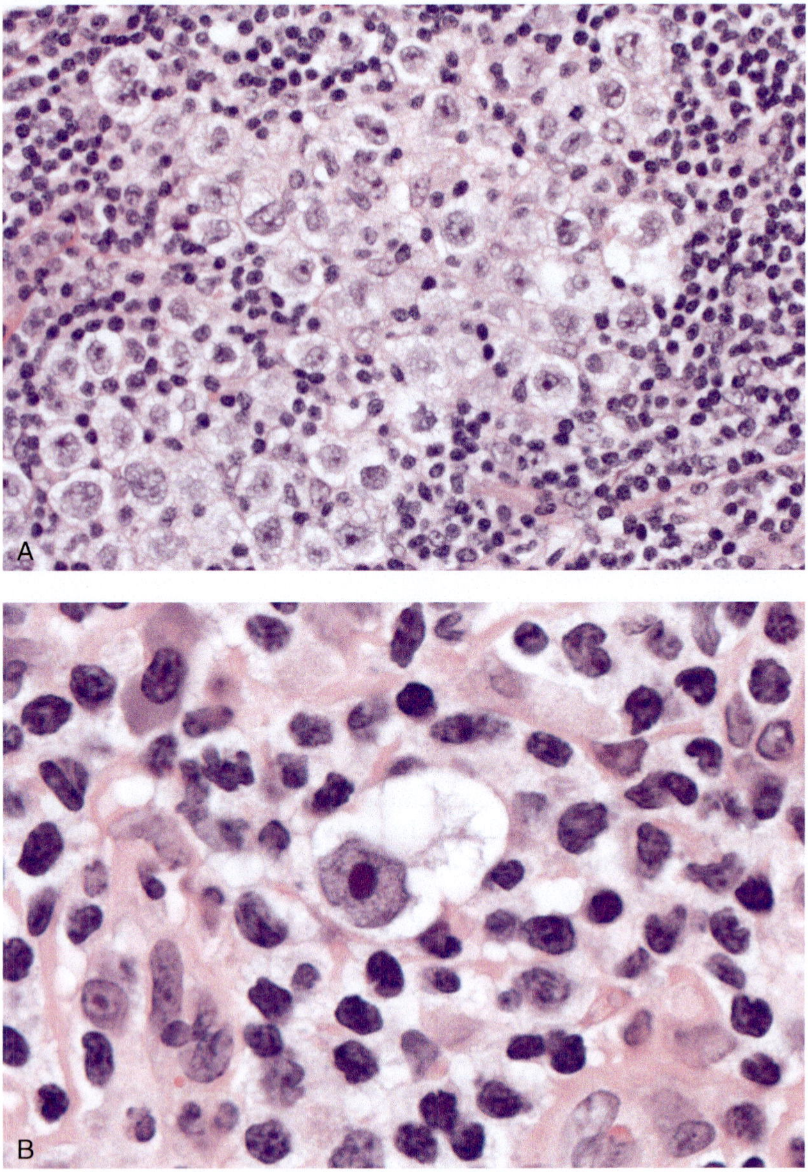

FIGURE 7.2 A, Cluster of lacunar cells in NSHL. B, Lacunar cell shows a prominent nucleolus, a space around the cell ("lacuna"), and wisps of cytoplasm.

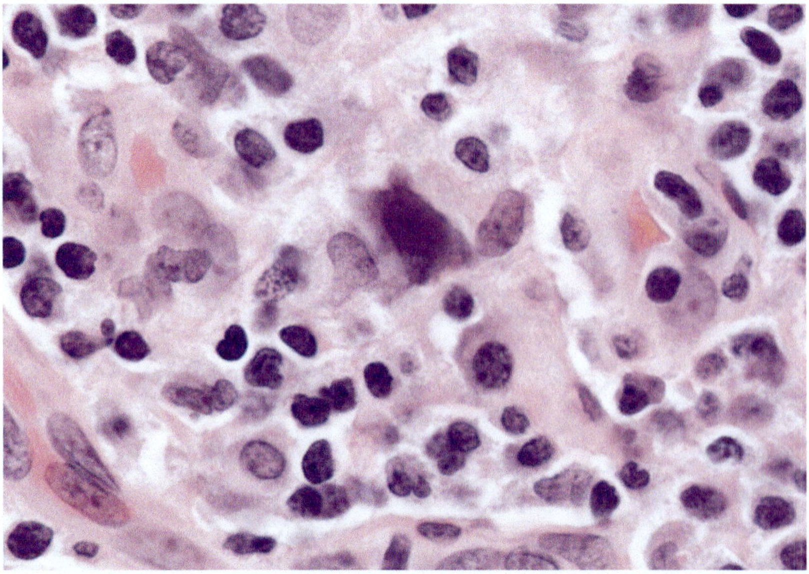

FIGURE 7.3 Mummified cell with eosinophilic nucleus with smudged appearance.

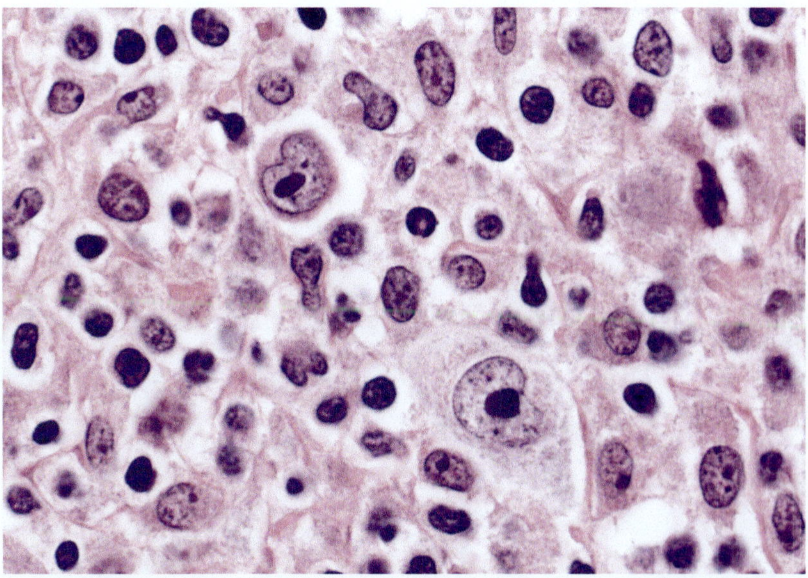

FIGURE 7.4 Hodgkin-type Hodgkin/Reed-Sternberg cells with prominent nucleoli.

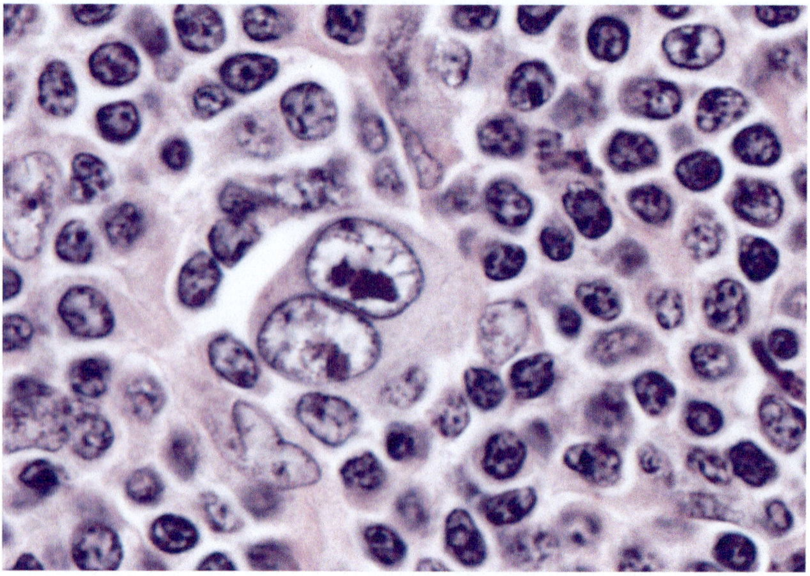

FIGURE 7.5 Classic Reed-Sternberg cell with binucleation and prominent nucleoli.

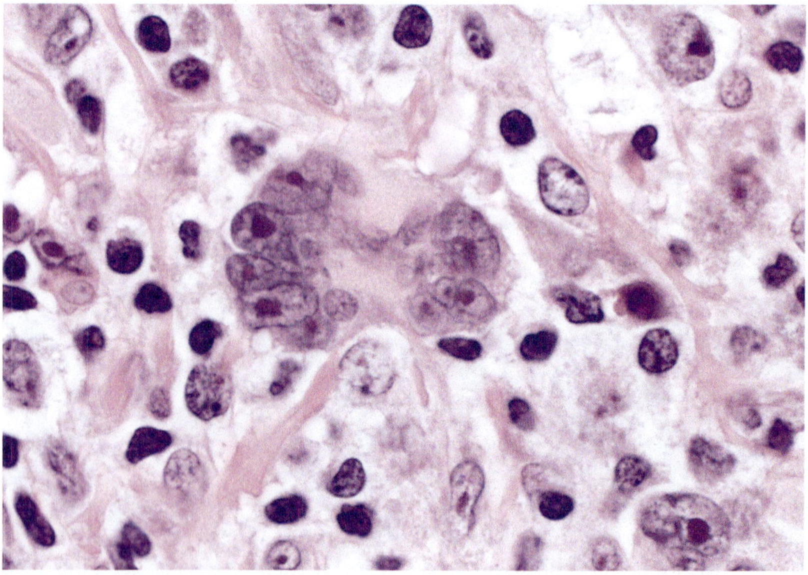

FIGURE 7.6 Multinucleated HRS cell.

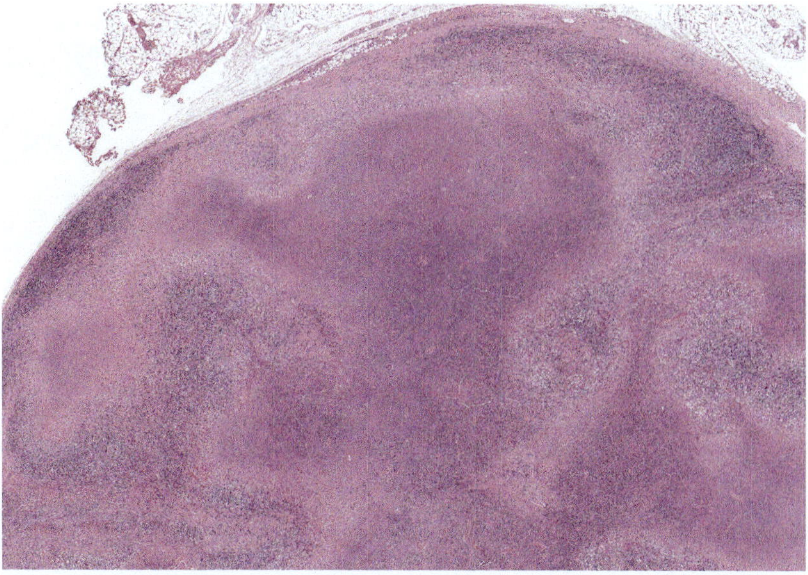

FIGURE 7.7 Syncytial variant of NSHL showing geographic areas of necrosis.

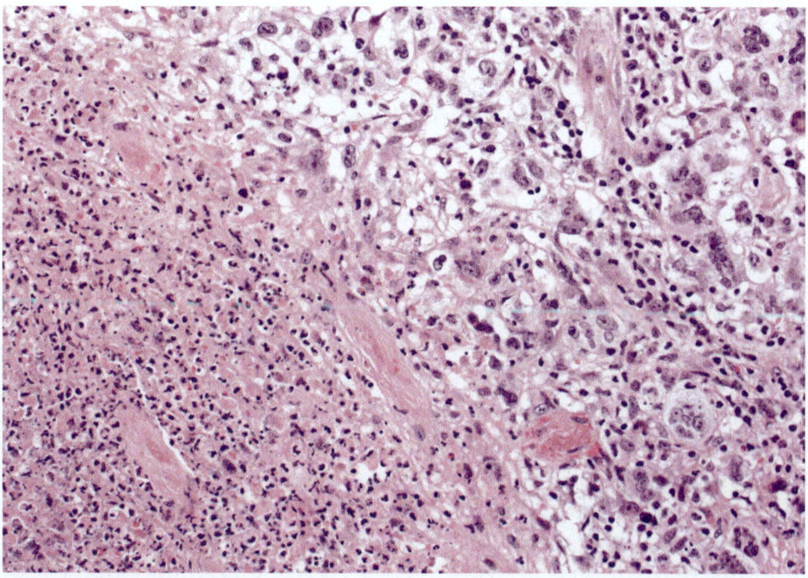

FIGURE 7.8 Necrosis in syncytial variant of NSHL (left) rimmed by HRS cells admixed with histiocytes.

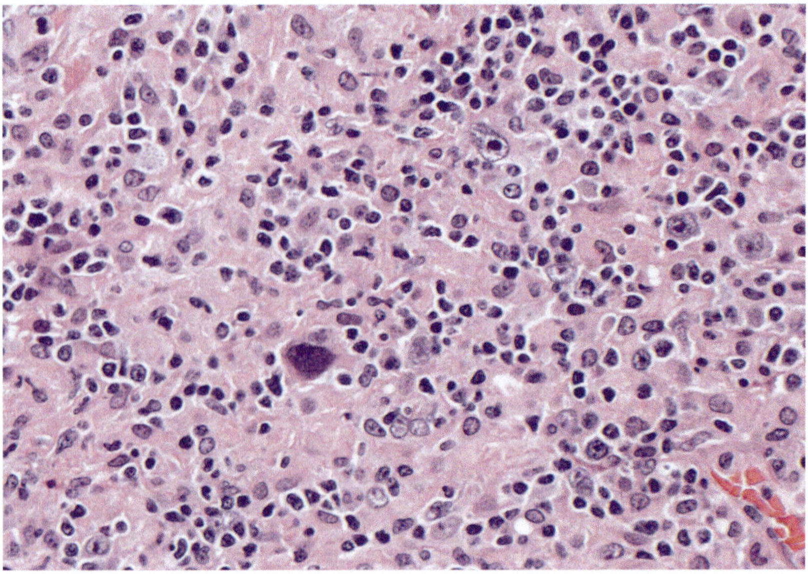

FIGURE 7.9 Mixed-cellularity Hodgkin lymphoma with scattered HRS cells (including a mummified cell), histiocytes, plasma cells, and small lymphocytes.

LDHL is vanishingly rare. Morphologically, it has a paucity of lymphocytes or mixed inflammatory cells. This makes it difficult to recognize as CHL since this disease, in many ways, is defined by the inflammatory background. In some cases, there is dense fibrosis and histiocytes with scattered neoplastic cells, and in other cases there are sheets of pleomorphic cells. The differential diagnosis on morphology alone includes diffuse large B-cell lymphoma (DLBCL), peripheral T-cell lymphoma, and nonhematopoietic neoplasms including sarcomas.

Phenotype

A useful basic battery of immunohistochemical studies in the evaluation of CHL includes CD20, CD3, PAX-5, CD30, and CD15. In difficult cases, an extended panel can be performed (Table 7.1). In virtually all cases, HRS cells are positive for CD30, usually in a membranous and Golgi-staining pattern (Figure 7.13A). CD15 is typically positive in fewer cells and may show only a Golgi staining pattern or may be negative (Figure 7.13B).[7] When interpreting immunohistochemical studies, it is important to remember that benign immunoblasts can be positive for CD30, and granulocytes (eosinophils/neutrophils) are positive for CD15. CD20 may mark a subset of cells, but usually only a fraction, and with variable intensity. CD20 is more often expressed in LRHL but may be present in the other subtypes.

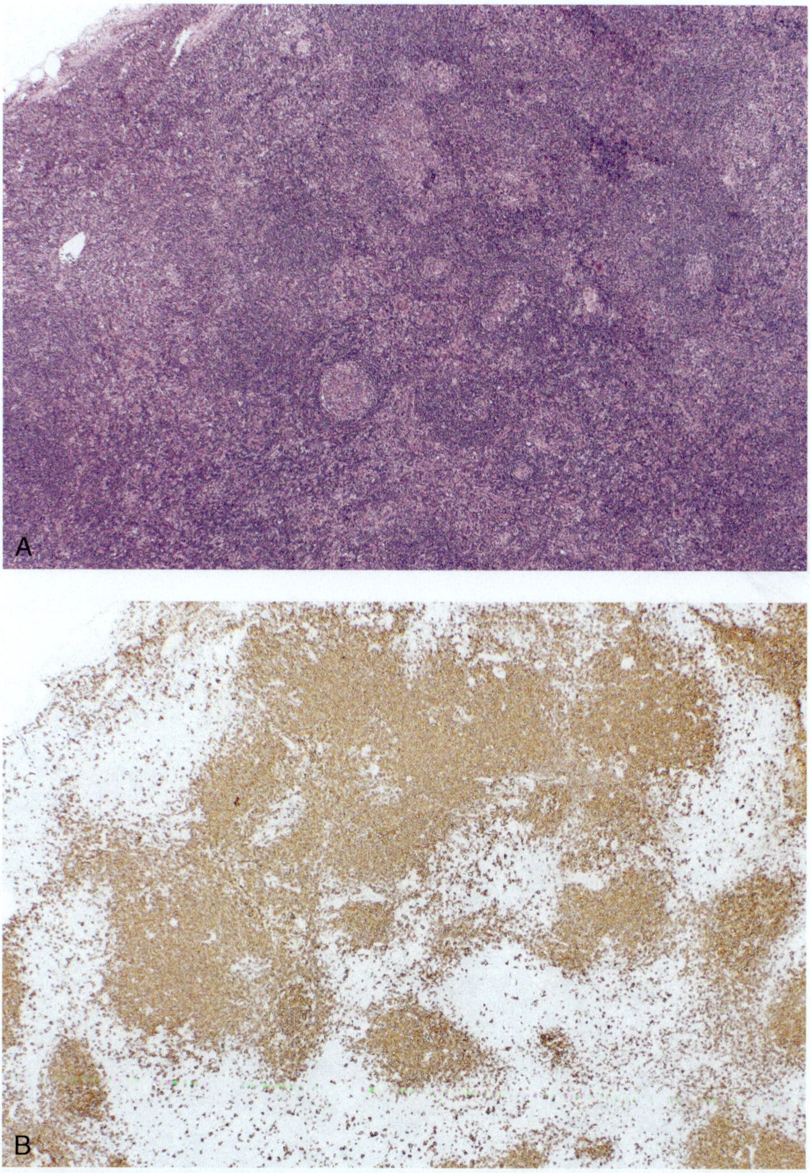

FIGURE 7.10 A, Lymphocyte-rich Hodgkin lymphoma showing distorted architecture by large nodules with expanded mantle zones and occasional small germinal centers. B, CD20 highlights the abnormal nodules rich in B cells.

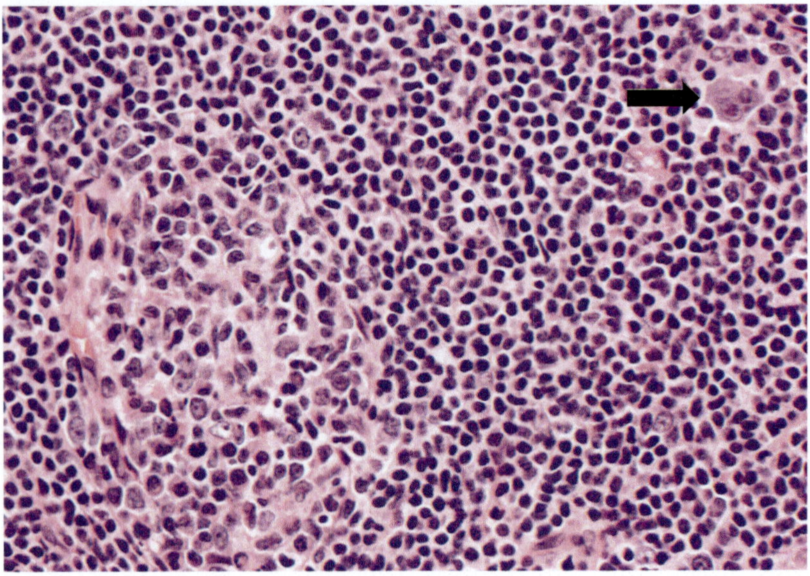

FIGURE 7.11 **Lymphocyte-rich Hodgkin lymphoma.** Regressively transformed germinal center and a Reed-Sternberg cell in the mantle zone (arrow).

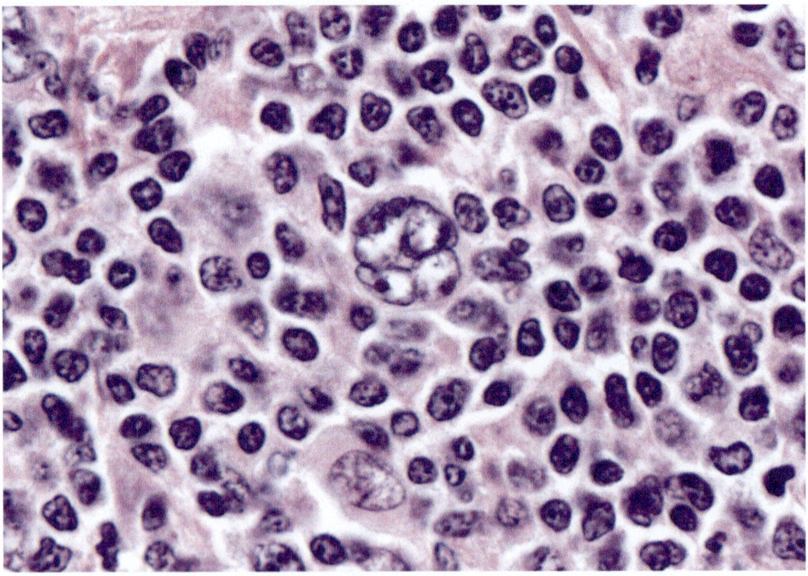

FIGURE 7.12 **HRS cell in LRHL that resembles lymphocyte-predominant cell.**

TABLE 7.1 Immunophenotypic Differences Between Classic Hodgkin Lymphoma and Nodular Lymphocyte predominant B-cell Lymphoma

Marker	CHL	NLPBL
CD20	–/+ (weak, variable)	+
CD30	+	–
CD15	+ (70%)	–
CD45 (LCA)	–	+
CD79a	–/+ (5%-10%)	+
PAX-5	+ (weak)	+
EMA	–	+/–
BOB.1	–/+	+
OCT-2	–/+	+
PU.1	–	+
MUM1	+	–
Fascin	+	–
EBER-ISH	+	–

Strong expression of CD20 may occur in a small percentage of cases and in itself is not sufficient to diagnose mediastinal gray zone lymphoma (see Chapter 5). PAX5 is a very important immunohistochemical stain because nearly all CHL cases are positive. Compared with the background small B cells, PAX5 is typically weaker on the HRS cells (Figure 7.13C). If PAX5 is negative, other diagnoses should be strongly considered including T-cell lymphomas. MUM1 is also positive in virtually all cases. The B-cell transcription factors are less commonly positive in CHL than NLPBL, where they are virtually always positive; however, it is important to know that OCT-2 and/or BOB.1 can be positive in CHL. PU.1 is the transcription factor that is least likely to be positive in CHL. Fascin is consistently positive in CHL, and if it is negative other diagnoses should be considered. However, fascin is positive in many entities and is not specific for CHL. Epstein-Barr encoding region in situ hybridization (EBER-ISH) is often positive in MCHL (75%), LDHL (75%), and in a smaller percentage of NSHL cases. It is nearly always positive in cases that are associated with immunodeficiency such as HIV infection or in the posttransplantation setting. Leukocyte common antigen (CD45/LCA) should be negative in CHL, but it may be difficult to interpret, as the background lymphocytes and histiocytes are positive. The background lymphocytes in CHL are usually CD3-positive T cells, typically with a marked predominance of CD4-positive over CD8-positive cells. HRS cells are negative for T-cell markers, although rare cases can show partial staining and this does not preclude the diagnosis (most commonly CD2 and CD4).[8] T cells usually predominate over background B cells in all subtypes except LRHL due to the presence of B-cell-rich follicles. CD3 will often show T-cell rosettes in LRHL, similar to what is seen in NLPBL.

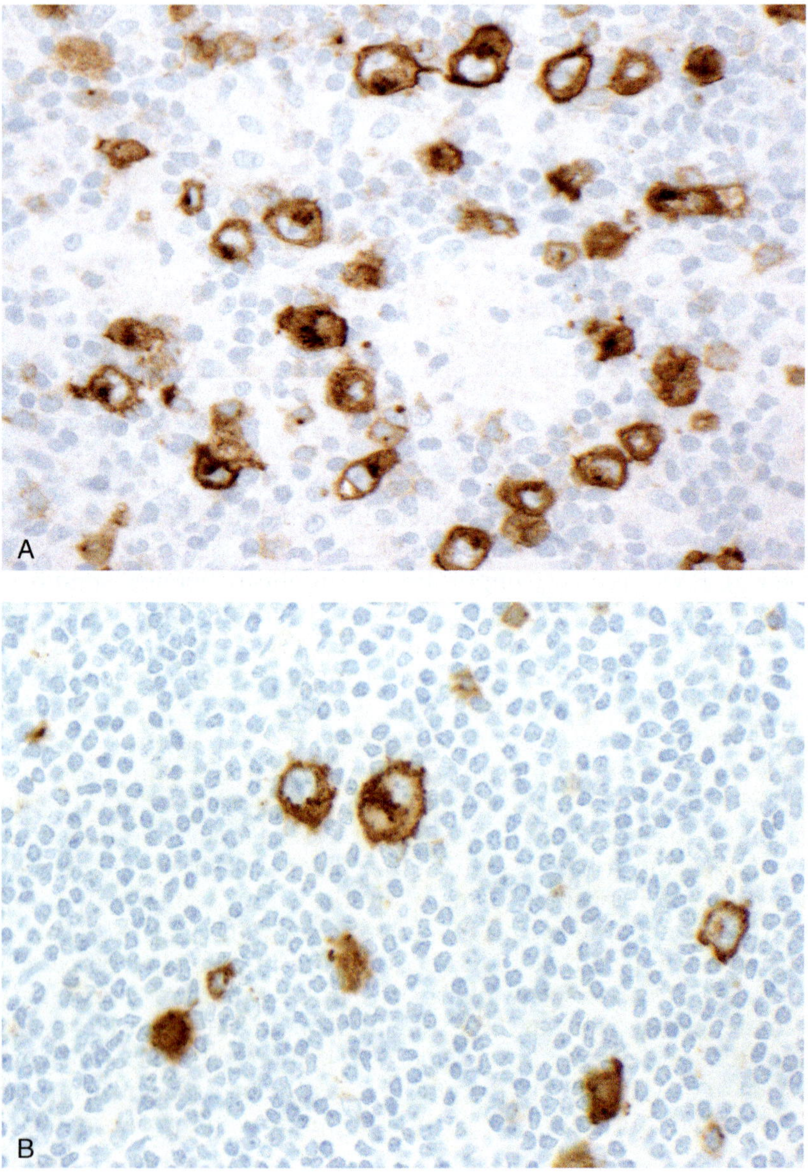

FIGURE 7.13 (*Continued*)

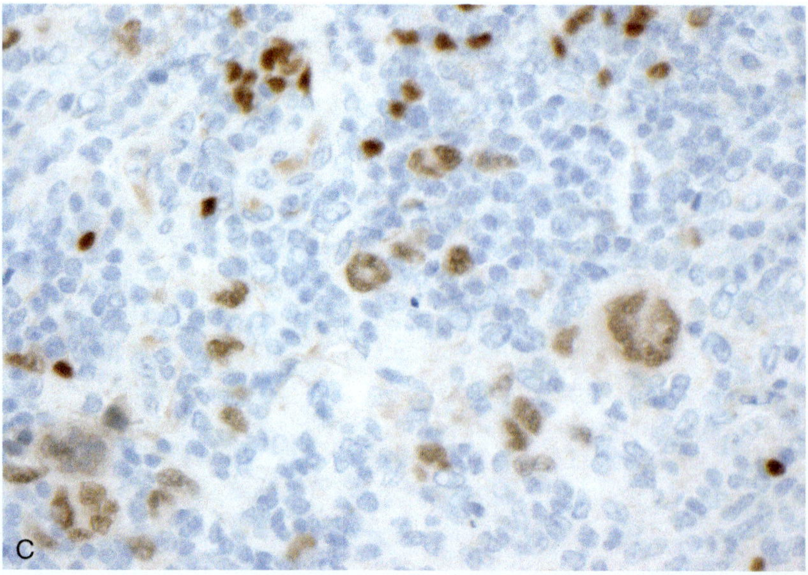

FIGURE 7.13 **Immunophenotype of CHL.** A, CD30 shows a membranous and Golgi staining pattern. B, CD15 typically marks fewer cells than CD30 and may show only Golgi staining in some cases. C, PAX5 weakly stains the HRS cells and more strongly marks the small B cells.

The differential diagnosis of CHL includes a number of entities, including both benign and neoplastic conditions (Table 7.2). Among the benign entities, EBV lymphadenitis (infectious mononucleosis) is a condition that may mimic CHL. EBV lymphadenitis often presents in a similar age group and may have significant systemic symptoms mimicking B symptoms. Elevations in liver enzymes, splenomegaly, and cytopenias may lead to clinical concern for lymphoma. Morphologically, EBV infection differs from CHL in that the lymph node architecture is typically distorted, but there is no effacement. It is characterized by a paracortical expansion, including numerous large mononuclear cells (some HRS-like) which are strongly staining with CD20 or CD3, as well as CD45. Rather than true HRS cells, they often resemble immunoblasts. EBER will show sheets of positive cells between the retained reactive follicles. CHL may also be confused with other infections including cat scratch disease and syphilis. Cat scratch disease will have large abscesses surrounded by histiocytes. Occasionally CHL will have syncytial areas that resemble cat scratch disease, but the center of these areas will contain necrosis as well as variable numbers of neutrophils (Figure 7.7). The HRS cells will be present among the histiocytes surrounding the necrosis (Figure 7.8). In syphilis, inguinal lymph nodes are more likely to be involved in isolation. This would be an unusual clinical presentation for CHL. The thickened capsule in syphilis can mimic CHL, but the parenchyma of the lymph node will contain prominent or florid follicular hyperplasia, which should not be seen in CHL. The capsule in syphilis will be infiltrated by plasma cells, but no HRS cells are seen.

TABLE 7.2 Differential Diagnosis of Classic Hodgkin Lymphoma

Benign entities
EBV lymphadenitis (infectious mononucleosis)
Cat scratch disease
Syphilis
Nodular lymphocyte predominant B-cell lymphoma
Mature B-cell lymphomas
EBV-positive diffuse large B-cell lymphoma, NOS
Primary mediastinal large B-cell lymphoma
Mediastinal gray zone lymphoma
Small B-cell lymphomas with Hodgkin-Reed/Sternberg-like cells
Mature T-cell lymphomas
Angioimmunoblastic T-cell lymphomas
Peripheral T-cell lymphoma, NOS
Anaplastic large cell lymphoma

CHL may be difficult to distinguish from NLPBL, particularly LRHL. LRHL is the only subtype of CHL in which small B cells are prominent in the background; therefore, the follicles in LRHL may be confused with the expanded nodules of small B cells in NLPBL. On morphology, the nodules of LRHL are often smaller and more moth-eaten in appearance than the ones in NLPBL, although this is difficult to appreciate on a core biopsy. In addition, NLPBL should generally not have germinal centers within the nodules. Rather, the residual reactive follicles are often pushed to the side of the node by the proliferation of large nodules. Importantly, the HRS cells in CHL cannot be reliably distinguished from LP cells seen in NLPBL based on cytologic features. However, in LRHL CD30 should be more strongly and uniformly expressed, while CD20 (if positive) is often weak and variable. CD45 will also be negative on the HRS cells in LRHL. Table 7.1 shows immunohistochemical stains and in situ studies that can be used to help differentiate CHL from NLPBL. It is important to remember, however, that no one stain will be decisive and ordering too many studies can lead to confusion.

Another important differential diagnosis to consider is EBV-positive DLBCL, not otherwise specified (NOS), which sometimes can morphologically resemble CHL (Figure 7.14), frequently expresses CD30, and can show a loss or weak expression of B-cell markers. In general, however, EBV-positive DLBCL, NOS shows stronger expression of B-cell markers than CHL, with multiple B-cell markers typically being positive (Figures 7.15 and 7.16). This differential can be very challenging, especially on limited tissue.

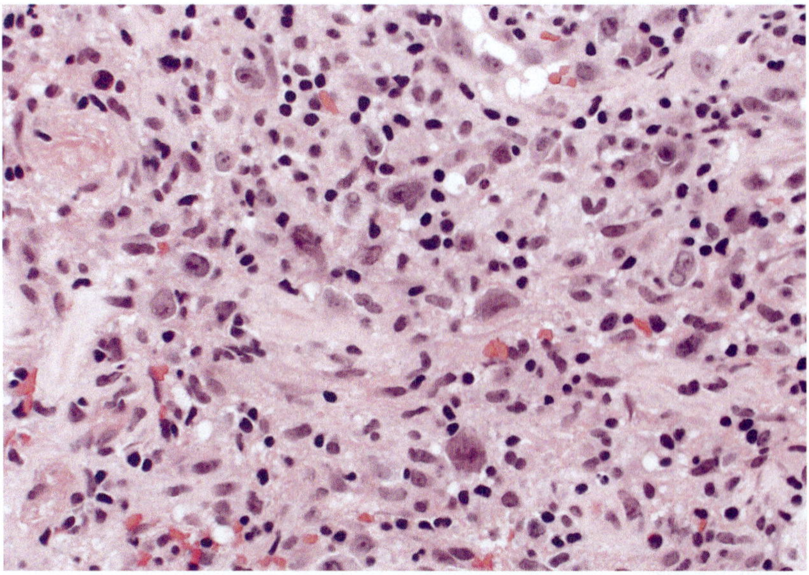

FIGURE 7.14 **EBV-positive diffuse large B-cell lymphoma, NOS.** Scattered HRS-like cells in a mixed inflammatory background, reminiscent of CHL.

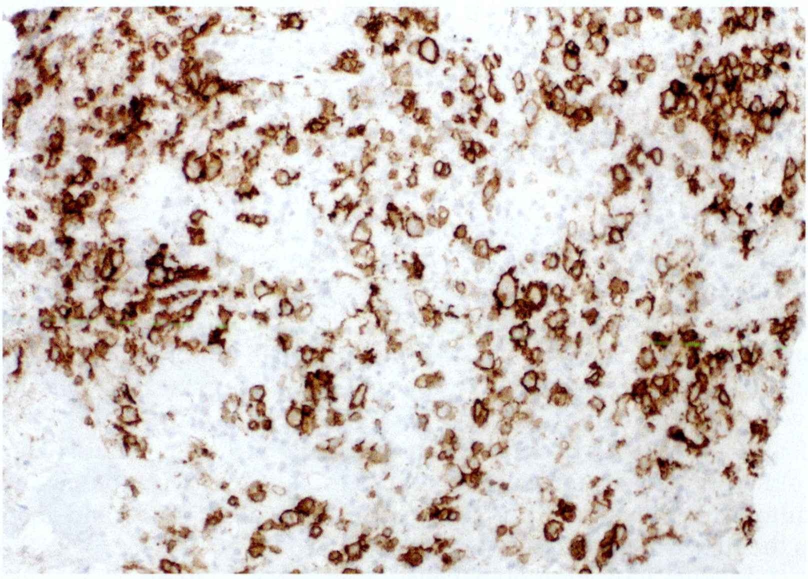

FIGURE 7.15 **EBV-positive diffuse large B-cell lymphoma, NOS.** The neoplastic cells are strongly positive for CD20. This case showed expression of multiple B-cell markers and CD45.

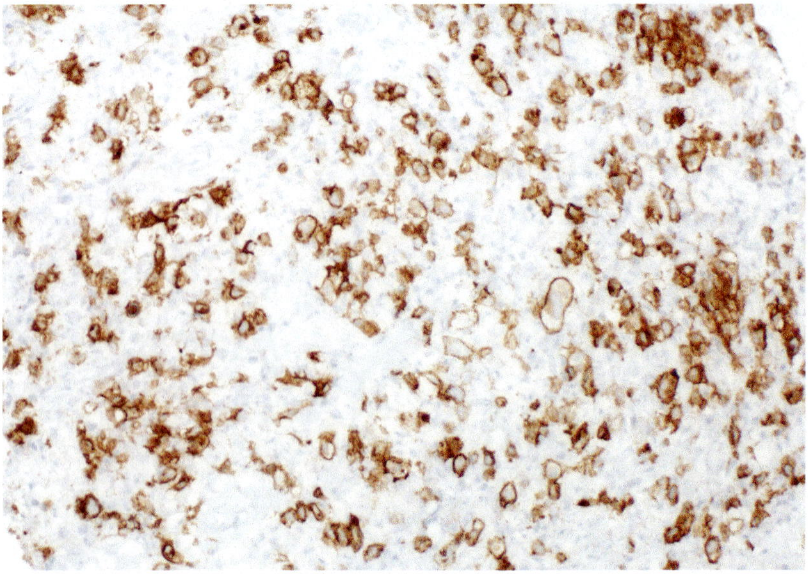

FIGURE 7.16 **EBV-positive diffuse large B-cell lymphoma, NOS.** The neoplastic cells are CD30 positive, a frequent finding in this entity.

CHL affects a similar patient population as primary mediastinal large B-cell lymphoma (PMBL) and is in the differential diagnosis in mediastinal mass biopsies, which are frequently limited and fibrotic. Morphologically, PMBL will have sclerosis that is alveolar/compartmentalizing rather than large nodules with dense fibrosis. Most importantly, the cases of PMBL will show sheets of large cells that are strongly positive for CD20. Another differential diagnosis that comes up in the mediastinum is mediastinal gray zone lymphoma, an extremely challenging entity on a limited biopsy, which is covered in more detail in Chapter 5.

Occasionally, small B-cell lymphomas may be confused with CHL when there are scattered HRS-like cells. This can occur in virtually any small B-cell non-Hodgkin lymphoma (NHL) but is most common in chronic lymphocytic leukemia/small lymphocytic lymphoma (CLL/SLL). It can also be seen in follicular lymphoma (FL), marginal zone lymphoma, and very rarely in mantle cell lymphoma (Figures 7.17-7.20).[9,10] The sheets of small and large CD20-positive B cells and lack of the characteristic mixed inflammatory background usually allows this distinction to be made with immunohistochemistry. CLL/SLL may transform to CHL, and in those cases the mixed inflammatory background should be present for definitive distinction from CLL with HRS cells.

Mature T-cell lymphomas (such as angioimmunoblastic T-cell lymphoma and peripheral T-cell lymphoma, NOS) are an important differential diagnosis in CHL, since they frequently contain HRS-like cells

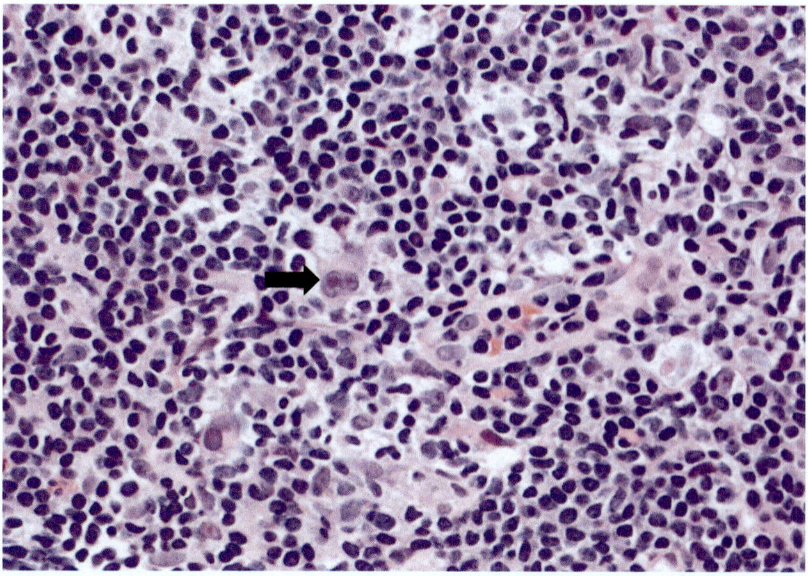

FIGURE 7.17 **Mantle cell lymphoma with HRS-like cells.** Scattered HRS-like cells (arrow) are seen in the background of small lymphoma cells in this rare case.

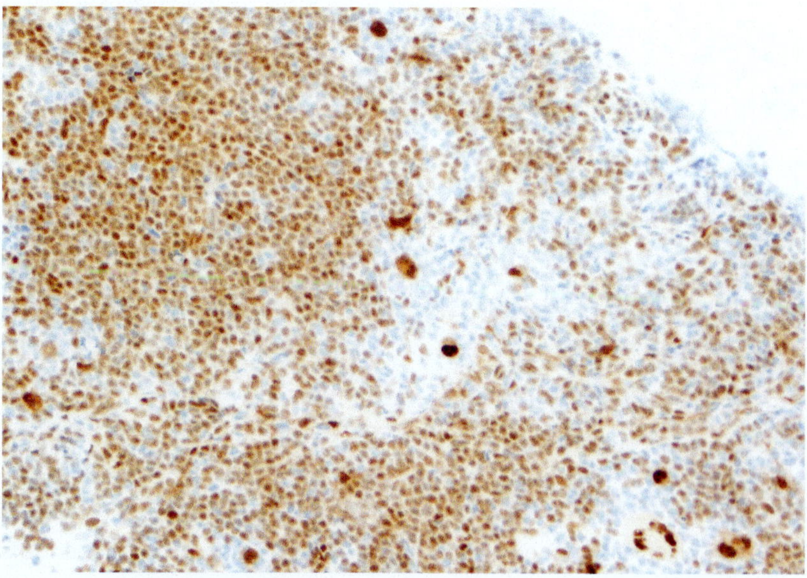

FIGURE 7.18 **Mantle cell lymphoma with HRS-like cells.** Cyclin D1 stains small and large HRS-like cells.

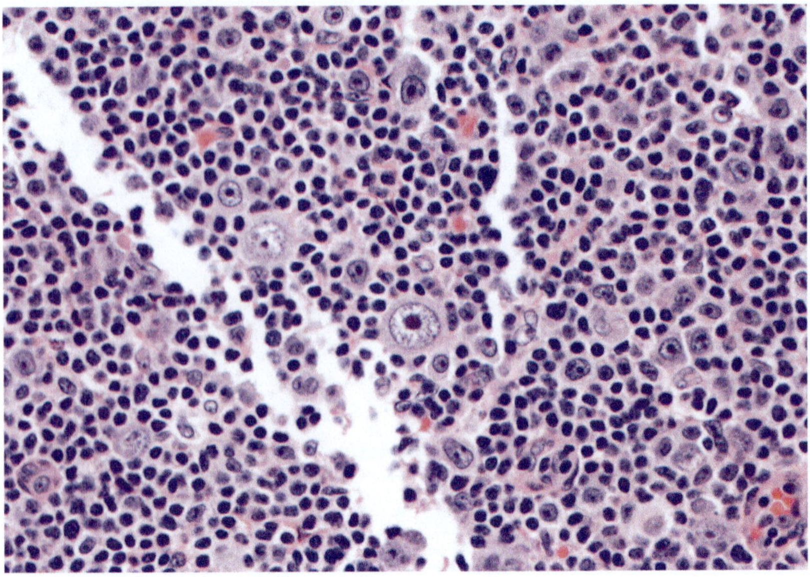

FIGURE 7.19 Marginal zone lymphoma with HRS-like cells.

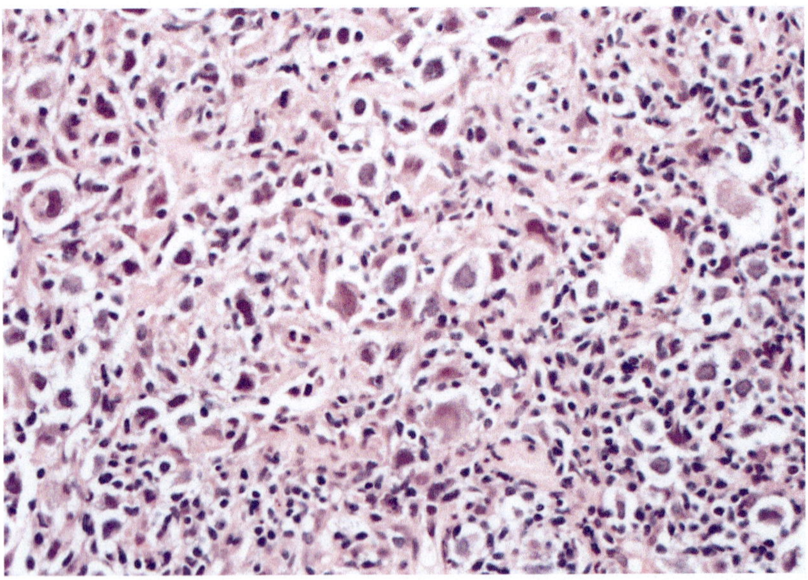

FIGURE 7.20 Follicular lymphoma with scattered cells resembling lacunar cells.

(Figure 7.21). Morphologically, angioimmunoblastic T-cell lymphoma will have a mixed inflammatory background that is similar to CHL including lymphocytes, eosinophils, histiocytes, and plasma cells. Increased numbers of high endothelial venules will be present (Figure 7.22). However, the T cells usually have cytologic atypia. Importantly, the HRS-like cells are typically positive for CD20 (strongly) and EBER (frequently). CD15 is usually, although not always, negative in the immunoblasts/HRS-like cells in T-cell lymphomas. In difficult cases, T-cell clonality studies are very helpful, as CHL should be negative for a clonal rearrangement.

Anaplastic large cell lymphoma (ALCL) is another mature T-cell lymphoma that can mimic CHL on small biopsies and can be particularly problematic in cases that have a rich inflammatory background. The lymphoma cells in ALCL can be virtually identical to HRS cells (Figure 7.23). If the case is ALK-positive, the distinction is clear; however, in ALK-negative cases other studies are needed. Nearly all ALCL cases are negative for PAX5, and nearly all CHL cases are positive for PAX5. If PAX5 is negative or equivocal, additional T-cell markers, and in selected cases T-cell and immunoglobulin gene rearrangement studies, may be helpful.

Genetics

The neoplastic cells in CHL have clonal immunoglobulin gene rearrangement.[11] Recurrent cytogenetic abnormalities in CHL, among others, are amplifications of the 9p24.1 locus, affecting *JAK2, PD-L1*, and *PD-L2*

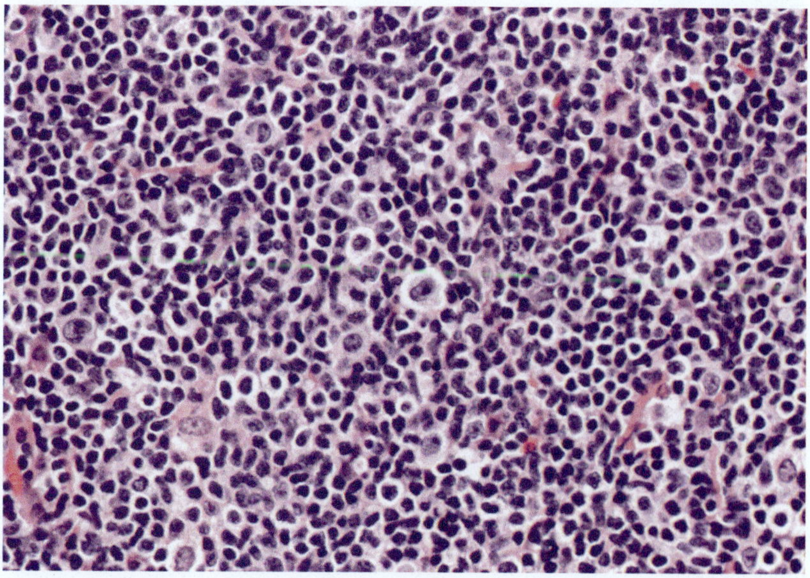

FIGURE 7.21 Peripheral T-cell lymphoma, NOS with scattered HRS-like cells.

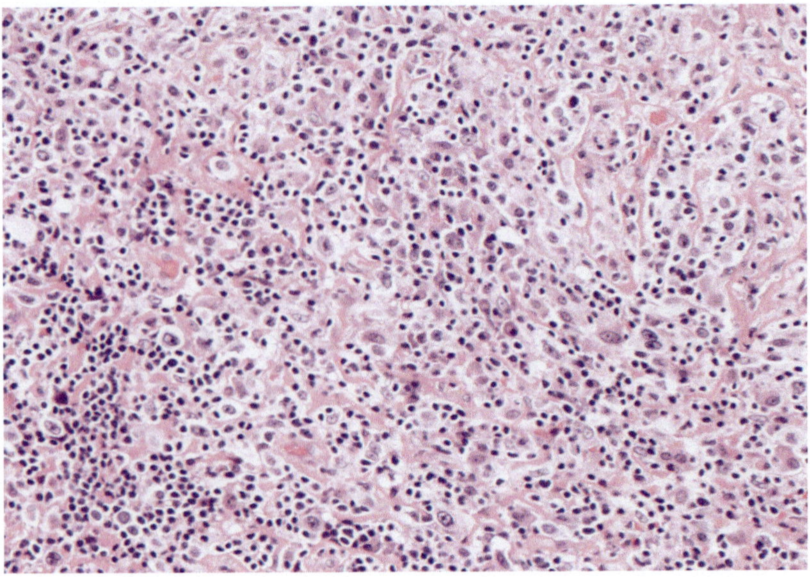

FIGURE 7.22 Angioimmunoblastic T-cell lymphoma with a mixed inflammatory infiltrate with occasional HRS-like cells.

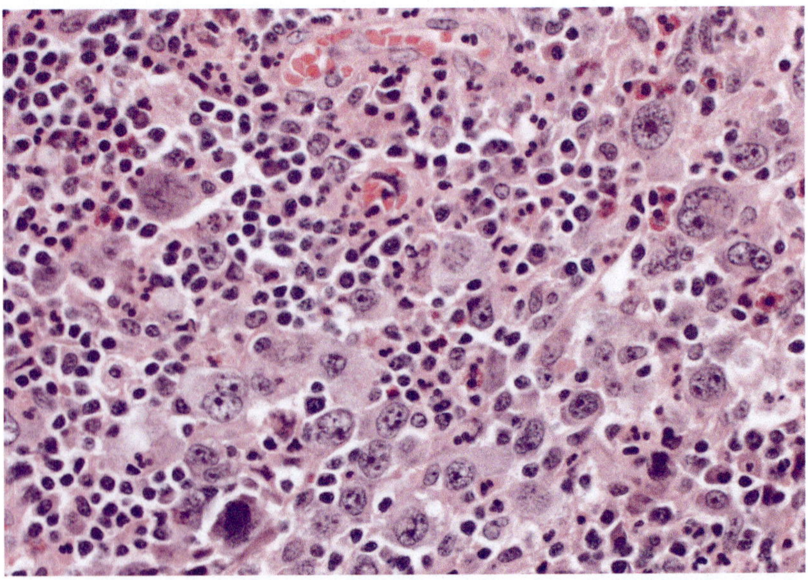

FIGURE 7.23 Anaplastic large cell lymphoma with a rich inflammatory background and HRS-like cells.

genes. The main genetic alterations in CHL include constitutive activation of NF-κB and JAK-STAT signaling pathways.[12,13]

NODULAR LYMPHOCYTE-PREDOMINANT B-CELL LYMPHOMA

NLPBL, a.k.a. nodular lymphocyte predominant Hodgkin lymphoma, is a relatively indolent B-cell neoplasm originating from germinal center B cells. NLPBL is much less common than CHL, comprising 5% of all Hodgkin lymphoma cases, and typically presents in young to middle-aged patients (fourth to sixth decade) with a slow-growing lymph node in a peripheral location.[14] Cervical, axillary, and inguinal lymph nodes are usually involved. B-symptoms are rare, and patients are usually diagnosed in low clinical stage (stage I or II). Radiation therapy is often sufficient for early-stage disease, while chemotherapy is given in advanced and/or bulky disease.[15] In the unusual cases that present with advanced disease (stage III or IV), spleen, liver, and bone marrow may be involved. The condition recurs in up to 20% of patients, irrespective of clinical stage. Recurrence, however, also does not necessarily warrant aggressive treatment, since even ,the patients with recurrence have a favorable outcome.[16] Moreover, a small subset of cases will transform into DLBCL.[17]

Morphology

NLPBL has at least six well-described morphologic patterns, frequently designated as patterns A-F (Figure 7.24).[18] Patterns A and B are most commonly encountered and are called "classic" patterns, while the other four, so-called variant patterns, are less common. Some cases show a

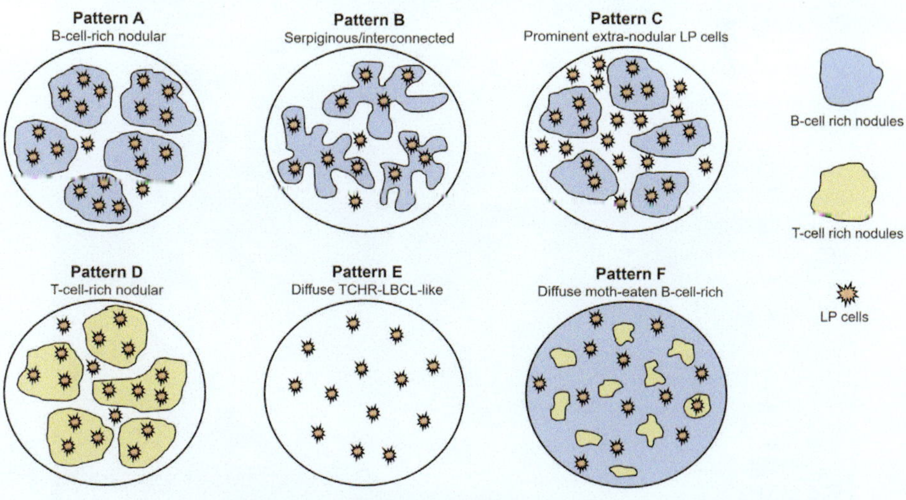

FIGURE 7.24 The patterns of nodular lymphocyte-predominant B-cell lymphoma with the most common patterns being A and B (so-called classic) and the least common being E and F (variant patterns).

combination of patterns with one dominant pattern. In the most common pattern (B-cell-rich nodular or pattern A), the lymph node architecture is effaced by macronodules composed of scattered small lymphocytes and epithelioid histiocytes (scattered singly or forming small clusters) (Figure 7.25). Admixed with these cells are large cells with hyperlobated

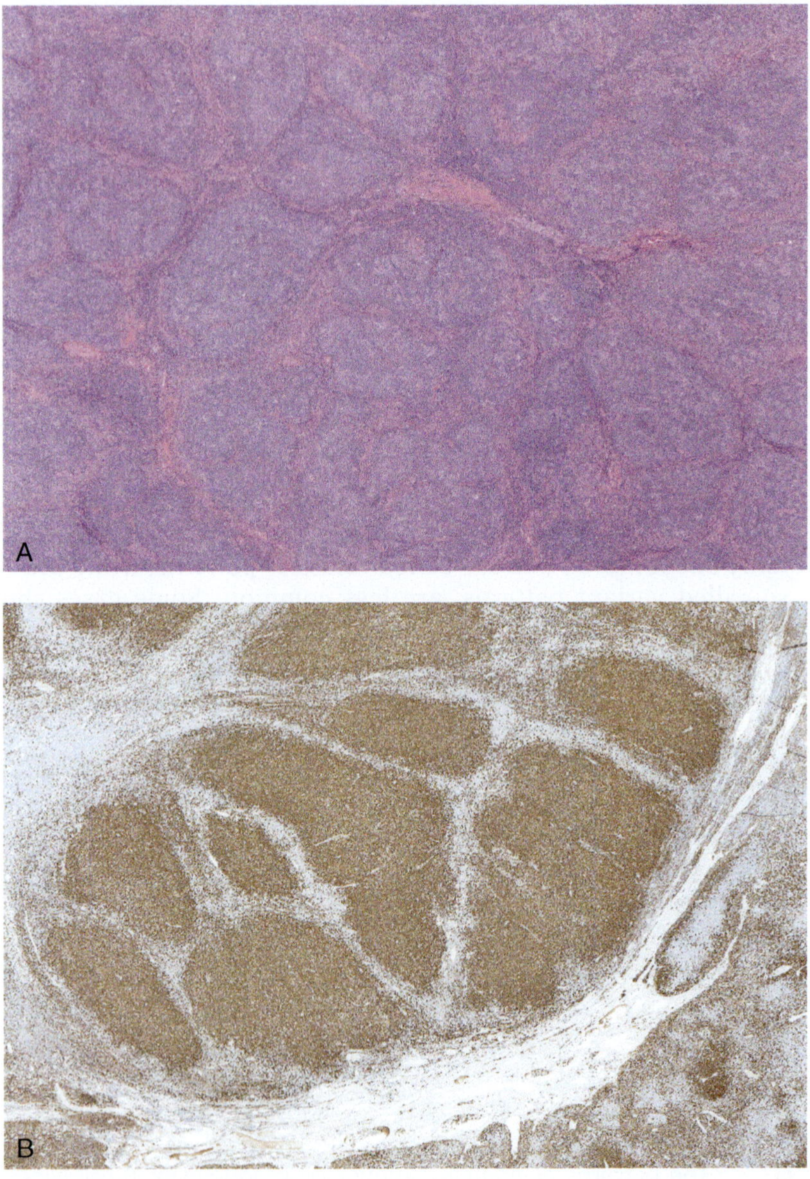

FIGURE 7.25 **Lymph node with NLPBL.** A, Classic (pattern A) is characterized by large nodules effacing the architecture. B, CD20 showing macronodules that fit together like puzzle pieces with residual lymph node architecture pushed to the edge.

nuclei, called lymphocyte-predominant (LP) cells or "popcorn" cells as they resemble a kernel of popped popcorn. They have vesicular chromatin, a thin nuclear membrane, and small nucleoli (Figure 7.26A). In addition to the typical popcorn appearance, LP cells can have round nuclei, and in some cases the neoplastic cells resemble HRS cells seen in CHL (Figure 7.26B). LP cells are usually scattered, but occasionally form

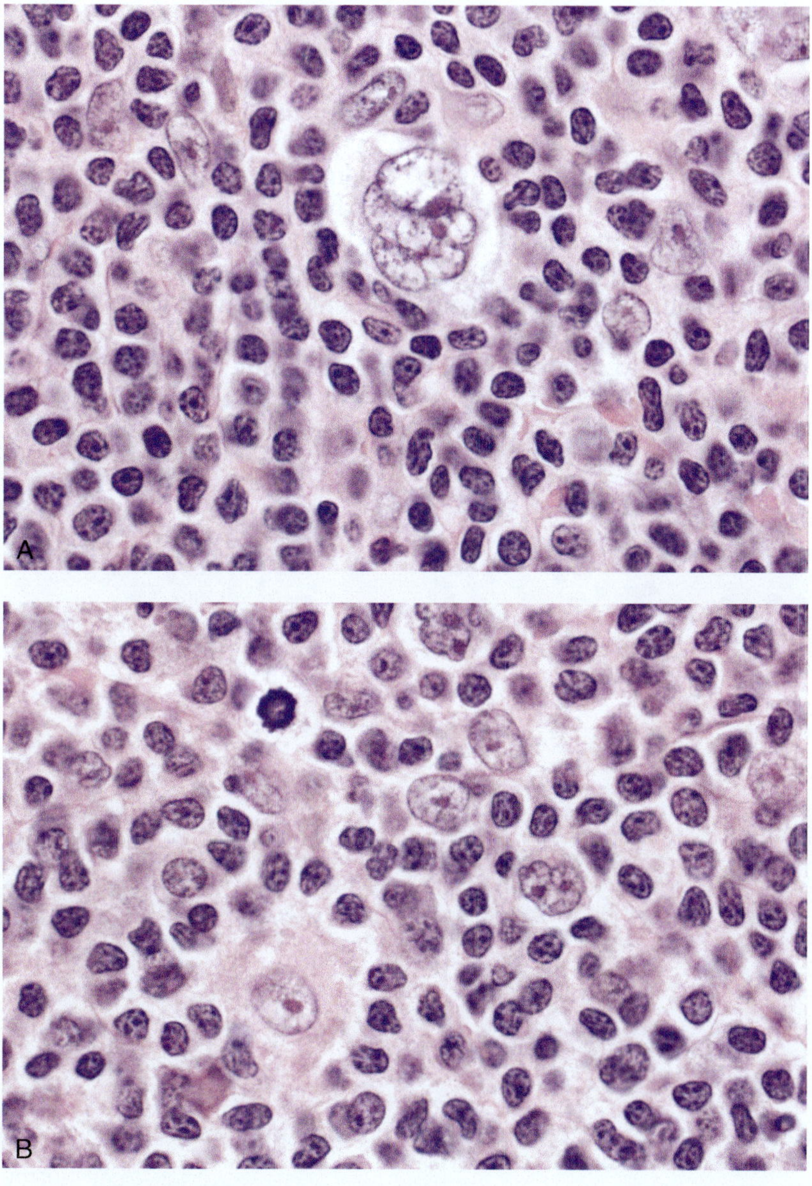

FIGURE 7.26 **Lymphocyte-predominant (LP) cell.** A, Classic appearance with multilobated nucleus reminiscent of popcorn. B, Mononuclear-type LP cells.

clusters and may be difficult to distinguish from the admixed histiocytes (Figure 7.27). Unlike CHL, it is unusual for NLPBL to have other mixed inflammatory cells, such as eosinophils and plasma cells, although it is possible. Rare cases can show prominent fibrosis. Other morphologic patterns include pattern B, in which the infiltrate is serpiginous rather than macronodular (Figure 7.28). Pattern C is similar to pattern A, in that the infiltrate is macronodular, but many LP cells are located outside of the nodules (Figure 7.29). Pattern D, so-called T-cell-rich nodular, is characterized by a macronodular infiltrate with decreased small B cells in the nodules/background and a predominance of small T cells. Diffuse pattern E is similar to T-cell/histiocyte-rich large B-cell lymphoma (so-called TCHR-LBCL-like pattern) but will usually have admixed small B cells in the background. Most of these cases have at least focal nodularity if the tissue is completely sampled. Seeing only pattern E is extremely rare. Lastly, a very rare pattern F, so-called diffuse moth-eaten B-cell-rich, is characterized by numerous B cells in the background, but there are no definitive nodules (Figure 7.30). Variant morphologic patterns should be mentioned in the report as they are associated with a higher relapse rate and more frequent transformation.[15] Cases that transform into DLBCL can show sheets of LP-like cells or cells resembling centroblasts or immunoblasts. Residual areas of NLPBL are frequently seen.

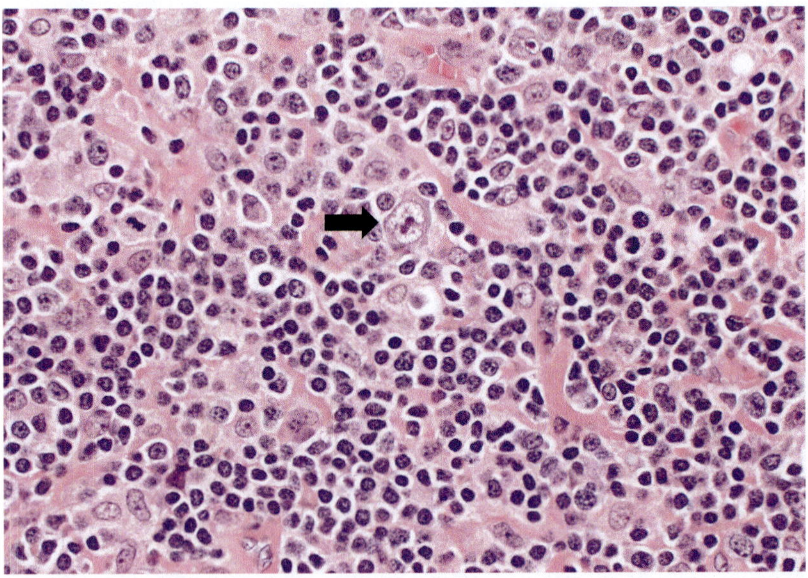

FIGURE 7.27 High magnification of NLPBL nodule showing the small lymphocytes, histiocytes, and occasional LP cells (arrow).

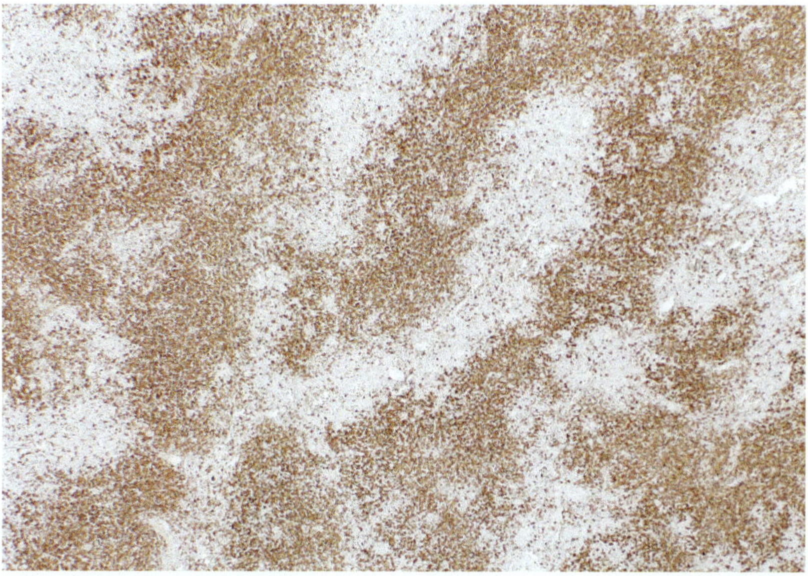

FIGURE 7.28 **NLPBL, pattern B.** CD20 immunostain showing a serpiginous pattern of B cells.

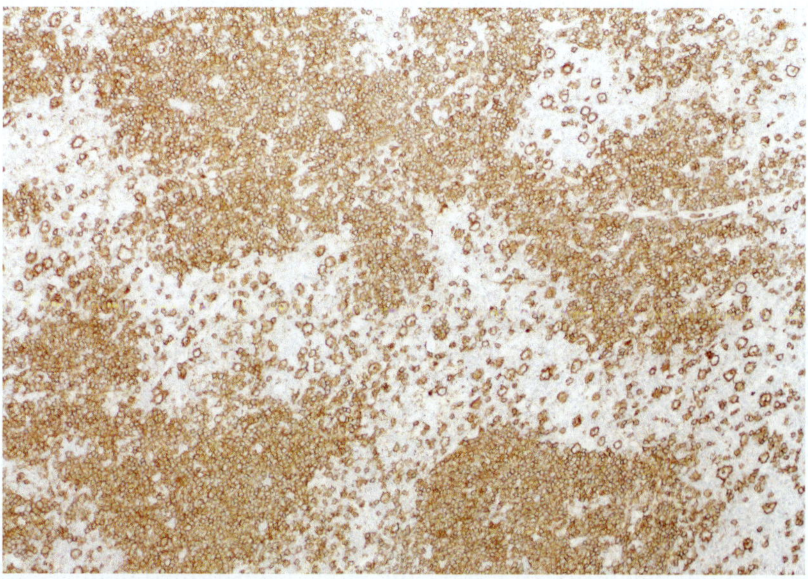

FIGURE 7.29 **NLPBL pattern C.** CD20 immunostain showing B-cell-rich nodules with numerous extranodular LP cells.

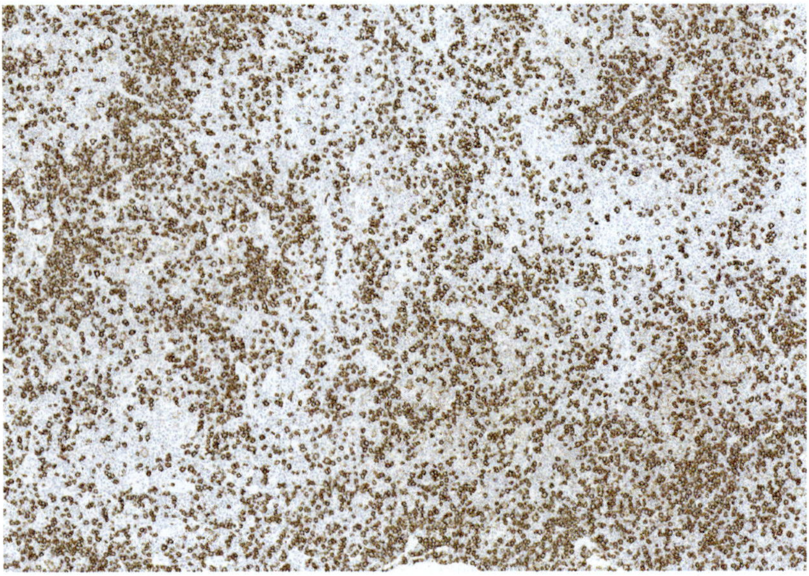

FIGURE 7.30 **NLPBL pattern F.** CD20 immunostain showing small clusters of B cells and scattered LP cells without distinct nodules.

Phenotype

In contrast to CHL, NLPBL shows strong expression of pan-B-cell markers including CD20 (Figure 7.31A), CD79A, PAX5, and a full battery of B-cell transcription factors (OCT-2, BOB.1, and PU.1).[19] CD30 may mark occasional cells but predominantly highlights admixed immunoblasts between the nodules. An important immunohistochemical stain in NLPBL is CD45/LCA. It strongly marks the LP cells in most cases (Figure 7.31B). BCL6 is also positive but is not specific. EMA is positive in a minority of cases. IgD marks LP cells more often in younger male patients.[20] EBER-ISH is almost always negative. Assessment of background cells is also important in this disease. CD3 and PD-1 will often show rosettes of small T lymphocytes around the LP cells. This finding is best appreciated in the classic nodular pattern or patterns in which the LP cells are not admixed with numerous T cells (Figure 7.32). IgD highlights the small mantle zone B cells within the nodules. The nodules can be highlighted with follicular dendritic cell markers including CD21 and CD23.

The differential diagnosis of NLPBL includes both benign and neoplastic conditions (Table 7.3). Follicular hyperplasia with progressive transformation of germinal centers (PTGC) is an important consideration in the differential diagnosis. In PTGC, the large, transformed nodules will be surrounded by numerous reactive follicles. This is really a low-power diagnosis since centroblasts or follicular dendritic cells may be mistaken for LP cells if the nodules are scrutinized on high magnification. PTGC does

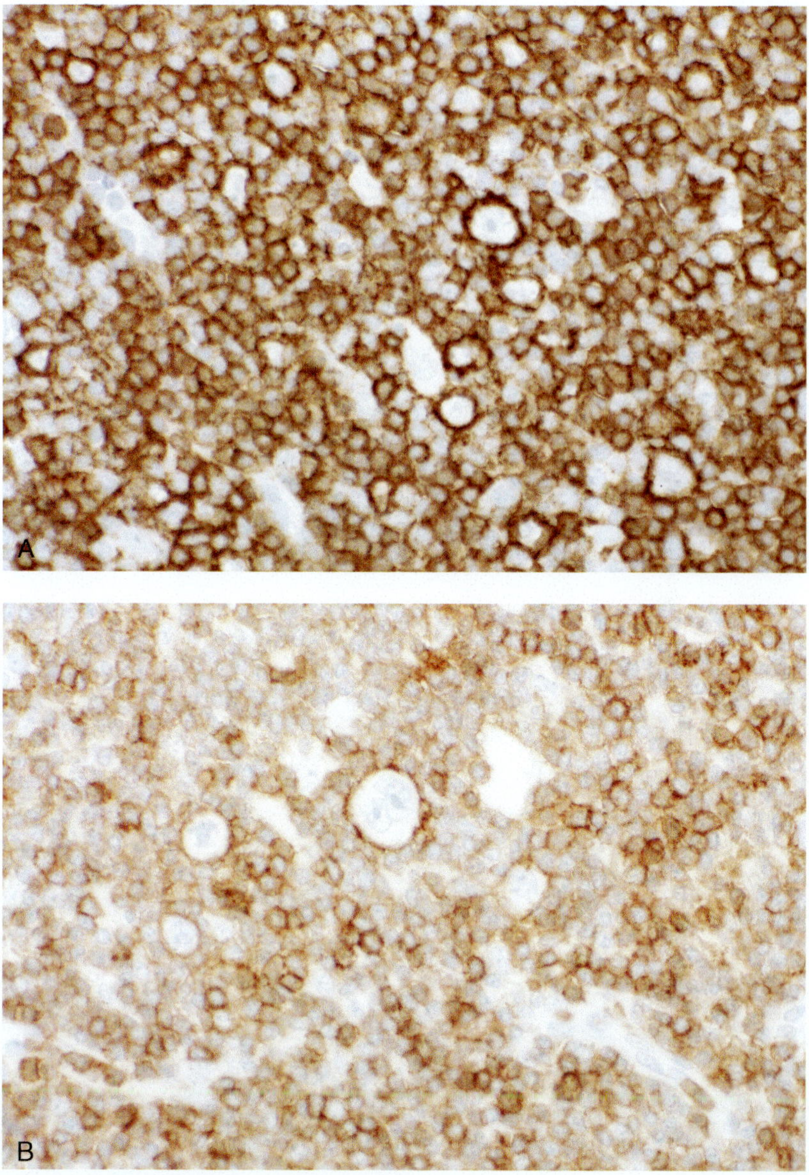

FIGURE 7.31 **Immunophenotype of NLPBL.** A, CD20 and (B) CD45 strongly marking LP cells and background small lymphocytes.

not have LP cells. As mentioned in Chapter 3, PTGC can precede, follow, or occur with NLPBL (in the same or separate lymph nodes), but there is no definitive evidence in the literature that PTGC carries increased risk of NLPBL. Differentiating PTGC from NLPBL is challenging on a small core biopsy, as the low-power architecture will not be evident.

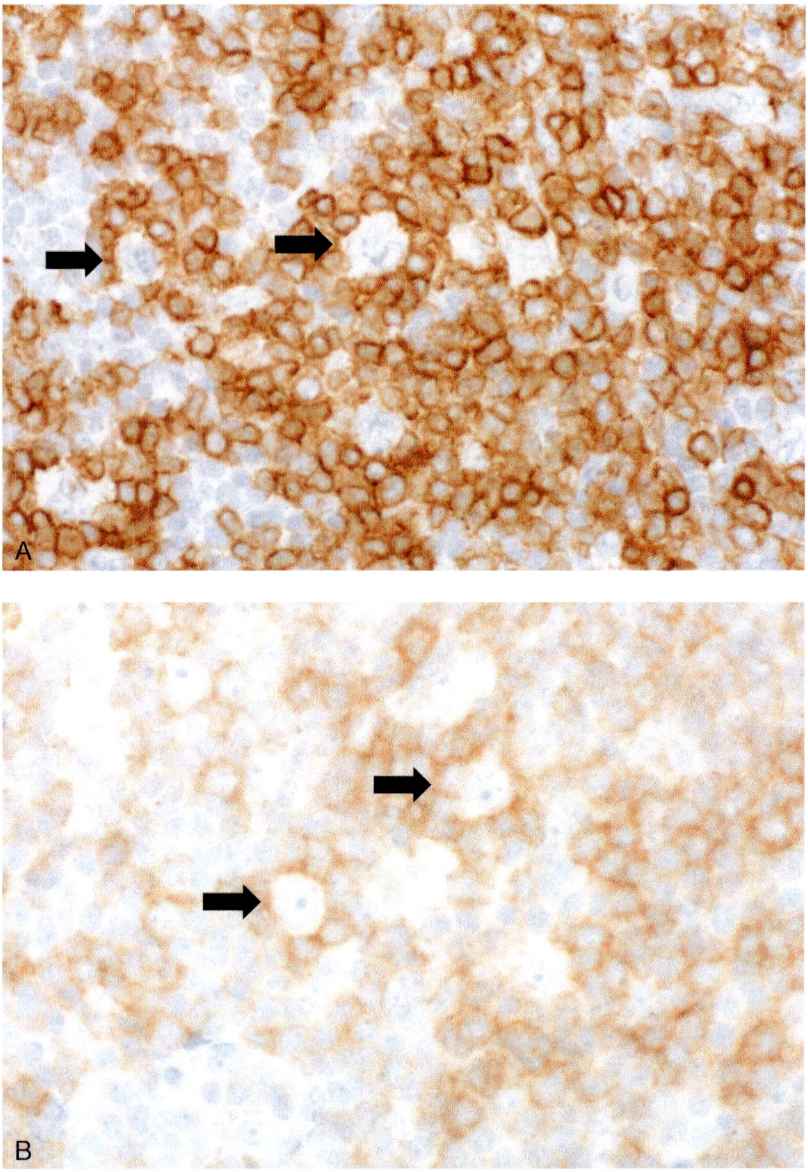

FIGURE 7.32 Background T cells in NLPBL marking with (A) CD3 and (B) PD-1 and showing T-cell rosettes around LP cells (arrows).

As discussed in the previous section on CHL, one of the most important differential diagnostic considerations among lymphomas is LRHL.

TCHR-LBCL is an important differential diagnosis that may be nearly impossible to distinguish on a core biopsy from the diffuse variant (pattern E) of NLPBL. The clinical presentation is helpful as TCHR-LBCL is more likely to present with widespread and high-stage disease. Morphologically, NLPBL tends to have some admixed small B cells in the background.

TABLE 7.3 Differential Diagnosis of Nodular Lymphocyte-predominant B-cell Lymphoma

Follicular hyperplasia with progressive transformation of germinal centers
Classic Hodgkin lymphoma, particularly lymphocyte-rich variant
Mature B-cell lymphomas
T-cell/histiocyte-rich large B-cell lymphoma
Floral variant of follicular lymphoma
Follicular T-cell lymphoma

Furthermore, as mentioned above, most cases of NLPBL with a diffuse pattern will have at least focal nodularity when the entire lymph node is examined. This is an important distinction clinically since TCHR-LBCL is an aggressive disease that requires more intensive treatment than NLPBL. With this differential in mind, it is generally not prudent to make a diagnosis of NLPBL on a core biopsy unless it is a recurrence. Exceptions to this apply if you can confidently make the diagnosis, which is often easier in the classic patterns. If the patient has a well-documented history of NLPBL and has recurrent disease that morphologically resembles TCHR-LBCL, the term "TCHR-LBCL-like" is recommended, as this is a variant pattern rather than a true transformation of the disease.

Other lymphomas are also in the differential diagnosis of NLPBL. The floral variant of FL has irregular neoplastic follicles that can resemble PTGC or NLPBL. The morphology of the lymphoma cells and the immunophenotype of the neoplastic follicles, which are usually CD10 and/or BCL6 positive, helps in distinguishing these entities. Of note, however, BCL2 may be negative in the floral variant of FL, as these cases are more often grade 3.

Some rare entities that can resemble NLPBL include T-cell lymphomas such as follicular T-cell lymphoma with PTGC-like morphology. This lymphoma can show occasional large, atypical B cells that could mimic LP cells. The immunophenotype and T-cell gene rearrangement studies should be helpful in distinguishing between these two diagnoses.

Genetics

The neoplastic LP cells have clonal IGH gene rearrangement, although as in CHL this may not be apparent in studies done on whole sections due to the small number of LP cells in the sample. By conventional cytogenetic analysis, cases of NLPBL usually have a complex karyotype. Rearrangement of *BCL6* is a relatively frequent abnormality. Recurrent mutations in NLPBL include *DUSP2, SGK1,* and *JUNB.*[21] One study showed that cases of NLPBL that transformed into DLBCL have frequent mutations affecting the PI3K pathway, the NF-κB pathway, and linker histones.[22]

REFERENCES

1. Alaggio R, Amador C, Anagnostopoulos I, et al. The 5th edition of the World Health Organization Classification of Haematolymphoid Tumours: Lymphoid Neoplasms. *Leukemia*. 2022;36(7):1720-1748.
2. Campo E, Jaffe ES, Cook JR, et al. The International Consensus Classification of Mature Lymphoid Neoplasms: a report from the Clinical Advisory Committee. *Blood*. 2022;140(11):1229-1253.
3. Ansell SM. Hodgkin lymphoma: a 2020 update on diagnosis, risk-stratification, and management. *Am J Hematol*. 2020;95(8):978-989.
4. Evens AM, Carter J, Loh KP, David KA. Management of older Hodgkin lymphoma patients. *Hematology Am Soc Hematol Educ Program*. 2019;2019(1):233-242.
5. Yosipovitch G. Chronic pruritus: a paraneoplastic sign. *Dermatol Ther*. 2010;23(6):590-596.
6. Fend F, Quintanilla-Martinez L. Hodgkin lymphoma. In: Hsi ED, ed. *Hematopathology*. 3rd ed. Elsevier; 2018.
7. Pinkus GS, Thomas P, Said JW. Leu-M1–a marker for Reed-Sternberg cells in Hodgkin's disease. An immunoperoxidase study of paraffin-embedded tissues. *Am J Pathol*. 1985;119(2):244-252.
8. Venkataraman G, Song JY, Tzankov A, et al. Aberrant T-cell antigen expression in classical Hodgkin lymphoma is associated with decreased event-free survival and overall survival. *Blood*. 2013;121(10):1795-1804.
9. Gomez-Gelvez JC, Smith LB. Reed-Sternberg-like cells in non-Hodgkin lymphomas. *Arch Pathol Lab Med*. 2015;139(10):1205-1210.
10. Bayerl MG, Bentley G, Bellan C, Leoncini L, Ehmann WC, Palutke M. Lacunar and Reed-Sternberg-like cells in follicular lymphomas are clonally related to the centrocytic and centroblastic cells as demonstrated by laser capture microdissection. *Am J Clin Pathol*. 2004;122(6):858-864.
11. Kuppers R, Kanzler H, Hansmann ML, Rajewsky K. Single cell analysis of Hodgkin/Reed-Sternberg cells. *Ann Oncol*. 1996;7(suppl 4):27-30.
12. Mathas S, Hartmann S, Kuppers R. Hodgkin lymphoma: pathology and biology. *Semin Hematol*. 2016;53(3):139-147.
13. Perry AM, Smith LB, Bagg A. Classic Hodgkin lymphoma–old disease, new directions: an update on pathology, molecular features and biological prognostic markers. *Acta Med Acad*. 2021;50(1):110-125.
14. Morton LM, Wang SS, Devesa SS, Hartge P, Weisenburger DD, Linet MS. Lymphoma incidence patterns by WHO subtype in the United States, 1992-2001. *Blood*. 2006;107(1):265-276.
15. Binkley MS, Rauf MS, Milgrom SA, et al. Stage I-II nodular lymphocyte-predominant Hodgkin lymphoma: a multi-institutional study of adult patients by ILROG. *Blood*. 2020;135(26):2365-2374.
16. Spinner MA, Varma G, Advani RH. Modern principles in the management of nodular lymphocyte-predominant Hodgkin lymphoma. *Br J Haematol*. 2019;184(1):17-29.
17. Kenderian SS, Habermann TM, Macon WR, et al. Large B-cell transformation in nodular lymphocyte-predominant Hodgkin lymphoma: 40-year experience from a single institution. *Blood*. 2016;127(16):1960-1966.
18. Fan Z, Natkunam Y, Bair E, Tibshirani R, Warnke RA. Characterization of variant patterns of nodular lymphocyte predominant Hodgkin lymphoma with immunohistologic and clinical correlation. *Am J Surg Pathol*. 2003;27(10):1346-1356.
19. Pinkus GS, Said JW. Hodgkin's disease, lymphocyte predominance type, nodular – a distinct entity? Unique staining profile for L&H variants of Reed-Sternberg cells defined by monoclonal antibodies to leukocyte common antigen, granulocyte-specific antigen, and B-cell-specific antigen. *Am J Pathol*. 1985;118(1):1-6.

20. Prakash S, Fountaine T, Raffeld M, Jaffe ES, Pittaluga S. IgD positive L&H cells identify a unique subset of nodular lymphocyte predominant Hodgkin lymphoma. *Am J Surg Pathol.* 2006;30(5):585-592.

21. Hartmann S, Schuhmacher B, Rausch T, et al. Highly recurrent mutations of SGK1, DUSP2 and JUNB in nodular lymphocyte predominant Hodgkin lymphoma. *Leukemia.* 2016;30(4):844-853.

22. Song JY, Egan C, Bouska AC, et al. Genomic characterization of diffuse large B-cell lymphoma transformation of nodular lymphocyte-predominant Hodgkin lymphoma. *Leukemia.* 2020;34(8):2238-2242.

8

LYMPHOPROLIFERATIVE DISORDERS ASSOCIATED WITH IMMUNODEFICIENCY

ANAMARIJA M. PERRY

In this group of disorders, classification of which did not substantially change in the 2022 International Consensus Classification (ICC) from the previous World Health Organization Classification, knowledge of patient's clinical history/context of immunosuppression is in many cases essential for making the diagnosis.[1,2] As emphasized in Chapter 1, clinical history of immunosuppression should be (ideally) provided with every tissue sample that is submitted to pathology. However, even if pertinent clinical history is not provided, some clinical and morphologic clues should raise the hematopathologist's suspicion for possible underlying immunosuppression. For example, a child with Epstein-Barr virus (EBV)-positive diffuse large B-cell lymphoma (DLBCL), a young adult with low-grade B-cell lymphoma, diagnosis of EBV-positive polymorphic B-cell lymphoproliferative disorder at any age, or plasmablastic lymphoma in young adult, to name a few, are all somewhat unusual clinical scenarios in "immunocompetent" individuals.

In this chapter, four categories of diseases will be covered, in essence reflecting different contexts of immune suppression–posttransplant lymphoproliferative disorders (PTLDs), lymphoproliferative disorders associated with primary immunodeficiency disorders (PIDs), iatrogenic lymphoproliferative disorders (ILDs), and lymphomas associated with human immunodeficiency virus (HIV) infection. All these categories share common morphologic and immunophenotypic characteristics, including histologic variability of lesions that range from nondestructive hyperplasias to polymorphic proliferations and frank lymphomas. Among lymphomas, the overwhelming majority are aggressive B-cell lymphomas. Also, polymorphic B-cell proliferations are encountered in all settings of immune suppression. Moreover, a substantial number of lymphomas (and virtually all polymorphic B-cell proliferations) are EBV driven, which reflects a patient's decreased T-cell repertoire needed to keep latent EBV infection "in check." It is important to mention that some individuals with no apparent cause of immune suppression develop EBV-positive lymphoproliferations (eg, EBV-positive mucocutaneous ulcer or EBV-positive polymorphic B-cell lymphoproliferative disorder, not otherwise specified [NOS]) that are typically associated with immunosuppressive states.[3,4] Many of these patients are elderly, and one theory is that immune senescence (ie, "decay" of immune system with aging) could be a possible explanation for these lesions.[5] However, this is a complex and evolving area.

How to approach these specimens/lymph nodes? The simple answer is, like any other lymph node specimen (see Chapter 1), with notable exception that in every specimen, no matter if benign appearing, polymorphic, or lymphoma, Epstein-Barr encoding region (EBER) in situ hybridization (ISH) should be performed. Another important question to address is how to formulate the diagnosis/what to include in the report. Three things should be in the front and center in the report (ie, in the diagnostic line and comment): (1) morphologic diagnosis; (2) EBV status (particularly if positive); and (3) context/cause of immunosuppression (eg, monomorphic PTLD, DLBCL, NOS, EBV-positive; or iatrogenic [methotrexate (MTX)-associated] lymphoproliferative disorder, polymorphic type, EBV-positive). By including this information in the report, all the important aspects of the case will be communicated to the clinical team.

POSTTRANSPLANT LYMPHOPROLIFERATIVE DISORDERS

PTLDs are lymphoid or plasmacytic proliferations that occur in people under immune suppression due to solid organ or allogeneic stem cell transplantation. Most PTLDs occur within the first year after transplantation, with the median time to development of several years. Overall, PTLD occurs in approximately 2% of transplanted individuals, but the incidence varies widely depending on the transplanted organ and degree of immunosuppression, among other factors, with the highest incidence in recipients of intestinal and multivisceral transplants (5%-20%) and the lowest in renal transplant (0.5%-1%).[6-10] Risk of PTLD after stem cell transplantation is <1% and typically occurs in the setting of T-cell depleting therapy.[11] EBV plays a major role in PTLD pathogenesis. Most PTLDs are EBV positive, with 20% to 40% of cases being EBV negative when EBER-ISH is performed. Among EBV-positive PTLDs, most are B-cell proliferations. EBV-negative PTLDs are characterized by a longer latency period after transplantation and are enriched for T/natural killer (NK)-cell proliferations. Another important risk factor for development of PTLD is seronegativity for EBV at the time of transplantation, which is one of the major reasons for the higher risk of PTLD in children who are more frequently EBV naïve. PTLD more commonly occurs in males with a male to female ratio of 2:1. Based on histologic and immunophenotypic findings, PTLDs are divided into four categories (Table 8.1): nondestructive, polymorphic, monomorphic, and classic

TABLE 8.1 **Histologic Categories of Posttransplant Lymphoproliferative Disorders**

Posttransplant Lymphoproliferative Disorders (PTLD)
Nondestructive PTLD
Plasmacytic hyperplasia
Infectious mononucleosis
Florid follicular hyperplasia
Polymorphic PTLD
Monomorphic PTLD
B-cell neoplasms
T/NK-cell neoplasms
Classic Hodgkin lymphoma PTLD

Hodgkin lymphoma (CHL) PTLD.[2] Clinical presentation varies, depending on the histologic type of PTLD. Nondestructive lesions arise most commonly in the head and neck, involving the lymph nodes, tonsils, and adenoids. Some patients present with an infectious mononucleosis-like syndrome. Polymorphic, monomorphic, and CHL PTLD present with lymphadenopathy or extranodal involvement, with the most common sites being gastrointestinal tract, lungs, and liver. In a subset of patients the allograft is involved by PTLD.[1,7,12] Management of PTLD depends on histologic subtype and clinical presentation and includes reduction of immunosuppression, single agent rituximab, chemotherapy, and antiviral medications. Nondestructive lesions and polymorphic PTLD usually respond well to more conservative management and overall have favorable prognosis. Patients with monomorphic PTLD usually require chemotherapy, and their prognosis is variable.[10,13]

Morphologic Subtypes of PTLD

Nondestructive PTLD

Three histologic types of nondestructive PTLD lesions are recognized, including plasmacytic hyperplasia (PH), infectious mononucleosis (IM), and florid follicular hyperplasia (FH). The common feature of all nondestructive lesions is a degree of architectural preservation of involved tissue. PH is characterized by preservation of tissue architecture with a prominent interfollicular proliferation of mature plasma cells. As the name implies, florid FH-PTLD is characterized by prominent hyperplastic follicles (Figure 8.1A). Lymph nodes involved by IM-PTLD are characterized by marked paracortical expansion with a polymorphous infiltrate including increased immunoblasts, B cells, and plasma cells among other

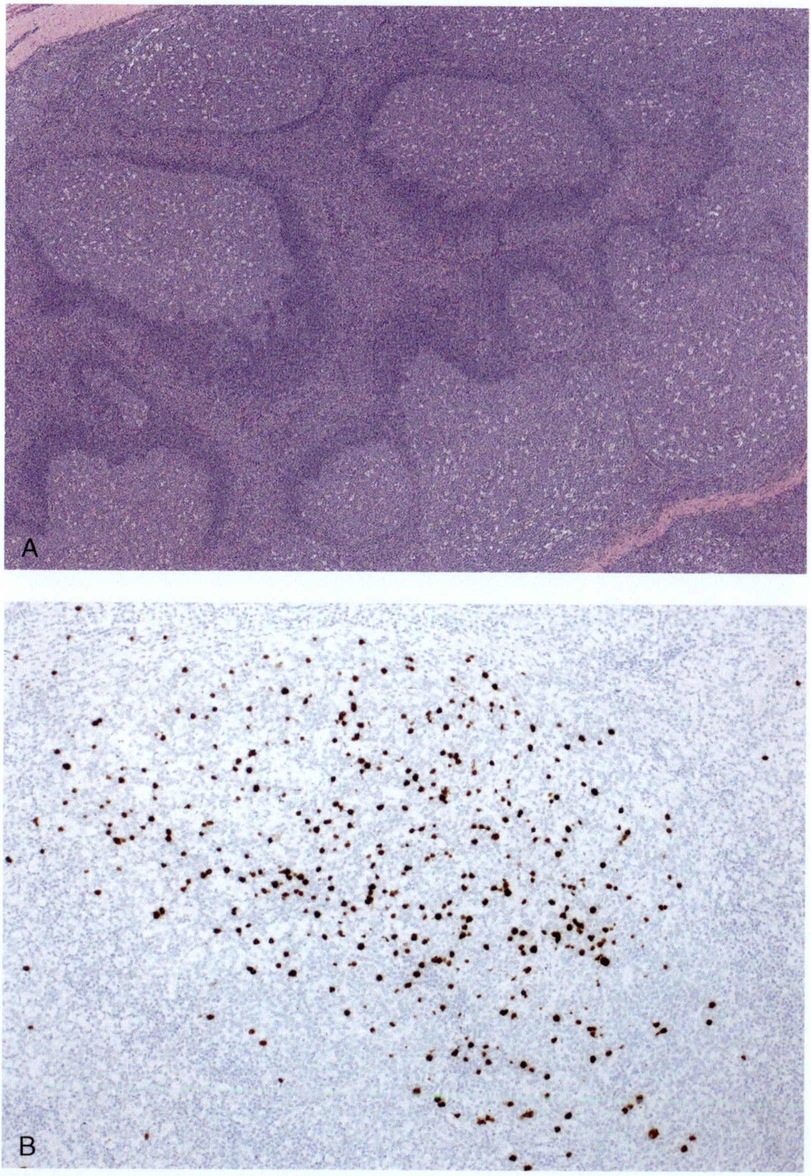

FIGURE 8.1 **Posttransplant lymphoproliferative disorder, florid follicular hyperplasia.** A, Large, expansile follicles are seen. B, EBER in situ hybridization stains numerous cells, primarily within follicles.

inflammatory cells (Figure 8.2A and B). The precise ratios of the different cell types is variable. Virtually all cases of IM-PTLD are EBV positive (Figure 8.3). Since the morphologic findings are otherwise nonspecific, EBV positivity is a distinguishing sign and (for all practical purposes) a

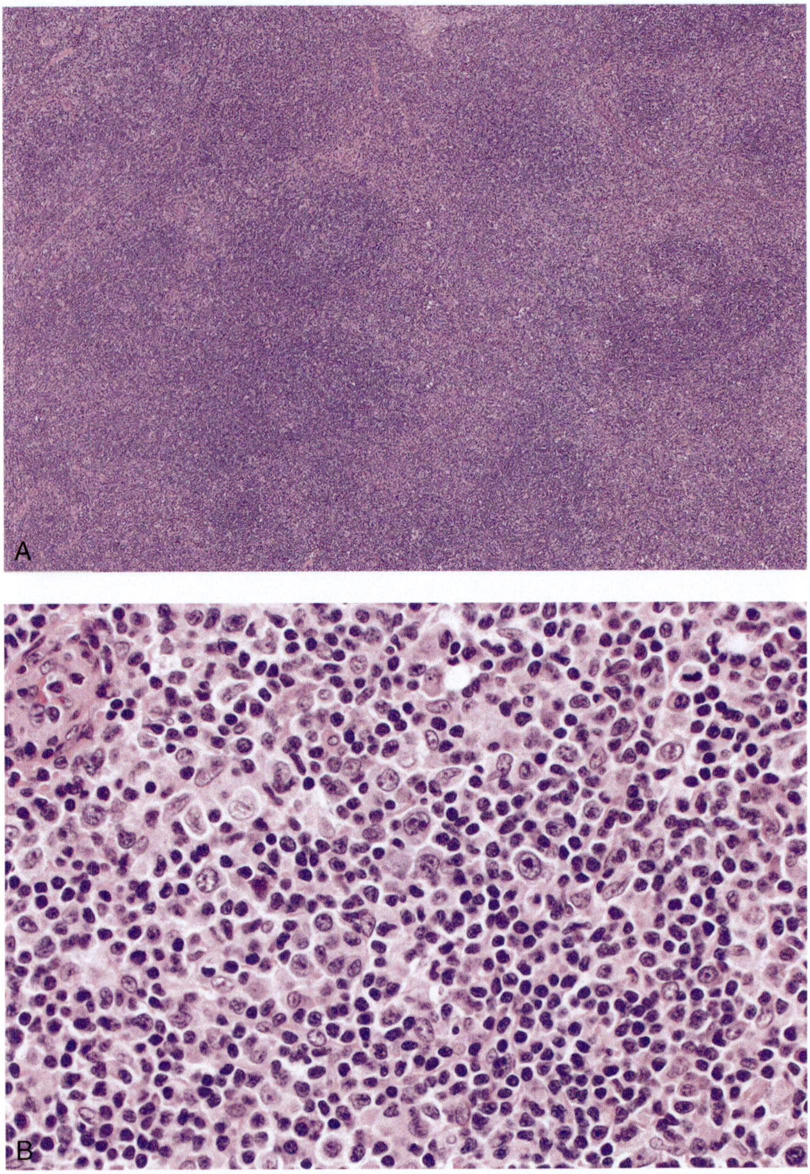

FIGURE 8.2 **Posttransplant lymphoproliferative disorder, infectious mononucleosis-like.** A, Lymph node architecture is partially preserved with marked paracortical expansion. B, Infiltrate is polymorphic with increased large immunoblasts.

diagnostic requirement for making a diagnosis of nondestructive PTLD in most instances, particularly in cases of FH and PH (Figure 8.1B).

Immunohistochemical stains can be used to highlight relatively preserved architecture in these cases and to demonstrate that plasma cells are polytypic in most cases of PH.[1]

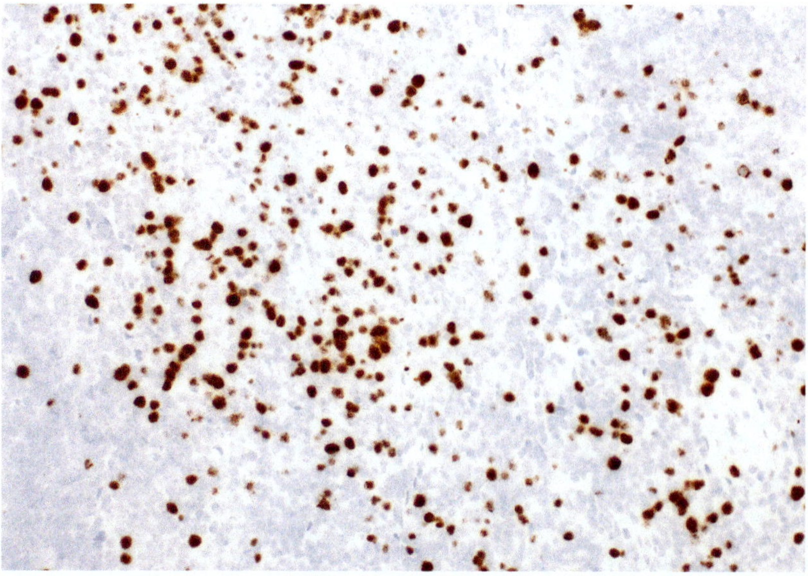

FIGURE 8.3 **Posttransplant lymphoproliferative disorder, infectious mononucleosis-like.** EBER in situ hybridization stains numerous cells of variable size.

Polymorphic PTLD

These lesions are more common in the younger patients who were EBV seronegative at the time of transplantation. Morphologically, lymph nodes show effaced architecture by diffuse destructive polymorphous infiltrate composed of variably sized and frequently irregular lymphocytes, plasma cells, histiocytes, and large cells including immunoblasts as well as plasmacytoid cells (Figure 8.4). Some cases show necrosis. Scattered Hodgkin-and Reed-Sternberg (HRS)-like cells are frequently seen. Occasional cases show areas with predominance of large cells and even display a spectrum between polymorphic and monomorphic PTLD. The distinction between these two histologic subtypes can be challenging and somewhat subjective, especially on a needle core biopsy. Generally, in cases that show predominance/sheets of immunoblasts or transformed cells, diagnosis of monomorphic PTLD is favored. Furthermore, this diagnosis should not be made in cases that fulfill the morphologic criteria for T-cell/histiocyte-rich large B-cell lymphoma, EBV-positive DLBCL, NOS (EBV-DLBCL), or peripheral T-cell lymphoma (PTCL), although these diseases technically have a "polymorphic" appearance.[1,6,14]

Immunohistochemical stains show variable numbers of variably sized B cells with expression of pan-B-cell markers, admixed with variable number of T cells. Plasma cells and large plasmacytoid cells are positive for the plasma cell marker CD138 and usually negative for CD20. CD30 stains proportion of cells in most cases, predominantly larger ones.

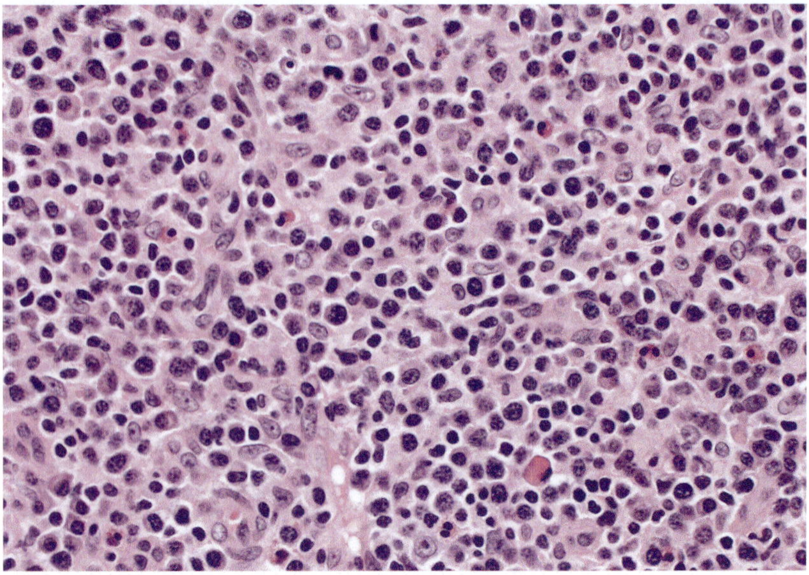

FIGURE 8.4 **Posttransplant lymphoproliferative disorder, polymorphic type.** Infiltrate is composed of lymphocytes, plasma cells, histiocytes, and larger cells, many consistent with immunoblasts.

Of note, HRS-like cells are usually CD20+, CD30+, and CD15-negative. Immunohistochemical stains or in situ hybridization for kappa and lambda demonstrate light chain restriction in some cases, which does not preclude the diagnosis. Immunoglobulin gene rearrangement studies should be discouraged in this setting as clonality is not akin to lymphoma in this setting. EBER-ISH is diffusely positive in majority of cases, staining spectrum of cell sizes, from small to large (Figure 8.5).[7]

Monomorphic PTLD

Monomorphic PTLD is the largest morphologic group, comprising 60% to 80% of all PTLD cases. This heterogeneous group includes the cases that fulfill the morphologic and immunophenotypic criteria for one of the B- or T/NK-cell neoplasms that occur in immunocompetent individuals and are described in detail throughout this book. Nearly 90% of cases are B-cell neoplasms.

Among B-cell neoplasms, DLBCL is by far the most common subtype. Morphologically, these cases are composed of sheets of large cells with centroblastic, immunoblastic, or occasionally anaplastic appearance (Figure 8.6). Some cases are more polymorphic and can show a degree of plasmacytic differentiation or scattered HRS-like cells, while others meet the criteria for EBV-DLBCL outside of the immunosuppression setting. As outlined above, cases of DLBCL with a polymorphic appearance can be very difficult to distinguish from polymorphic PTLD. EBER-ISH is

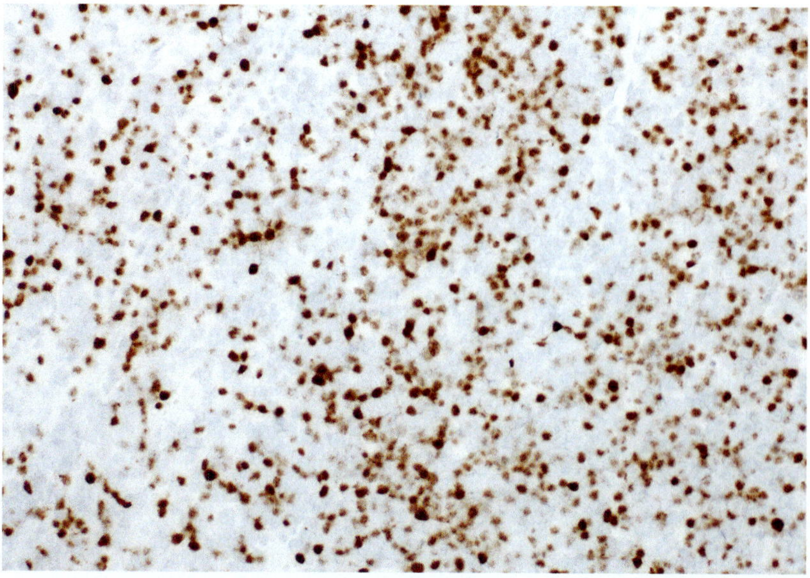

FIGURE 8.5 **Posttransplant lymphoproliferative disorder, polymorphic type.** EBER in situ hybridization stains numerous cells. Nearly all of these cases are EBV positive.

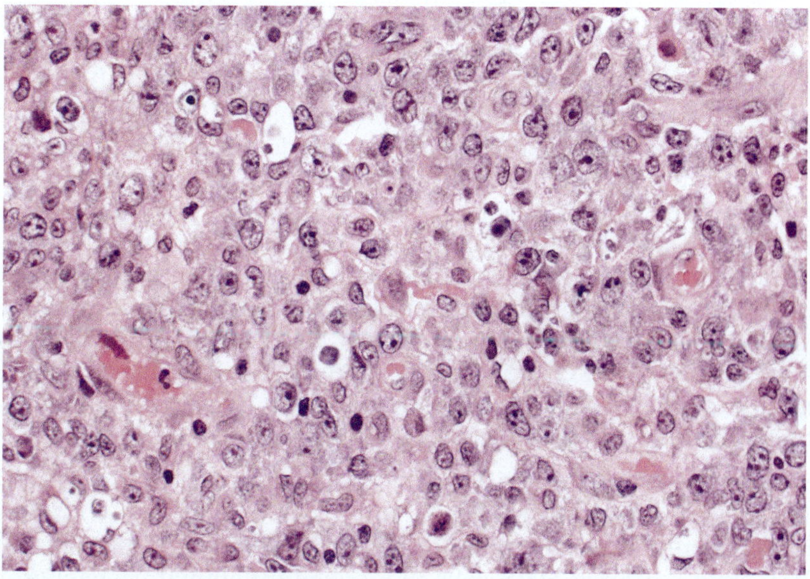

FIGURE 8.6 **Posttransplant lymphoproliferative disorder, monomorphic type, diffuse large B-cell lymphoma, NOS.** Sheets of large lymphoma cells with open chromatin and one to several small nucleoli are seen.

positive in over 50% of cases. By immunohistochemistry, the lymphoma expresses pan-B-cell markers and most cases are of non–germinal center B-cell like (non–GCB) subtype by Hans algorithm, particularly the cases that are EBV positive. In contrast, the cases that show GCB subtype are usually EBV negative. A subset of cases shows variable CD30 positivity.[1,7,10]

Burkitt lymphoma (BL) occasionally occurs in the posttransplantation setting. These cases commonly occur in children. Morphologically, they show sheets of medium-sized, monotonous lymphoma cells with scattered tingible body macrophages. They have typical BL immunophenotype (CD10+, BCL6+, BCL2−) and very high proliferation index, and overall approximately 70% are EBV positive (Figure 8.7A and B).[15,16]

Other morphologic subtypes that are occasionally seen are plasmacytoma-like lesions, which arise in nodal and extranodal sites and show sheets of mature-appearing plasma cells. Approximately 40% of these cases are EBV positive.[17,18] Rarely, plasmablastic lymphoma can occur in this setting and, according to relatively limited data in the literature, approximately 60% show EBV positivity.[19]

EBV-negative low-grade B-cell lymphomas occur in transplanted individuals but are not considered PTLD. Exceptions are EBV-positive extranodal marginal zone lymphoma of mucosa-associated lymphoid tissue (MALT lymphoma), as well as rare cases of EBV-positive nodal marginal zone lymphoma.[1,20,21]

T/NK-cell neoplasms occur in the posttransplantation setting but are much less common comprising approximately 10% to 15% of monomorphic PTLD cases. Most arise late after transplantation (>5 years) and are EBV negative. The most common morphologic subtype is PTCL, NOS (Figure 8.8). Other primarily nodal types of mature T-cell lymphoma PTLDs include anaplastic large cell lymphoma, ALK positive and ALK negative. Of note, although primarily extranodal in presentation, hepatosplenic T-cell lymphoma is a relatively common T-cell neoplasm to occur in the posttransplantation setting. The immunophenotype of T-cell lymphomas is the same as that of their counterparts that arise in the immunocompetent patients, with approximately one-third of cases being EBV positive. The most important differential diagnosis is polymorphic PTLD. Immunohistochemical stains are helpful in resolving this differential. Caution should be taken not to overinterpret T-cell clonality studies, as T-cell clones can be seen in cases that are not T-cell lymphomas in the posttransplantation setting (eg, B-cell PTLD).[1,22]

Classic Hodgkin Lymphoma PTLD

CHL is a very rare form of PTLD and a challenging one to diagnose. Morphologically, it most commonly appears like mixed cellularity subtype of CHL, with scattered HRS cells in a mixed inflammatory background. However, other morphologic subtypes of CHL were also described. By immunohistochemistry, the lymphoma cells are positive for CD30, CD15, and PAX5 and are negative for CD45. EBER-ISH is positive in virtually

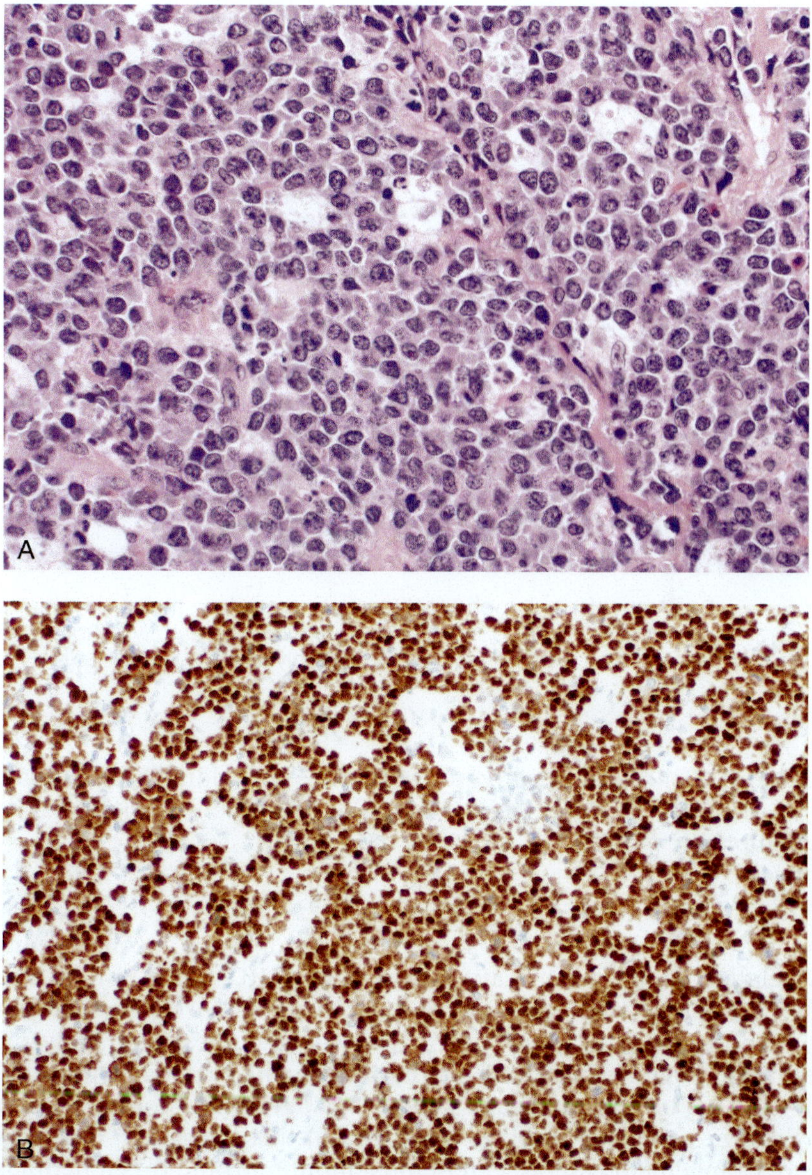

FIGURE 8.7 **Posttransplant lymphoproliferative disorder, monomorphic type, Burkitt lymphoma.** A, Lymphoma cells are medium sized with mild nuclear irregularity and inconspicuous to small nucleoli. Scattered tingible body macrophages impart "starry-sky" appearance. B, Lymphoma cells are strongly positive for EBV by EBER in situ hybridization. This case showed simple karyotype with *MYC* rearrangement.

all cases. Strict criteria must be used for CHL in this setting as the differential diagnosis includes EBV-DLBCL. Another important differential diagnosis is with polymorphic PTLD with HRS-like cells. In contrast to HRS cells seen in CHL, these HRS-like cells are positive for CD20,

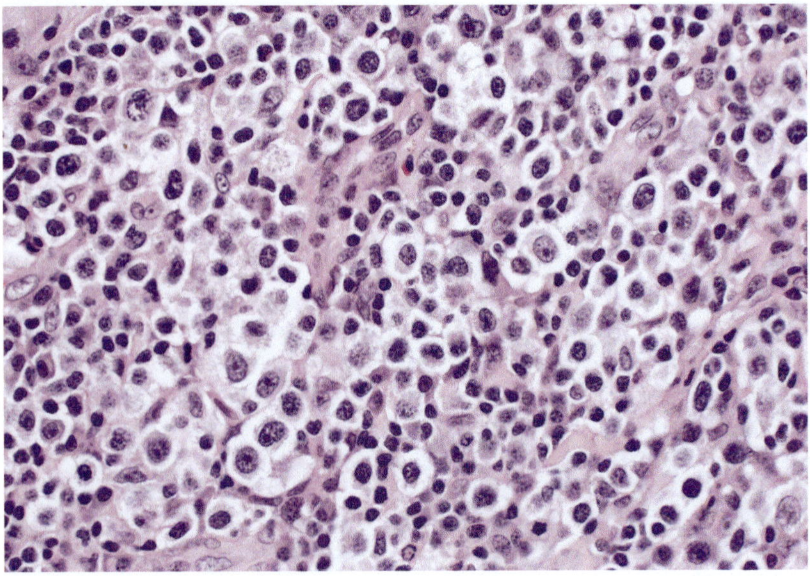

FIGURE 8.8 **Posttransplant lymphoproliferative disorder, monomorphic type, peripheral T-cell lymphoma, NOS.** Sheets of medium-sized to large lymphoma cells are seen with abundant pale cytoplasm. This case showed only rare EBV-positive cells.

CD30, and CD45 and negative for CD15.[23,24] In addition, EBV staining will be restricted to RS cells in CHL and should be in various cell types in polymorphic PTLD.

Genetics

Gene rearrangement studies should be discouraged in the setting of EBV-related lymphoproliferative disorders (LPDs). In nondestructive PTLD, molecular studies for B- and T-cell gene rearrangement usually show a polyclonal pattern.[1,12,14,25-27] Molecular studies may show clonal B-cell immunoglobulin gene (IG) rearrangement in polymorphic PTLD, while there is usually no T-cell gene rearrangement. Clonal cytogenetic abnormalities are seen in up to one-third of these cases.[14,28-30] Clonal IG gene rearrangement can be seen in most monomorphic B-cell neoplasms, while T-cell neoplasms show clonal T-cell gene rearrangement. In monomorphic, as well as polymorphic, PTLD, EBV is present in the clonal episomal form. *MYC* rearrangement can be detected in some cases of DLBCL, subset of plasmablastic lymphomas, and most cases of BL.[7,16,19] Next-generation sequencing showed that polymorphic PTLD shows fewer mutations than DLBCL PTLD. Moreover, DLBCL in the post-transplantation setting showed more frequent mutations in *TP53*.[31] Gene expression profiling studies showed differences between EBV-positive and EBV-negative PTLD cases, with EBV-positive cases showing viral response signature.[32]

LYMPHOPROLIFERATIVE DISORDERS ASSOCIATED WITH PRIMARY IMMUNODEFICIENCY DISORDERS

Individuals with inborn errors of immunity (ie, primary immunodeficiency disorders/syndromes, PIDs) have an overall 10 to 200 times higher risk of developing lymphoma than the general population. PIDs are classified according to the International Union of Immunological Societies (IUIS) Classification, and currently 10 categories of inborn errors of immunity exist, with multiple diseases in each category, nearly all of which are genetically defined.[33] This is a rapidly developing and expanding area, beyond the scope of this text, but the included reference provides the current classification of these complex disorders. Several points, however, are worth emphasizing. These are very rare conditions and not all are associated with increased lymphoma risk. The most common specimen that pathologists could encounter in this context is from a patient with common variable immunodeficiency (CVID), which is by far the most common entity associated with increased lymphoma risk. Other entities are extremely rare disorders, most of which a pathologist in an average size general practice will never encounter. Some of the most common PIDs associated with lymphoproliferative disorders include ataxia telangiectasia, severe combined immunodeficiency (SCID), hyper-IgM syndrome, Wiskott-Aldrich syndrome, Nijmegen syndrome, and autoimmune lymphoproliferative syndrome (ALPS). In most PIDs, lymphomas are diagnosed in childhood, with notable exception of patients with CVID who usually develop lymphomas as young adults or even later in life. In some patients, diagnosis of LPD/lymphoma is a first clue to underlying immunodeficiency.[1,6,34]

Clinically, patients present with constellation of signs, symptoms, and laboratory abnormalities characteristic of their respective disorder. Susceptibility to infections is one of the hallmarks of PIDs. Patients who develop lymphoproliferative disorder usually present with lymphadenopathy or involvement of extranodal sites (eg, gastrointestinal tract, lungs), and occasionally with hepatosplenomegaly. Patients with some disorders (SCID, for example) develop EBV-driven IM-like syndrome, which is typically fulminant and often fatal. Although lymph node and tissue biopsies in these patients are done primarily to rule out lymphoproliferative disorders, some common (or disease-specific) histologic features are observed in benign lymph nodes of patients with PID and should be recognized (discussed below).[6,7]

Morphology

Benign Changes in Lymph Nodes

Although not specific, some histologic features are characteristically seen in the lymph nodes of patients with PID and reflect, in part, underlying immunologic defect. As noted above, pathologists will most frequently encounter lymph nodes from patients with CVID. They are characterized by FH, frequently with poorly defined germinal centers, sometimes lacking mantle zones. These should not be mistaken for nodules of follicular lymphoma. Most importantly, these patients will have markedly decreased to absent plasma cells, a finding best appreciated in the medullary cords. Of note, nodular lymphoid hyperplasia in the gastrointestinal tract is frequently seen in patients with CVID. Another disease that has a somewhat characteristic histologic appearance is hyper-IgM syndrome where there is an underlying defect in heavy chain switching, so the patients' B cells only have either IgM or IgD. In the lymph nodes, only primary follicles are seen, with no secondary follicles with germinal centers. Other changes that can be seen in lymph nodes of patients with PID include general lymphocyte depletion, sometimes with Castleman-like "burn-out" appearance of follicles, which can also be seen in advanced HIV infection (see Chapter 3). Plasma cells are usually prominent in lymphocyte-depleted lymph nodes. Moreover, increase in histiocytes or granulomatous inflammation is frequently seen. In these cases, special stains for fungi and mycobacteria should be done to evaluate for infection.[35-38]

Lymphoproliferative Disorders

Similar to the spectrum of PTLD, LPDs in patients with PID represent a spectrum from nondestructive to polymorphous proliferations, to frank lymphomas. Another common thread with PTLD is that many LPDs in these patients are EBV driven.

Among proliferations that are "nonlymphomas," EBV-driven IM-like proliferation and ALPS will be highlighted in this text. Patients with inborn errors of immunity that lead to profound decrease/absence of T cells (ie, SCID and X-linked lymphoproliferative syndrome, type 1) are at the highest risk to develop fulminant EBV-driven IM-like syndrome. Changes in lymph nodes seen in IM are described in detail in Chapter 3. Patients with PID frequently show markedly polymorphous infiltrate in lymph nodes with frequent immunoblasts and some HRS-like cells. In addition to lymphoid organs, other organ systems (such as GI tract) can be involved. This is an aggressive condition with relatively high mortality.

ALPS is the so-called phenocopy of PID in the IUIS Classification and is characterized by mutations in *FAS* gene (most commonly) and defective lymphocyte apoptosis, resulting in accumulation of TCR-alpha/beta, CD4/CD8 double-negative T cells in lymphoid tissues and peripheral blood. Typical clinical findings include lymphadenopathy, splenomegaly, and autoimmune cytopenias. Lymph nodes in ALPS show paracortical expansion by a population of atypical T cells that are larger than normal small lymphocytes and have more dispersed chromatin and occasional small nucleoli (Figure 8.9A and B). Scattered mitotic figures may be seen. T cells are positive for CD3, CD57, and CD45RA and negative for CD45RO, as well as CD4/CD8 double negative (Figure 8.9C-E).[1,39] The most important diagnostic pitfall in these cases is T-lymphoblastic leukemia/lymphoma (T-ALL/LBL), given the paracortical distribution of the infiltrate and double-negative T-cell population. However, T cells in ALPS are mature,

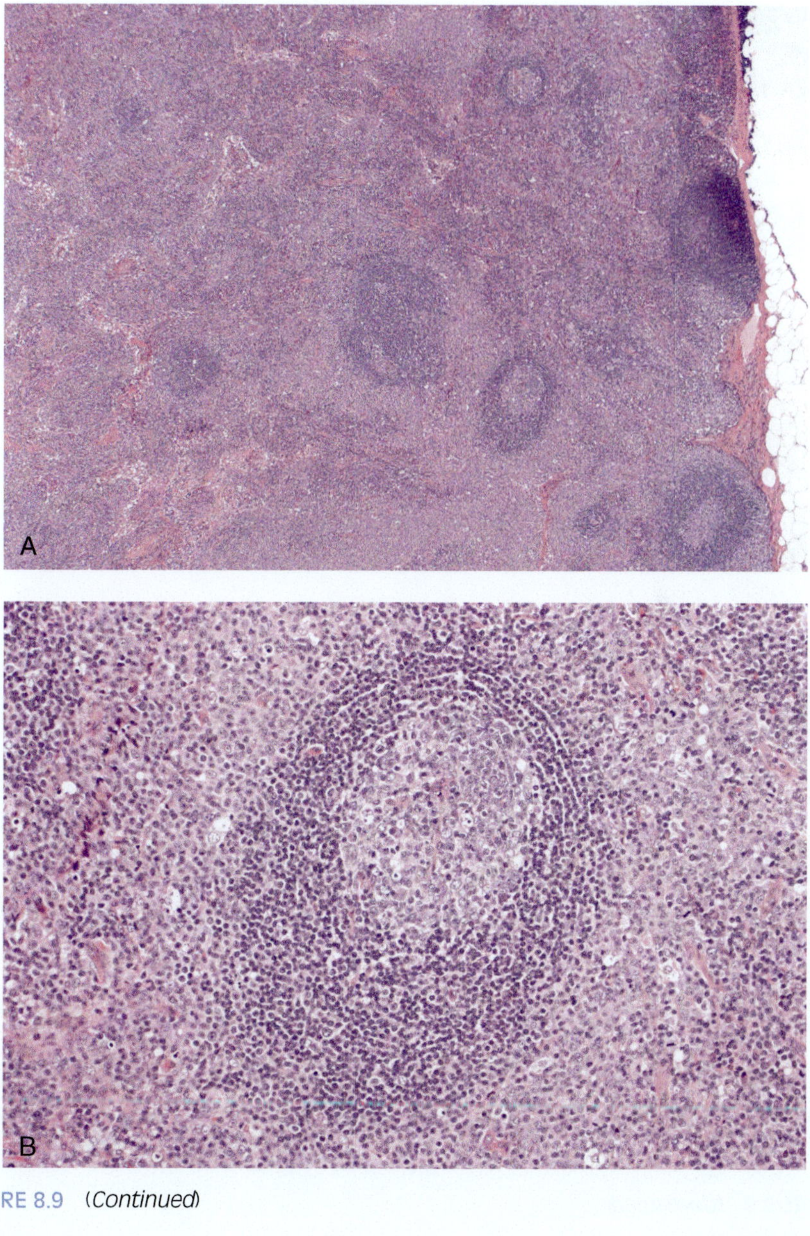

FIGURE 8.9 (*Continued*)

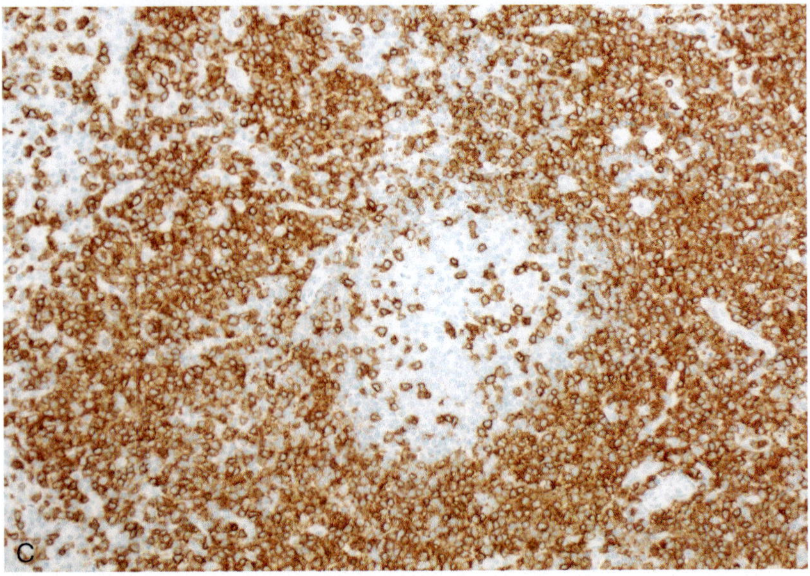

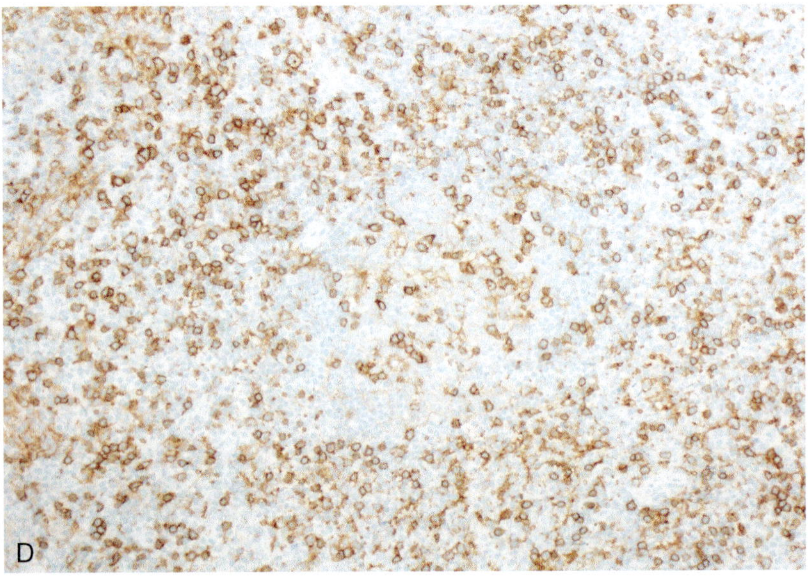

FIGURE 8.9 (*Continued*)

which is best demonstrated by flow cytometry. Other differential diagnosis is with mature T-cell lymphomas, but in contrast to these, T cells in ALPS are polyclonal and show no other aberrancies. Moreover, mature T-cell lymphomas are vanishingly rare in children (even in children with PID) and this diagnosis should be made very cautiously in this age group. Lastly, like any primarily paracortical proliferation, diagnosis of ALPS can be very challenging on a needle core biopsy, especially with no clinical history. Excisional biopsy is a preferred specimen in these circumstances.

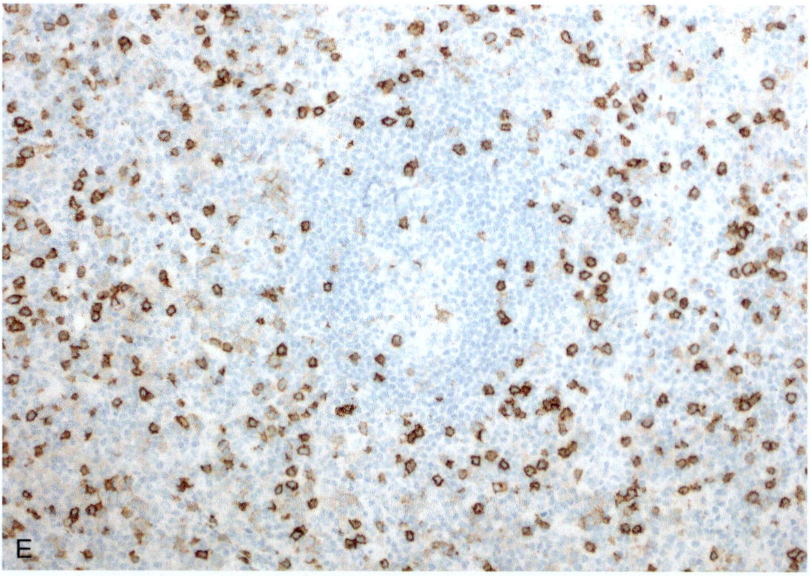

FIGURE 8.9 **Autoimmune lymphoproliferative syndrome.** A, Lymph node with expanded paracortex by pale-appearing infiltrate and some follicular hyperplasia. B, Atypical cells in paracortex are larger than small lymphocytes, with finer nuclear chromatin and more abundant cytoplasm. Immunohistochemical stains demonstrate that the paracortical infiltrates are composed of T cells that are positive for CD3 (C), but with substantial number being CD4 (D) and CD8 (E) double negative.

Patients with PIDs can develop polymorphic B-cell LPDs, which are similar to those seen in PTLD and are typically EBV positive.

Among lymphomas, approximately 80% are non-Hodgkin lymphomas (NHLs), the most common by far being DLBCL. Some cases show more polymorphous appearance and HRS-like cells, features commonly seen in DLBCL arising in patients with immunodeficiency. Other relatively common NHLs in this setting include lymphomatoid granulomatosis (LyG), BL, MALT lymphoma (in CVID), and follicular lymphoma. In addition to LyG, which is EBV-driven lymphoma, EBV is usually positive in a subset of DLBCL and BL cases.[40-43]

CHL comprises approximately 15% of lymphoma cases in patients with PID, with mixed cellularity being the most common subtype. Majority of these cases are EBV positive.[44]

Lastly, it is worth mentioning that patients with ataxia telangiectasia are at increased risk of developing T-ALL/LBL, as well as T-prolymphocytic leukemia, entities described in detail in Chapters 4 and 6, respectively.[45]

IATROGENIC LYMPHOPROLIFERATIVE DISORDERS

ILDs are a heterogeneous group of diseases that arise after therapy with immunosuppressive/immunomodulatory drugs, mostly in patients with autoimmune diseases (eg, rheumatoid arthritis [RA], systemic lupus erythematosus, dermatomyositis, inflammatory bowel disease, etc). Patients with autoimmune diseases have a baseline increased risk of developing lymphoma, and in RA that risk is 2 to 20 times higher compared with the general population. Among the drugs that are associated with ILD, the risk associated with MTX has been most strongly established. Other implicated drugs include antimetabolites (azathioprine and 6-mercaptopurine), tumor necrosis factor (TNF) antagonists (eg, infliximab, adalimumab, etanercept), interleukin-6 antagonists, and antibodies against CD11a, CD25, and CD121. The data in the literature regarding increased lymphoma risk in patients receiving TNF antagonists are somewhat confounding and complicated by the fact that many of those patients also received MTX, but overall agreement is that some increase in risk does exist.[1,46-49]

In this relatively rare group of disorders, the best characterized are ILDs that occur in people with RA who were treated with MTX. Most patients are elderly (median 7th decade) and they are more commonly seen in females, consistent with more common occurrence of autoimmune diseases in women. Most people have longstanding RA, with the average time from first administration of MTX to development of LPD of approximately 3 years. Patients present with lymphadenopathy and frequent extranodal involvement, with the most commonly involved sites being gastrointestinal tract, skin, and soft tissue. Approximately 40% of cases are EBV positive, with different prevalence depending on the histologic subtypes. Treatment involves cessation of the implicated drug, which leads to remission in 20% to 30% of patients who were on MTX. Regression is more commonly seen in EBV-positive cases and with polymorphic histology. Most patients, however, require chemotherapy.[1,7,50-53]

Among ILDs, the most common histologic subtypes include DLBCL (50%-75%), CHL (10%-20%), and polymorphic LPD (10%-15%). However, other proliferations do occur, including reactive hyperplasias, Hodgkin-like lesions, B-cell lymphomas (eg, follicular lymphoma, BL), and T/NK-cell lymphomas (eg, PTCL, hepatosplenic T-cell lymphoma). It is important to emphasize that, when dealing with reactive hyperplasias and low-grade/small B-cell lymphomas, one should be cautious to classify these as ILDs in the absence of considerable EBV positivity, as the EBV-negative cases are likely not immunodeficiency related.[3] Another well-recognized entity that is worth mentioning is EBV-positive mucocutaneous ulcer. This relatively indolent entity presents as ulcer in skin and mucosal sites.[4,7]

Morphologic and immunophenotypic findings of lymphomas occurring in this setting are similar to those in immunocompetent patients. Polymorphic proliferations are reminiscent of those seen in PTLD (Figure 8.10A and B). Several morphologic and immunophenotypic characteristics are worth mentioning. Some cases of DLBCL show HRS-like cells, and approximately 40% to 50% are EBV positive. Among CHL cases, most show morphology consistent with mixed cellularity, and malignant cells are EBV positive in 80% of cases. The most important histologic pitfall is differentiating CHL from Hodgkin-like lesions, which show

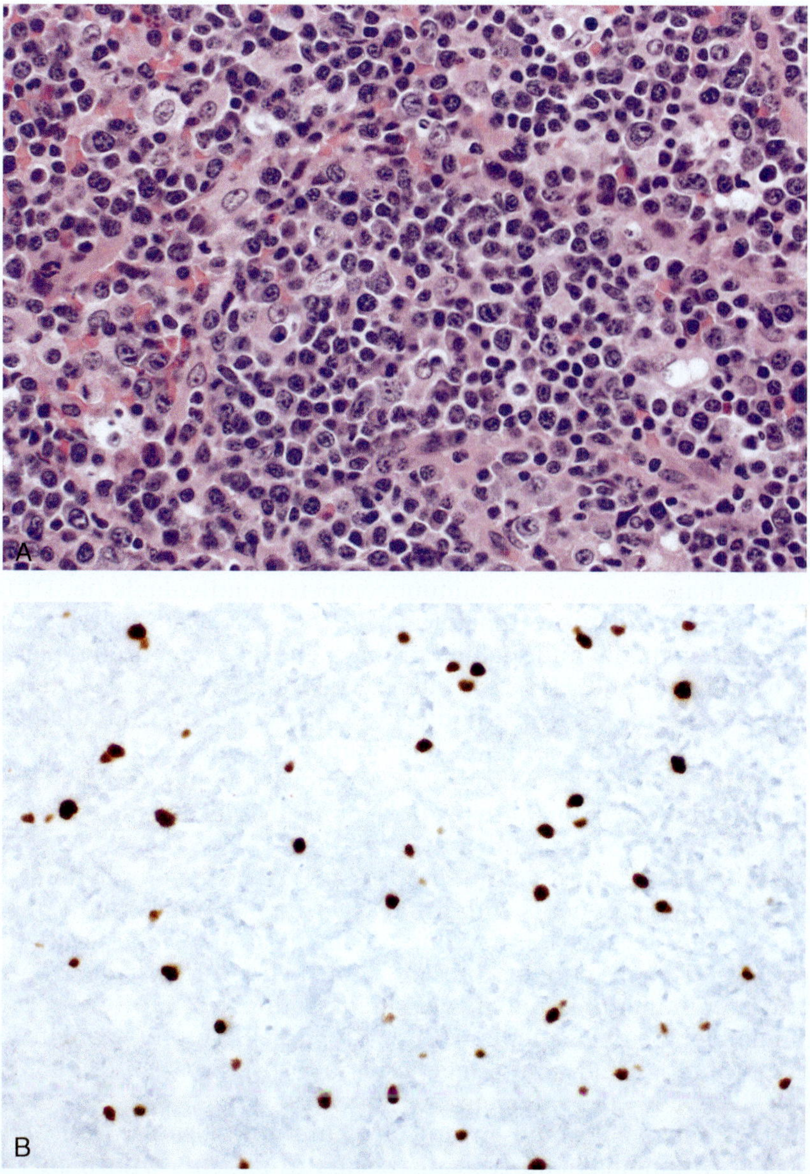

FIGURE 8.10 **Iatrogenic (methotrexate-associated) lymphoproliferative disorder, polymorphic type.** A, Infiltrate is composed of small lymphocytes, numerous plasma cells and plasmacytoid cells, histiocytes, and occasional larger lymphoid cells. B, EBER in situ hybridization is positive mostly in larger cells.

HRS-like cells in the polymorphous background and are morphologically more similar to polymorphic LPDs. Clinically, Hodgkin-like lesions are mostly extranodal, while CHL occurs in lymph nodes in majority of cases. Immunohistochemistry is most helpful, with HRS cells being positive for CD30 and CD15 and usually negative for CD20 and CD45. In contrast,

HRS-like cells are CD30+, CD20+, CD45+, and CD15 negative. Of note, most polymorphic LPDs are EBV positive.[7,46,54]

LYMPHOMAS ASSOCIATED WITH HIV INFECTION

Lymphomas are relatively common neoplasms in people infected with HIV and in some cases are acquired immunodeficiency syndrome–defining illness. Even though the risk of NHL decreased with the use of antiretroviral therapy (ART), it remains 11-fold higher in HIV-positive individuals compared with the general population. Moreover, incidence of CHL, which usually occurs in HIV-positive people with higher CD4 T-cell counts, increased with ART.[55] Factors contributing to pathogenesis of lymphomas associated with HIV infection include declining CD4 T-cell counts, inconsistent or no ART, coinfection with other viruses including EBV, human herpesvirus 8 (HHV8), and hepatitis B and C, as well as loss of EBV-specific immunity.[56] The most common lymphomas that occur in the setting of HIV infection are aggressive B-cell lymphomas, which are frequently EBV positive. Lymphomas in HIV can be divided into those that also occur in immunocompetent individuals (ie, DLBCL, BL, and CHL) and those that primarily (but not exclusively) occur in HIV-positive patients and include primary effusion lymphoma, plasmablastic lymphoma, and HHV8-positive DLBCL, NOS. These entities are described in more detail in Chapter 5 of this book, and only important characteristics of more common lymphomas, pertinent to the context of HIV infection, will be reviewed here. Clinically, lymphomas in HIV are frequently extranodal and patients present in advanced clinical stages, but prognosis has improved in the era of ART.

DLBCL is the most common NHL in HIV-positive individuals, and it usually occurs in patients with lower CD4 T-cell counts. Involvement of extranodal sites (eg, central nervous system, gastrointestinal tract) is very common, and many patients present with high clinical stage. The morphology and immunophenotype are similar to those of DLBCL occurring in immunocompetent patients. Frequently, B-cell lymphomas with high-grade morphology that do not meet criteria for BL are seen (Figure 8.11). EBV is positive in approximately 30% of cases.[1,57]

BL is relatively common and accounts for 20% to 30% of HIV-associated lymphomas and typically occurs in patients with higher CD4 T-cell counts. The morphology and immunophenotype are similar to those seen in immunocompetent patients (Figure 8.12). Some cases, however, show plasmacytoid differentiation, an unusual morphologic finding in HIV-associated BL. EBV is positive in up to 50% of cases, and *MYC* rearrangement is present in most cases.[1,58]

Plasmablastic lymphoma is a relatively common neoplasm in the setting of HIV infection, while it is a very rare lymphoma in immunocompetent individuals. It typically occurs in patients with poorly controlled HIV with high viral load and low CD4 T-cell counts. This lymphoma most commonly involves extranodal sites including oral cavity (pathognomonic site

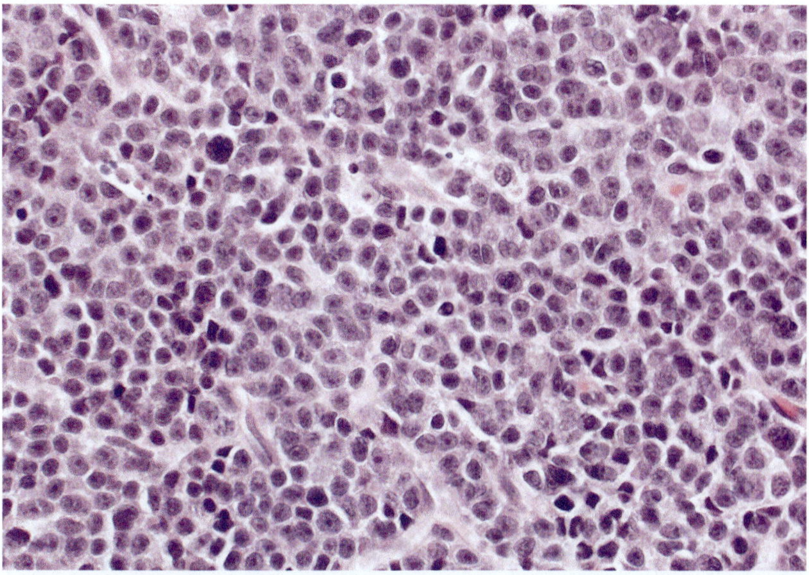

FIGURE 8.11 **High-grade B-cell lymphoma, HIV associated.** Lymphoma cells are medium sized with fine ("blasty") chromatin and small nucleoli.

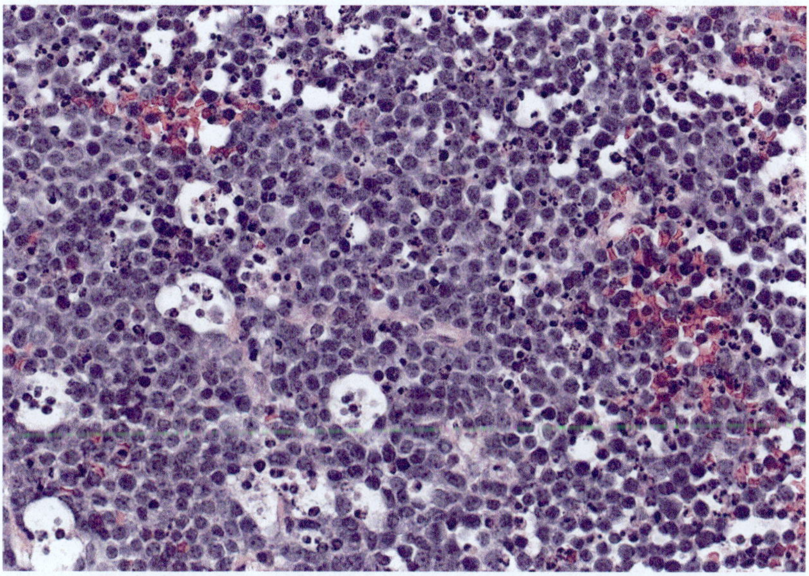

FIGURE 8.12 **Burkitt lymphoma, HIV associated.** "Starry-sky" pattern and typical monotonous morphology are seen in this case.

in patients with HIV), gastrointestinal tract, skin, and soft tissue; however, lymph nodes are frequently involved too. Majority of cases are EBV positive (approximately 70% or more in some studies), and *MYC* rearrangement can be seen in approximately half of cases (Figure 8.13A and B).[59,60]

CHL incidence in HIV-infected people has increased since the advent of ART, as these patients tend to have higher CD4 T-cell counts. Prevalence of morphologic subtypes has also changed, with nodular sclerosis being the most common subtype, while in the pre-ART era mixed cellularity and lymphocyte depletion were classic subtypes associated with HIV infection. Clinically, the majority of patients present in advanced

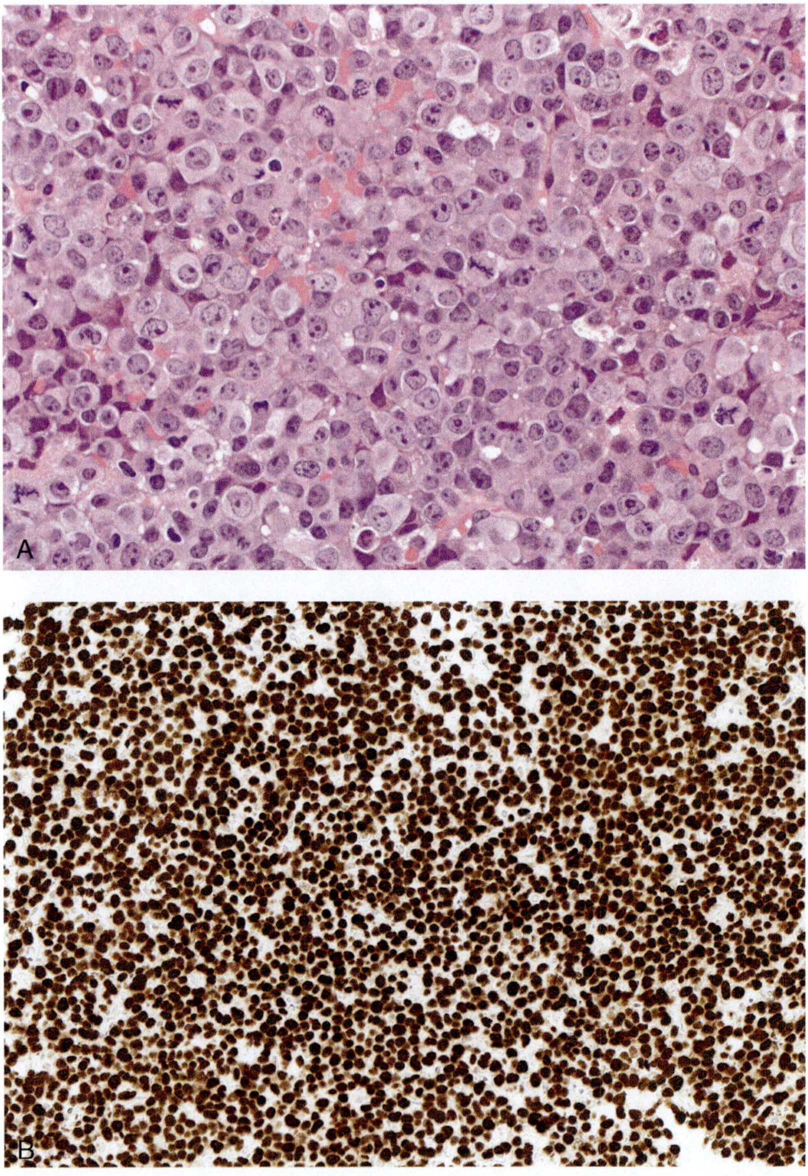

FIGURE 8.13 **Plasmablastic lymphoma, HIV associated.** A, Sheets of plasmablastic cells are seen with large eccentric nuclei, prominent nucleoli, and abundant cytoplasm. B, EBER in situ hybridization shows diffuse positivity in lymphoma cells.

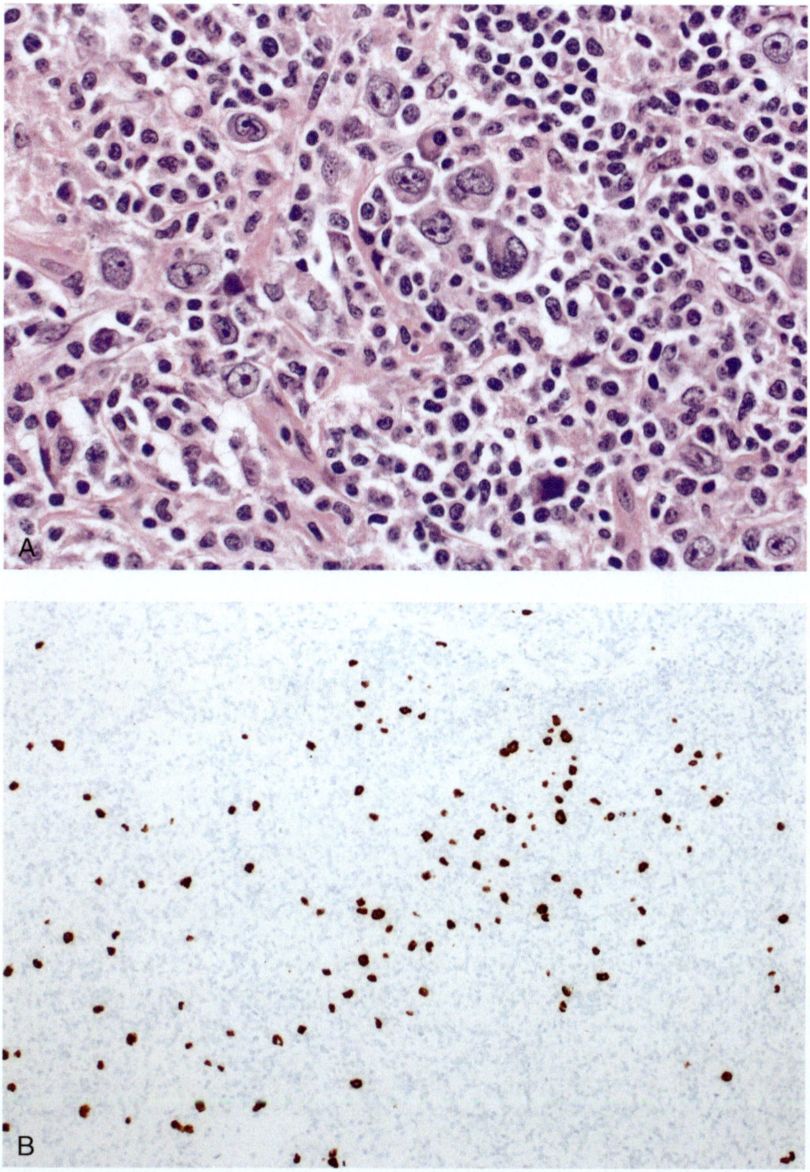

FIGURE 8.14 **Classic Hodgkin lymphoma, HIV associated.** A, Scattered Hodgkin cells are seen in the polymorphous background. B, EBER in situ hybridization is positive in neoplastic Hodgkin cells.

stages of disease, with frequent involvement of extranodal sites including bone marrow, liver, and spleen. The morphologic and immunophenotypic features are similar to those seen in immunocompetent patients. Of note, EBER-ISH is positive in HRS cells in virtually all cases of HIV-associated CHL (Figure 8.14A and B).[61]

Occasionally, polymorphic PTLD-like proliferations can be seen in HIV-positive individuals. These have been reported to occur in nodal and extranodal sites, and majority are EBV-positive.[62]

REFERENCES

1. Swerdlow SH, Campo E, Harris NL, et al. *WHO Classification of Tumours of Haematopoietic and Lymphoid Tissues*. IARC; 2017.
2. Campo E, Jaffe ES, Cook JR, et al. The International Consensus Classification of Mature Lymphoid Neoplasms: a report from the Clinical Advisory Committee. *Blood*. 2022;140(11):1229-1253.
3. Natkunam Y, Gratzinger D, Chadburn A, et al. Immunodeficiency-associated lymphoproliferative disorders: time for reappraisal? *Blood*. 2018;132(18):1871-1878.
4. Dojcinov SD, Venkataraman G, Raffeld M, Pittaluga S, Jaffe ES. EBV positive mucocutaneous ulcer—a study of 26 cases associated with various sources of immunosuppression. *Am J Surg Pathol*. 2010;34(3):405-417.
5. Mancuso S, Carlisi M, Santoro M, Napolitano M, Raso S, Siragusa S. Immunosenescence and lymphomagenesis. *Immun Ageing*. 2018;15:22.
6. Jaffe ESAD, Campo E, Harris NL, Quintanilla-Martinez L. *Hematopathology*. 2nd ed. Elsevier; 2017.
7. Medeiros LJ. *Ioachim's Lymph Node Pathology*. 5th ed. Wolters Kluwer; 2021.
8. Caillard S, Lelong C, Pessione F, Moulin B; French PTLD Working Group. Post-transplant lymphoproliferative disorders occurring after renal transplantation in adults: report of 230 cases from the French Registry. *Am J Transplant*. 2006;6(11):2735-2742.
9. Clarke CA, Morton LM, Lynch C, et al. Risk of lymphoma subtypes after solid organ transplantation in the United States. *Br J Cancer*. 2013;109(1):280-288.
10. Jagadeesh D, Woda BA, Draper J, Evens AM. Post transplant lymphoproliferative disorders: risk, classification, and therapeutic recommendations. *Curr Treat Options Oncol*. 2012;13(1):122-136.
11. Fujimoto A, Suzuki R. Epstein-Barr virus-associated post-transplant lymphoproliferative disorders after hematopoietic stem cell transplantation: pathogenesis, risk factors and clinical outcomes. *Cancers (Basel)*. 2020;12(2):328.
12. Nelson BP, Nalesnik MA, Bahler DW, Locker J, Fung JJ, Swerdlow SH. Epstein-Barr virus-negative post-transplant lymphoproliferative disorders: a distinct entity? *Am J Surg Pathol*. 2000;24(3):375-385.
13. Abbas F, El Kossi M, Shaheen IS, Sharma A, Halawa A. Post-transplantation lymphoproliferative disorders: current concepts and future therapeutic approaches. *World J Transplant*. 2020;10(2):29-46.
14. Tsao L, Hsi ED. The clinicopathologic spectrum of posttransplantation lymphoproliferative disorders. *Arch Pathol Lab Med*. 2007;131(8):1209-1218.
15. Mbulaiteye SM, Clarke CA, Morton LM, et al. Burkitt lymphoma risk in U.S. solid organ transplant recipients. *Am J Hematol*. 2013;88(4):245-250.
16. Zimmermann H, Reinke P, Neuhaus R, et al. Burkitt post-transplantation lymphoma in adult solid organ transplant recipients: sequential immunochemotherapy with rituximab (R) followed by cyclophosphamide, doxorubicin, vincristine, and prednisone (CHOP) or R-CHOP is safe and effective in an analysis of 8 patients. *Cancer*. 2012;118(19):4715-4724.
17. Engels EA, Clarke CA, Pfeiffer RM, et al. Plasma cell neoplasms in US solid organ transplant recipients. *Am J Transplant*. 2013;13(6):1523-1532.

18. Trappe R, Zimmermann H, Fink S, et al. Plasmacytoma-like post-transplant lymphoproliferative disorder, a rare subtype of monomorphic B-cell post-transplant lymphoproliferation, is associated with a favorable outcome in localized as well as in advanced disease: a prospective analysis of 8 cases. *Haematologica*. 2011;96(7):1067-1071.
19. Zimmermann H, Oschlies I, Fink S, et al. Plasmablastic posttransplant lymphoma: cytogenetic aberrations and lack of Epstein-Barr virus association linked with poor outcome in the prospective German Posttransplant Lymphoproliferative Disorder Registry. *Transplantation*. 2012;93(5):543-550.
20. Cassidy DP, Vega F, Chapman JR. Epstein-Barr virus-positive extranodal marginal zone lymphoma of bronchial-associated lymphoid tissue in the posttransplant setting: an immunodeficiency-related (posttransplant) lymphoproliferative disorder? *Am J Clin Pathol*. 2017;149(1):42-49.
21. Cheung CY, Lau WH, Cheuk W. Epstein-Barr virus-associated nodal marginal zone lymphoma: part of the spectrum of posttransplant lymphoproliferative disorder? *Int J Surg Pathol*. 2019;27(1):94-97.
22. Swerdlow SH. T-cell and NK-cell posttransplantation lymphoproliferative disorders. *Am J Clin Pathol*. 2007;127(6):887-895.
23. Rosenberg AS, Klein AK, Ruthazer R, Evens AM. Hodgkin lymphoma post-transplant lymphoproliferative disorder: a comparative analysis of clinical characteristics, prognosis, and survival. *Am J Hematol*. 2016;91(6):560-565.
24. Pitman SD, Huang Q, Zuppan CW, et al. Hodgkin lymphoma-like posttransplant lymphoproliferative disorder (HL-like PTLD) simulates monomorphic B-cell PTLD both clinically and pathologically. *Am J Surg Pathol*. 2006;30(4):470-476.
25. Nelson BP, Wolniak KL, Evens A, Chenn A, Maddalozzo J, Proytcheva M. Early posttransplant lymphoproliferative disease: clinicopathologic features and correlation with mTOR signaling pathway activation. *Am J Clin Pathol*. 2012;138(4):568-578.
26. Lones MA, Mishalani S, Shintaku IP, Weiss LM, Nichols WS, Said JW. Changes in tonsils and adenoids in children with posttransplant lymphoproliferative disorder: report of three cases with early involvement of Waldeyer's ring. *Hum Pathol*. 1995;26(5):525-530.
27. Vakiani E, Nandula SV, Subramaniyam S, et al. Cytogenetic analysis of B-cell posttransplant lymphoproliferations validates the World Health Organization classification and suggests inclusion of florid follicular hyperplasia as a precursor lesion. *Hum Pathol*. 2007;38(2):315-325.
28. Kaplan MA, Ferry JA, Harris NL, Jacobson JO. Clonal analysis of posttransplant lymphoproliferative disorders, using both episomal Epstein-Barr virus and immunoglobulin genes as markers. *Am J Clin Pathol*. 1994;101(5):590-596.
29. Knowles DM, Cesarman E, Chadburn A, et al. Correlative morphologic and molecular genetic analysis demonstrates three distinct categories of posttransplantation lymphoproliferative disorders. *Blood*. 1995;85(2):552-565.
30. Capello D, Rossi D, Gaidano G. Post-transplant lymphoproliferative disorders: molecular basis of disease histogenesis and pathogenesis. *Hematol Oncol*. 2005;23(2):61-67.
31. Menter T, Juskevicius D, Alikian M, et al. Mutational landscape of B-cell post-transplant lymphoproliferative disorders. *Br J Haematol*. 2017;178(1):48-56.
32. Morscio J, Dierickx D, Ferreiro JF, et al. Gene expression profiling reveals clear differences between EBV-positive and EBV-negative posttransplant lymphoproliferative disorders. *Am J Transplant*. 2013;13(5):1305-1316.
33. Bousfiha A, Jeddane L, Picard C, et al. Human inborn errors of immunity: 2019 update of the IUIS phenotypical classification. *J Clin Immunol*. 2020;40(1):66-81.
34. Gratzinger D, Jaffe ES, Chadburn A, et al. Primary/congenital immunodeficiency: 2015 SH/EAHP workshop report-Part 5. *Am J Clin Pathol*. 2017;147(2):204-216.

35. Unger S, Seidl M, Schmitt-Graeff A, et al. Ill-defined germinal centers and severely reduced plasma cells are histological hallmarks of lymphadenopathy in patients with common variable immunodeficiency. *J Clin Immunol.* 2014;34(6):615-626.
36. Facchetti F, Blanzuoli L, Ungari M, Alebardi O, Vermi W. Lymph node pathology in primary combined immunodeficiency diseases. *Springer Semin Immunopathol.* 1998;19(4):459-478.
37. Sander CA, Medeiros LJ, Weiss LM, Yano T, Sneller MC, Jaffe ES. Lymphoproliferative lesions in patients with common variable immunodeficiency syndrome. *Am J Surg Pathol.* 1992;16(12):1170-1182.
38. Lougaris V, Badolato R, Ferrari S, Plebani A. Hyper immunoglobulin M syndrome due to CD40 deficiency: clinical, molecular, and immunological features. *Immunol Rev.* 2005;203:48-66.
39. Matson DR, Yang DT. Autoimmune lymphoproliferative syndrome: an overview. *Arch Pathol Lab Med.* 2020;144(2):245-251.
40. Smith T, Cunningham-Rundles C. Lymphoid malignancy in common variable immunodeficiency in a single-center cohort. *Eur J Haematol.* 2021;107(5):503-516.
41. Kebudi R, Kiykim A, Sahin MK. Primary immunodeficiency and cancer in children; a review of the literature. *Curr Pediatr Rev.* 2019;15(4):245-250.
42. Cunningham-Rundles C, Cooper DL, Duffy TP, Strauchen J. Lymphomas of mucosal-associated lymphoid tissue in common variable immunodeficiency. *Am J Hematol.* 2002;69(3):171-178.
43. Leechawengwongs E, Shearer WT. Lymphoma complicating primary immunodeficiency syndromes. *Curr Opin Hematol.* 2012;19(4):305-312.
44. Said JW. Immunodeficiency-related Hodgkin lymphoma and its mimics. *Adv Anat Pathol.* 2007;14(3):189-194.
45. Taylor AM, Metcalfe JA, Thick J, Mak YF. Leukemia and lymphoma in ataxia telangiectasia. *Blood.* 1996;87(2):423-438.
46. Bagg A, Dunphy CH. Immunosuppressive and immunomodulatory therapy-associated lymphoproliferative disorders. *Semin Diagn Pathol.* 2013;30(2):102-112.
47. Hasserjian RP, Chen S, Perkins SL, et al. Immunomodulator agent-related lymphoproliferative disorders. *Mod Pathol.* 2009;22(12):1532-1540.
48. Wong AK, Kerkoutian S, Said J, Rashidi H, Pullarkat ST. Risk of lymphoma in patients receiving antitumor necrosis factor therapy: a meta-analysis of published randomized controlled studies. *Clin Rheumatol.* 2012;31(4):631-636.
49. Mariette X, Tubach F, Bagheri H, et al. Lymphoma in patients treated with anti-TNF: results of the 3-year prospective French RATIO registry. *Ann Rheum Dis.* 2010;69(2):400-408.
50. Takada H, Kaneko Y, Nakano K, et al. Clinicopathological characteristics of lymphoproliferative disorders in 232 patients with rheumatoid arthritis in Japan: a retrospective, multicenter, descriptive study. *Mod Rheumatol.* 2022;32(1):32-40.
51. Tokuhira M, Saito S, Okuyama A, et al. Clinicopathologic investigation of methotrexate-induced lymphoproliferative disorders, with a focus on regression. *Leuk Lymphoma.* 2018;59(5):1143-1152.
52. Ichikawa A, Arakawa F, Kiyasu J, et al. Methotrexate/iatrogenic lymphoproliferative disorders in rheumatoid arthritis: histology, Epstein-Barr virus, and clonality are important predictors of disease progression and regression. *Eur J Haematol.* 2013;91(1):20-28.
53. Kurita D, Miyoshi H, Ichikawa A, et al. Methotrexate-associated lymphoproliferative disorders in patients with rheumatoid arthritis: clinicopathologic features and prognostic factors. *Am J Surg Pathol.* 2019;43(7):869-884.

54. Loo EY, Medeiros LJ, Aladily TN, et al. Classical Hodgkin lymphoma arising in the setting of iatrogenic immunodeficiency: a clinicopathologic study of 10 cases. *Am J Surg Pathol.* 2013;37(8):1290-1297.

55. Gibson TM, Morton LM, Shiels MS, Clarke CA, Engels EA. Risk of non-Hodgkin lymphoma subtypes in HIV-infected people during the HAART era: a population-based study. *AIDS.* 2014;28(15):2313-2318.

56. Hubel K. The changing landscape of lymphoma associated with HIV infection. *Curr Oncol Rep.* 2020;22(11):111.

57. Lilly AJ, Fedoriw Y. Human immunodeficiency virus-associated lymphoproliferative disorders. *Surg Pathol Clin.* 2019;12(3):771-782.

58. Davi F, Delecluse HJ, Guiet P, et al. Burkitt-like lymphomas in AIDS patients: characterization within a series of 103 human immunodeficiency virus-associated non-Hodgkin's lymphomas. Burkitt's Lymphoma Study Group. *J Clin Oncol.* 1998;16(12):3788-3795.

59. Mai B, Wang W, Lin M, et al. HIV-associated plasmablastic lymphoma in the era of HAART: a single-center experience of 21 patients. *AIDS.* 2020;34(12):1735-1743.

60. Castillo J, Pantanowitz L, Dezube BJ. HIV-associated plasmablastic lymphoma: lessons learned from 112 published cases. *Am J Hematol.* 2008;83(10):804-809.

61. Carbone A, Gloghini A, Serraino D, Spina M. HIV-associated Hodgkin lymphoma. *Curr Opin HIV AIDS.* 2009;4(1):3-10.

62. Nador RG, Chadburn A, Gundappa G, Cesarman E, Said JW, Knowles DM. Human immunodeficiency virus (HIV)-associated polymorphic lymphoproliferative disorders. *Am J Surg Pathol.* 2003;27(3):293-302.

9

HISTIOCYTIC AND DENDRITIC CELL NEOPLASMS

KYLE D. PERRY and ANJANAA VIJAYANARAYANAN

Histiocytic and dendritic cell neoplasms are very rare tumors that can arise in lymph nodes, soft tissue, or virtually any organ. In the setting of a needle core biopsy, they can easily be misdiagnosed if not considered as a diagnostic possibility after more common entities have been excluded.

Histologically, these tumors are composed of histiocytoid or spindled cells that expand the lymph node sinuses or efface the lymph node architecture as a sheet-like or storiform proliferation, frequently associated with inflammatory cells. It is important to remember that this morphology is not particularly unique and that more common neoplasms should be considered and excluded. In particular, when encountering these proliferations in a lymph node biopsy, it is important to first assess the patient's clinical history and perform immunohistochemical stains to rule out a metastatic carcinoma (by a pancytokeratin stain), melanoma (by SOX10 stain), or germ cell tumor (by SALL4 stain). Furthermore, it is also important to remember that what might be clinically and radiologically designated as a "lymph node" could represent a soft tissue lesion. Many soft tissue tumors can present with a background or peripheral population of inflammatory cells, including angiomatoid fibrous histiocytoma, schwannoma, liposarcoma, myxoinflammatory fibroblastic sarcoma, and inflammatory rhabdomyoblastic tumor, among other possibilities. When considering one of the neoplasms described in this chapter, a prudent histiocytic/dendritic panel might include CD68, CD163, S100, CD1a, langerin, BRAFV600E stain, factor XIIIa, cyclinD1, OCT2, CD21, CD23, and CD35. However, the specific stains needed will be heavily guided by the morphologic features and differential diagnostic considerations. When assessing these immunohistochemical stains, it is critical to confirm that the positive cells are the actual neoplastic cells seen on the hematoxylin and eosin stain as many poorly differentiated neoplasms can have an incidental population of associated histiocytes or other inflammatory cells. Table 9.1 summarizes and compares immunophenotypic characteristics of different entities covered in this chapter.

TABLE 9.1 Comparison of Typical Immunophenotypes Between Histiocytic and Dendritic Cell Neoplasms

	S-100	CD1a	Langerin	CD68	CD163	CD21/CD23
Rosai-Dorfman disease	+	–	–	+	+	–
Histiocytic sarcoma	–/+	–	–	+	+	–
FDC sarcoma	–/+	–	–	–/+	–	+
IDC sarcoma	+	–	–	–/+	–/+	–
LCH	+	+	+	+/–	–	–

FDC, follicular dendritic cell; IDC, interdigitating dendritic cell; LCH, Langerhans cell histiocytosis.

ROSAI-DORFMAN DISEASE

Rosai-Dorfman disease (RDD; a.k.a. sinus histiocytosis with massive lymphadenopathy) is a histiocytic neoplasm that primarily involves lymph nodes and manifests with lymphadenopathy. Although traditionally considered a benign/reactive entity, the 2022 International Consensus Classification included it under "Histiocytic and dendritic cell neoplasms" due to identification of recurrent clonal abnormalities in this disease (see below).[1] Approximately a third of patients will have concurrent constitutional symptoms, including night sweats, fever, and weight loss. RDD involves extranodal sites in up to 40% of patients. This disease can present as a solitary entity, or it may arise in association with another disease process, such as a concurrent autoimmune, malignant, or hereditary disease.

There are number of approaches to treating RDD. As up to 50% of cases can spontaneously resolve, some clinicians opt for observation. Chemotherapy can be administered in refractory or relapsed cases. Refractory patients may benefit from molecular study to determine if they have a MAPK pathway mutation such as *KRAS* that would be amenable to targeted therapy. As noted, most patients have stable disease or regress; however, rare cases may have an aggressive course.[2,3]

Morphology

Lymph nodes affected by RDD typically show marked dilation/expansion of the sinuses by large histiocytes with abundant pale cytoplasm and vesicular nuclei with conspicuous central nucleoli. Histiocytes are admixed with plasma cells and lymphocytes. Many histiocytes show engulfed intact small lymphocytes and plasma cells, which is known as emperipolesis (Figures 9.1 and 9.2). Unlike histiocytic sarcoma, the RDD histiocytes do not exhibit substantial nuclear atypia.

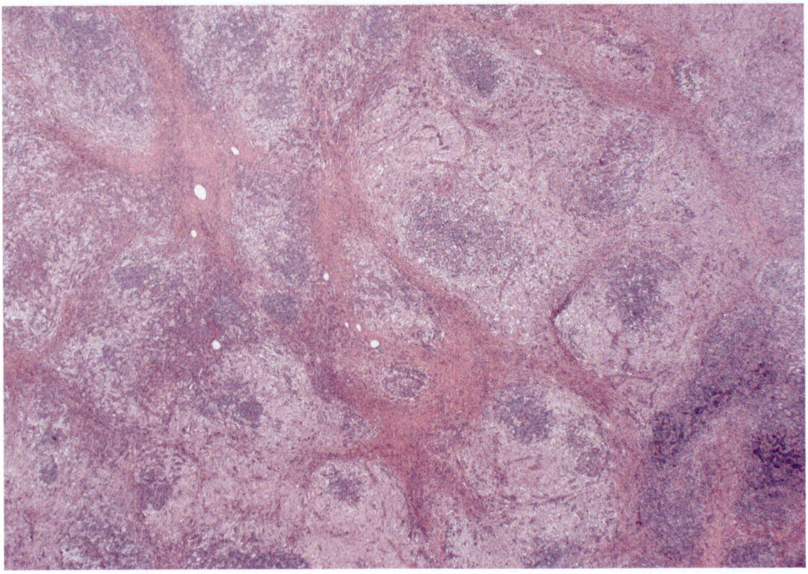

FIGURE 9.1 **Rosai-Dorfman disease.** Sinuses are markedly expanded by proliferation of histiocytes and inflammatory cells.

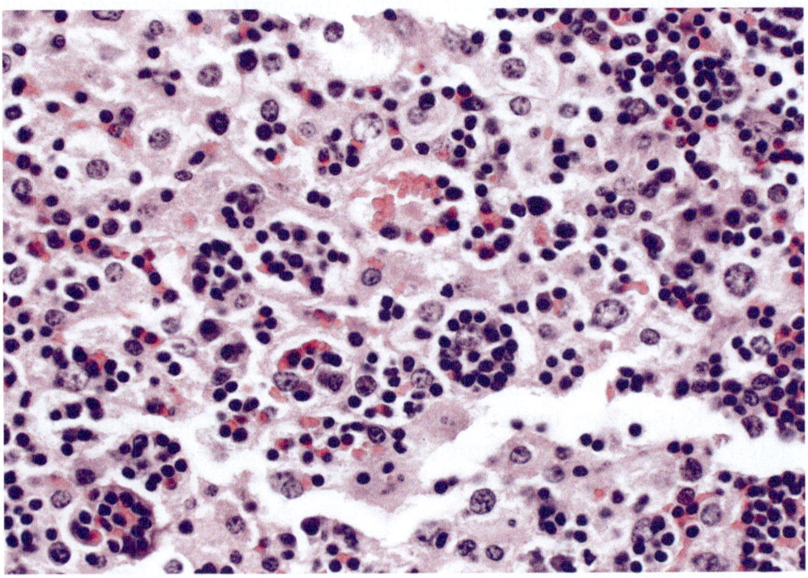

FIGURE 9.2 **Histiocytes in Rosai-Dorfman disease show emperipolesis.**

Phenotype

The histiocytes mark for usual macrophage markers CD68 and CD163, as well as OCT2, a marker of monocytic cells.[4] In addition, there is both cytoplasmic and nuclear staining for S100 (Figure 9.3). The RDD cells

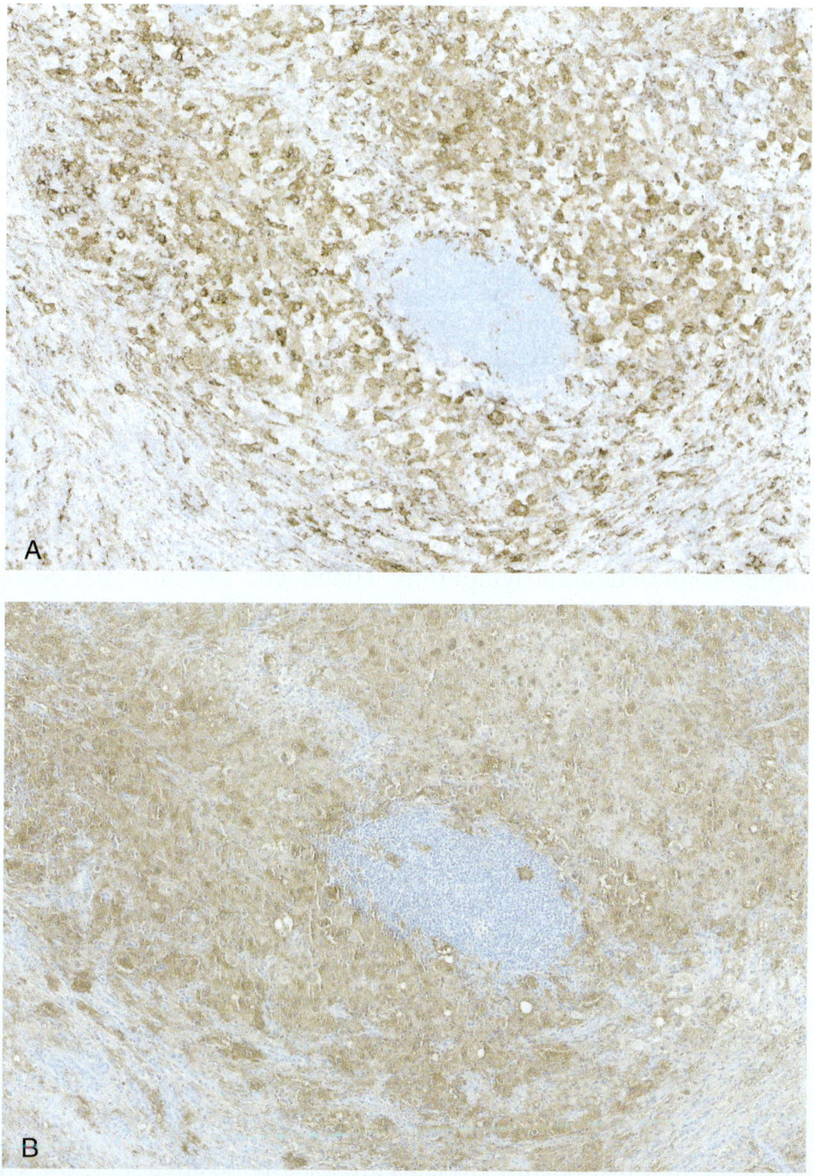

FIGURE 9.3 **Rosai-Dorfman disease.** Histiocytes are positive for CD68 (A) and S100 (B).

are negative for CD1a and langerin, which helps differentiate them from Langerhans cell histiocytosis (LCH). Reactive sinus histiocytes can express S100, so it is critical to identify the characteristic morphology of the histiocytes before proceeding to phenotyping to avoid overdiagnosis. Cyclin D1 is overexpressed in RDD cells, which can also be a helpful feature.[5]

Genetics

Approximately a third of RDD cases have mutually exclusive mutations in the *KRAS* and *MAP2K1* genes, highlighting the critical role of the MAPK pathway in this disease. The diagnosis, however, is typically made on morphologic and immunohistochemical grounds.[6]

HISTIOCYTIC SARCOMA

Histiocytic sarcoma (HS) is a malignant neoplasm composed of histiocytes. This tumor most commonly occurs in the 6th decade of life, although the age range is broad. The most common sites of involvement are gastrointestinal tract, nasal cavity, deep soft tissue, and lung. However, cases of HS that primarily involve the lymph nodes have been reported. A subset of patients with HS has an underlying hematolymphoid neoplasm that undergoes transdifferentiation to a histiocytic sarcoma. These include chronic lymphocytic leukemia/small lymphocytic lymphoma (CLL/SLL), follicular lymphoma, mantle cell lymphoma, marginal zone lymphoma, and B-lymphoblastic leukemia/lymphoma. Histiocytic sarcoma that occurs in these patients often shares identical immunoglobulin gene rearrangement with the underlying lymphoma in spite of not expressing typical B-cell antigens. Clinically, HS is an aggressive neoplasm and usually responds poorly to therapy.[7-9]

Morphology

Morphologically, HS is composed of sheets of large epithelioid histiocytes. Importantly, the neoplastic cells exhibit atypical (and sometimes even anaplastic) cytologic features such as enlarged nuclei and prominent nucleoli, which help in differentiating them from benign "inflammatory" histiocytes (Figures 9.4 and 9.5). Background inflammatory cells such as neutrophils, eosinophils, and plasma cells can be present.[8,10] When evaluating an HS, one should also adequately sample the specimen and remain vigilant for a coexisting lymphoma or other hematopoietic neoplasm. An example of HS arising in a patient with CLL/SLL is shown in Figure 9.6.

Phenotype

Similar to benign histiocytes, HS cells are usually positive for CD4, CD68, CD163, PU.1, and lysozyme (Figure 9.7). When interpreting these immunohistochemical stains, it is critical to confirm that the positive cells are not "incidental" histiocytes that are associated with some other type of malignancy, such as undifferentiated pleomorphic sarcoma. In addition to histiocytic markers, HS can show weak staining for S100, as opposed to IDC sarcoma, which shows strong staining. Unlike Langerhans cell histiocytosis or sarcoma, the tumor cells are usually negative for CD1a and langerin. Furthermore, HS lacks follicular dendritic markers (CD21, CD23, and CD35), which helps in excluding FDC sarcoma.[7,8]

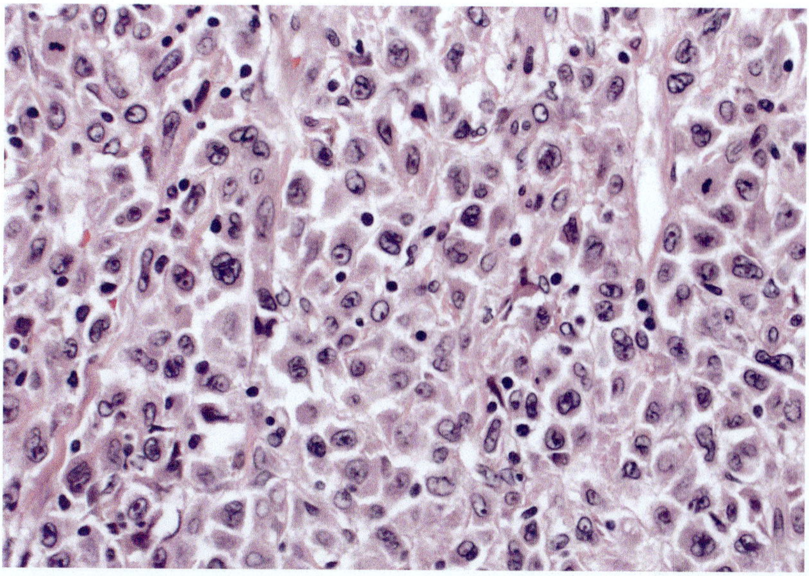

FIGURE 9.4 **Histiocytic sarcoma.** Malignant histiocytes are enlarged with nuclear atypia and focally prominent nucleoli.

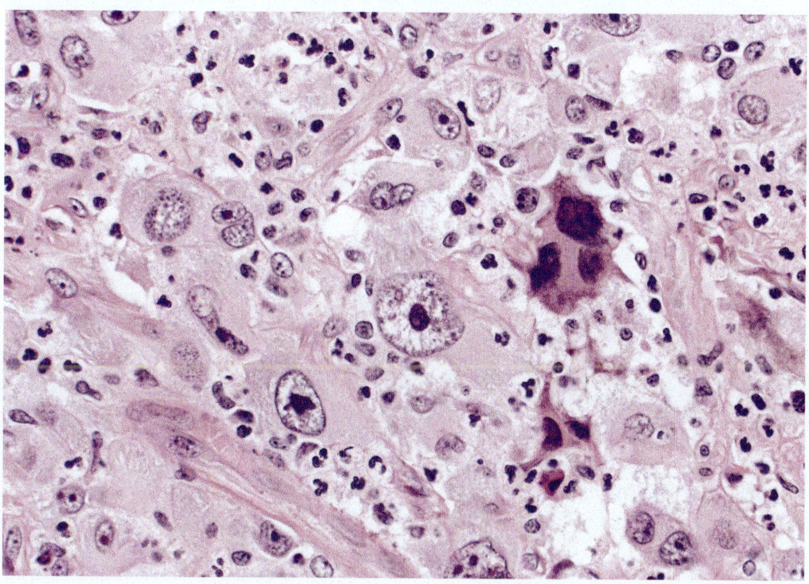

FIGURE 9.5 **Another case of histiocytic sarcoma with anaplastic features.**

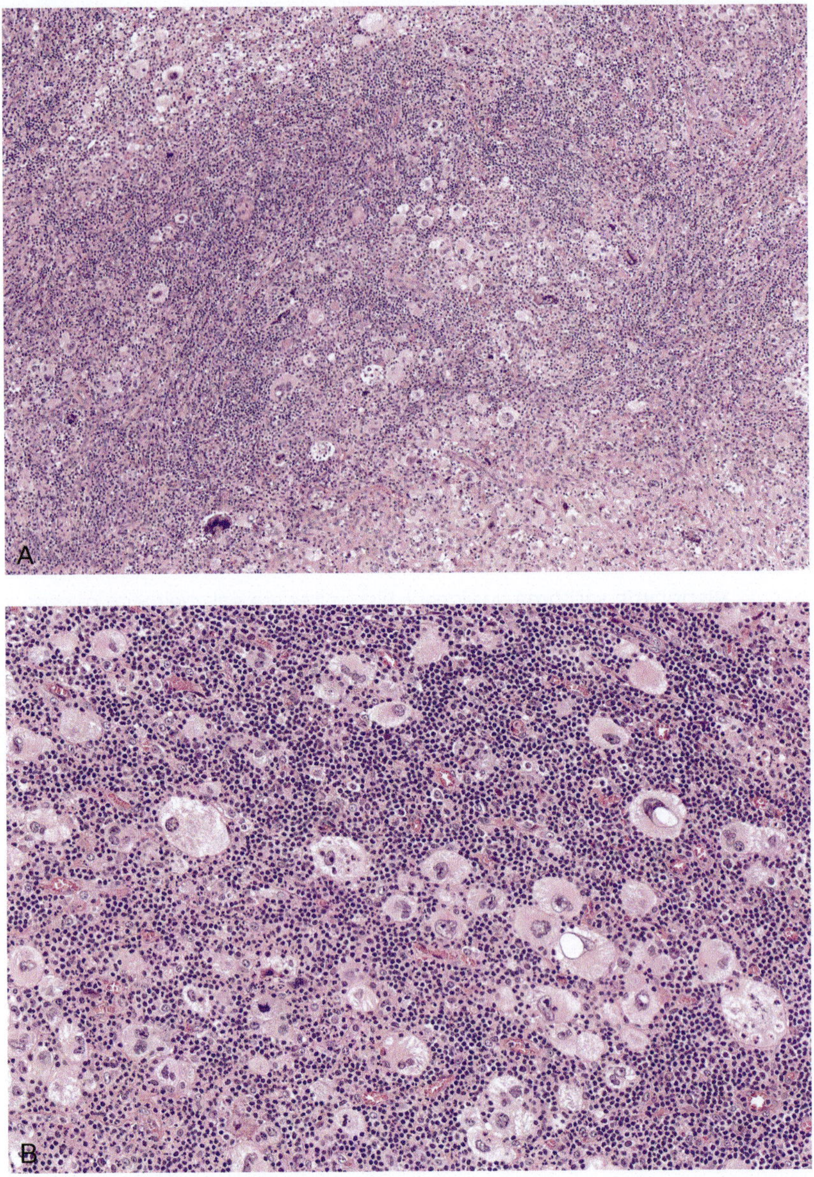

FIGURE 9.6 **Histiocytic sarcoma in patient with chronic lymphocytic leukemia/small lymphocytic lymphoma (SLL).** Scattered and clustered malignant histiocytic cells (A) are seen in the background of SLL in this lymph node (B).

Genetics

Approximately 40% to 50% of histiocytic sarcomas have been found to have mutations in genes that are part of the RAS-MAPK pathway, including *MAP2K1, CBL, BRAF, PTPN11, KRAS, NRAS,* and *MAP2K1.*[11] About a

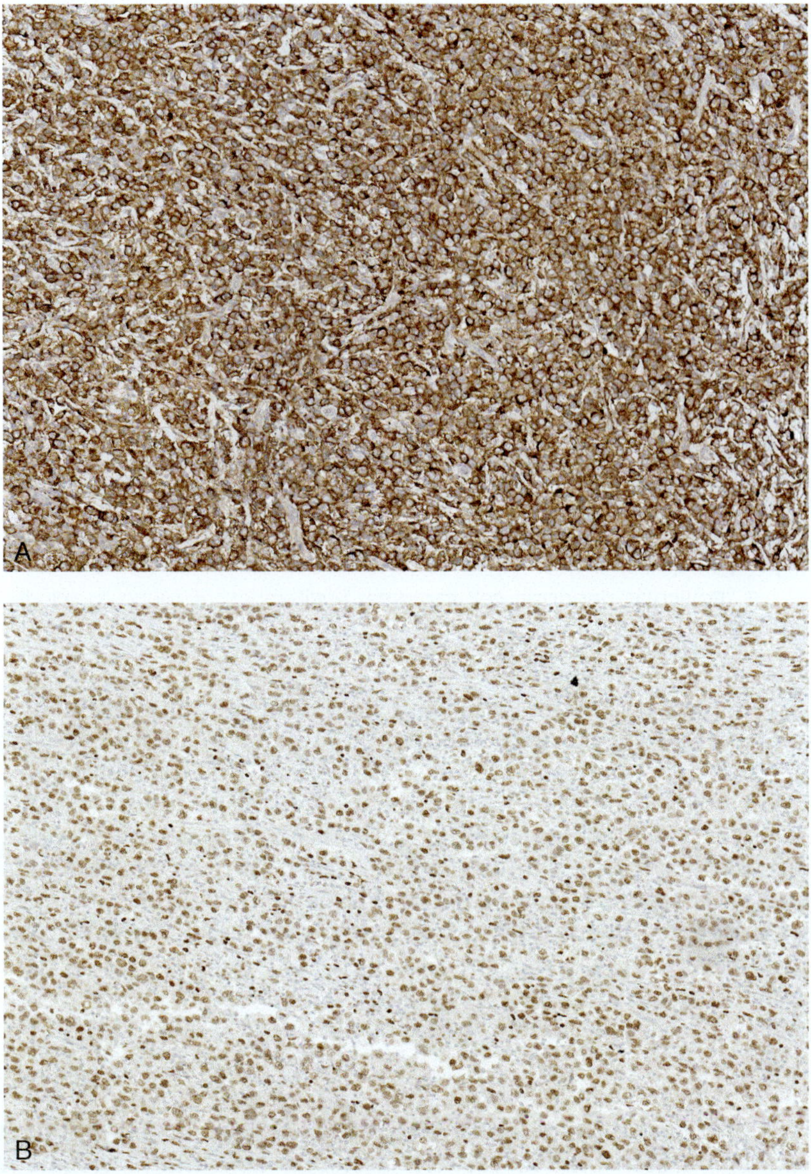

FIGURE 9.7 Histiocytic sarcoma is positive for CD163 (A) and PU.1 (B).

fifth of cases were also found to have mutations involving the PI3K-AKT-MTOR pathway, including the *MTOR, PTEN, PIK3CA*, and *PIK3R1* genes.[12]

FOLLICULAR DENDRITIC CELL SARCOMA

Follicular dendritic cells (FDCs) are mesenchymal-derived sustentacular cells that largely reside in the germinal centers and support humoral immunity.[13] They have a characteristic appearance with round to rectangular

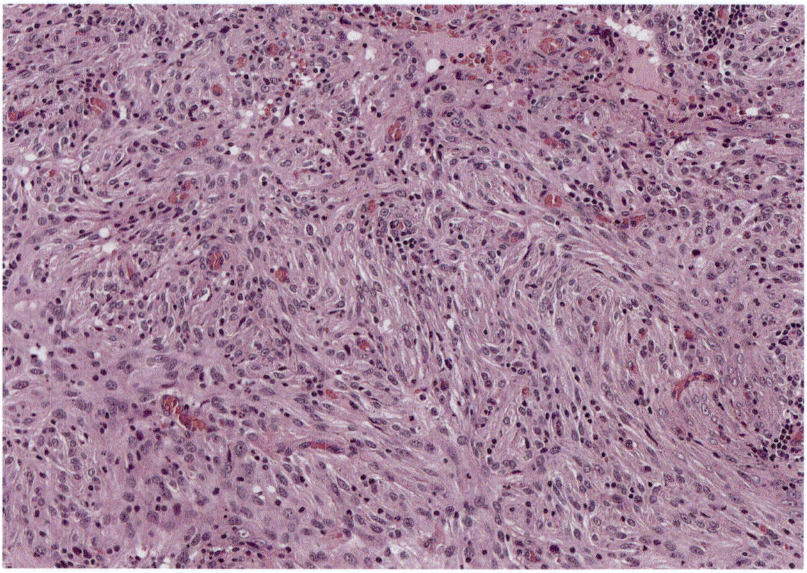

FIGURE 9.8 **Follicular dendritic cell sarcoma.** Proliferation of round to spindle cells forming fascicles.

nuclei and open chromatin with small central eosinophilic nucleoli. FDC sarcoma is a rare neoplasm derived from FDCs that may present as nodal disease, soft tissue masses, or both. The median age of presentation is in the 5th or 6th decade of life, and some patients present with weight loss and/or fever.[14] A minority of FDC sarcomas will arise in the setting of hyaline vascular Castleman disease (HVCD) and must be distinguished from reactive proliferations of FDCs that can occur in HVCD.[2,15] These tumors are typically considered to be either low or intermediate grade. Nearly 30% of FDC sarcomas recur, and approximately 30% of patients experience metastasis. More aggressive behavior has been associated with age $<$ 40 years or an abdominal presentation.[13]

Morphology

Microscopically, the lymph node is effaced by a spindle cell proliferation that exhibits a storiform to vaguely fascicular appearance (Figure 9.8). The cells typically exhibit indistinct cytoplasmic borders, and perivascular whorling can be identified. Small lymphocytes are usually seen in the background. Nucleoli are relatively inconspicuous. While the nuclei typically exhibit mild to moderate nuclear atypia, scattered pleomorphic cells can be present (Figure 9.9).[10]

Phenotype

The tumor cells are positive for FDC markers such as CD21, CD23, and CD35, as well as clusterin (Figure 9.10). Positive staining for one or more of these markers will typically distinguish FDC sarcoma from an angiomatoid

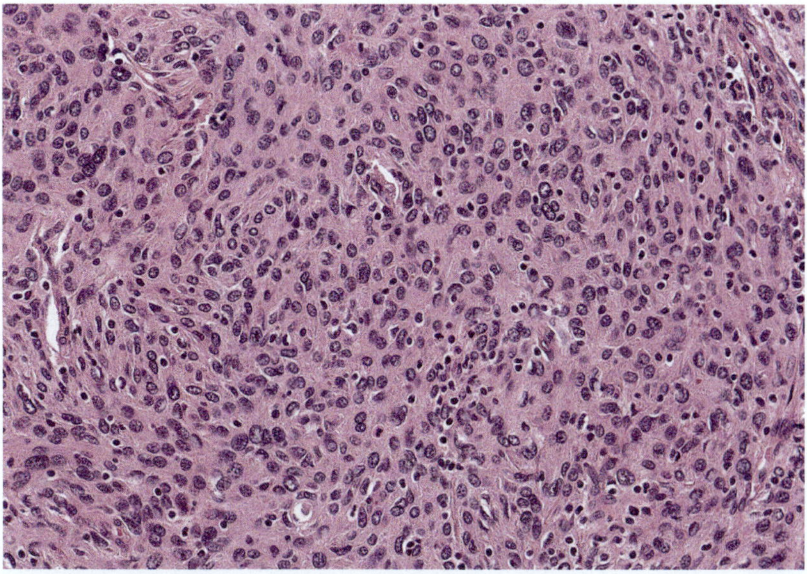

FIGURE 9.9 **Follicular dendritic cell sarcoma.** The neoplastic cells have relatively bland appearance with mild nuclear atypia and inconspicuous nucleoli.

fibrous histiocytoma, which can exhibit a perilesional lymphoid cuff and similar morphologic features. CD68 and S100 can show focal staining that could possibly result in misidentification as a histiocytic neoplasm (such as histiocytic sarcoma). Dedifferentiated liposarcoma, which also exhibits a storiform architecture and inflammatory background, lacks staining for CD21, CD23, or CD35 and is positive for MDM2.

Genetics

By conventional cytogenetic studies, these tumors exhibit a relatively complex karyotype. While one study showed *BRAF* V600E mutations in a minority of cases (about 20%), the consistency of this finding remains to be established.[16,17]

INTERDIGITATING DENDRITIC CELL SARCOMA

Interdigitating dendritic cells (IDCs) are typically found in the paracortex of the lymph node and are involved with antigen presentation to T lymphocytes.[18] Interdigitating dendritic cell sarcoma is an extremely rare neoplasm that usually affects adults over 40 years of age. While the lymph node is the most frequent location, the tumor can also involve extranodal sites such as the gastrointestinal tract, lung, kidney, larynx, skin, and nasopharynx.[19] In some cases, IDC sarcoma can arise from a previous low-grade B-cell lymphoma (so-called transdifferentiation).[20] The reported median survival is around 1 year; however, the clinical course of this disease can vary widely.

Morphology

Typically, IDC sarcomas are composed of large spindled cells with a vague fascicular to diffuse pattern. The cells contain vesicular nuclei with relatively inconspicuous nucleoli. Background lymphocytes and histiocytes are typically present, and even focal granulomatous inflammation has rarely been reported.[21]

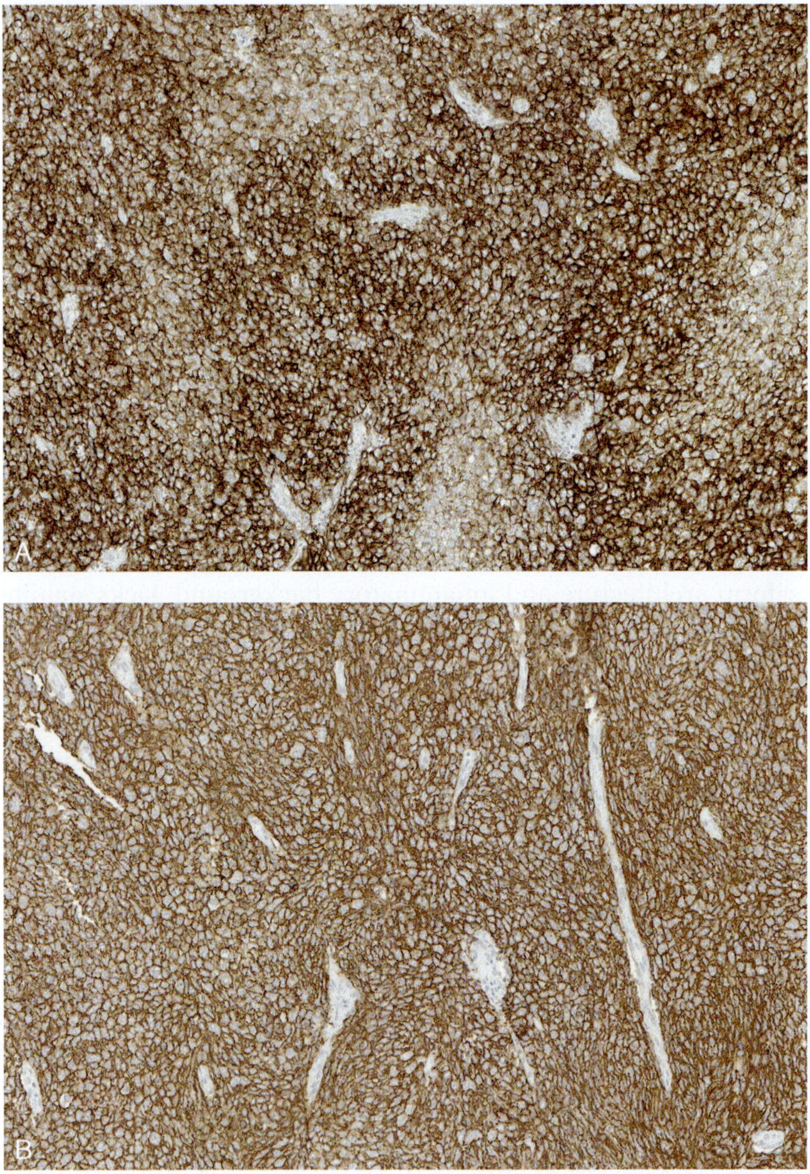

FIGURE 9.10 *(Continued)*

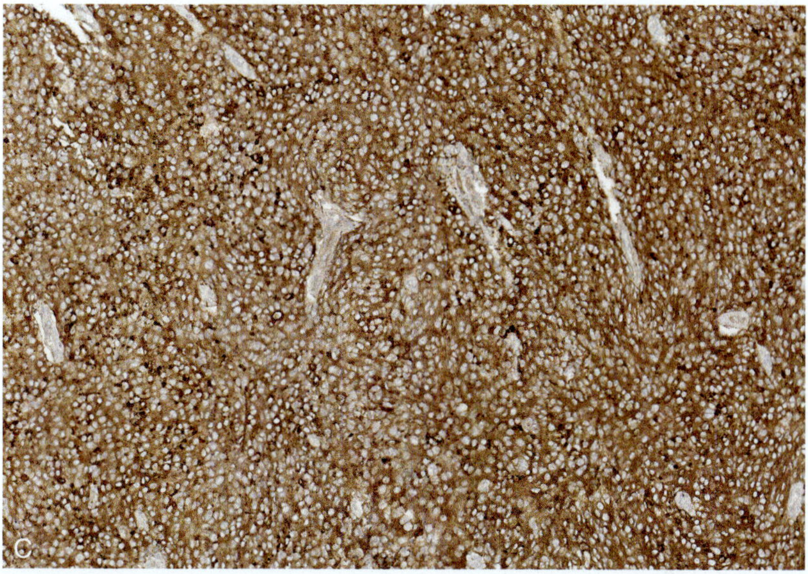

FIGURE 9.10 Follicular dendritic cell sarcoma stains positive for CD21 (A), CD23 (B), and clusterin (C).

Phenotype

IDC sarcomas typically exhibit strong diffuse staining for S100 without staining of CD1a or Langerin. About 20% of cases will show some staining with CD68 or CD163. This can sometimes make a differential diagnosis with histiocytic sarcoma somewhat problematic; however, histiocytic sarcomas will typically exhibit less prominent or negative S100 staining and usually have a more epithelioid-type morphology. Although these tumors can exhibit a whorling architecture reminiscent of FDC sarcoma, they are negative for CD21, CD23, and CD35. Unlike spindle cell melanomas, interdigitating dendritic cell sarcomas do not express SOX10 protein.[10,19]

Genetics

A consistent cytogenetic abnormality has not been identified in IDC sarcomas. A small subset was shown to exhibit mutations in *BRAF* V600E.[2]

LANGERHANS CELL HISTIOCYTOSIS AND LANGERHANS CELL SARCOMA

LCH is a proliferation of Langerhans-type cells (likely myeloid dendritic cells) that can involve various sites including the skin, lymph nodes, bone, and gastrointestinal tract. Patients are typically young children in the first decade of life, although it can arise in virtually any age. Lymph node involvement is typically found in pediatric patients who have systemic disease, but isolated involvement of lymph nodes can also occur. Patients with systemic disease will also exhibit constitutional symptoms such as fever, lymphadenopathy, hepatosplenomegaly, and pancytopenia.[2,22,23] A concurrent or association of LCH with other lymphomas (eg, classic Hodgkin lymphoma, diffuse large B-cell lymphoma, angioimmunoblastic T-cell lymphoma) has been well documented in the literature. In these cases the preferred terminology is "tumor-associated LCH." These cases likely represent reactive proliferation of Langerhans cells, as they lack mutations typically associated with LCH (ie, *BRAF* V600E and *MAP2K1*).[24-26] The clinical behavior and associated treatment for LCH vary widely depending on the extent of disease. Patients with localized disease may see spontaneous resolution while infants with involvement of numerous organs have a poor prognosis. Patients with systemic disease often receive chemotherapy while localized disease can often be treated surgically. Treatment with recently developed MAPK pathway inhibitors has shown some promising results.[2,10,27]

Langerhans cell sarcoma (LCS) is an extremely rare tumor (even when compared with soft tissue tumors). Incidence is estimated at 2 per 100,000,000. Patients typically present with systemic disease at diagnosis and are usually older (median age 50 years) than patients with LCH. These tumors often present in the lymph nodes and have a poor prognosis, with a median survival of <30 months.[28,29]

Morphology

Lymph nodes involved by LCH show variable degree of architectural effacement. Langerhans cells are typically initially seen in the sinuses, which can be mildly to markedly expanded (Figure 9.11). This is a helpful feature distinguishing LCH from a more common, benign mimicker, dermatopathic lymphadenopathy, which will have proliferation of reactive Langerhans cells in the paracortex. The LCH infiltrate emanates from the sinuses and can disrupt the lymph node architecture to the point of total effacement. Langerhans cells show pale pink cytoplasm and have folded, vesicular nuclei with grooves often referred to as "coffee bean" nuclei. Occasional multinucleated giant cells are seen. Significant nuclear atypia is typically not present. Admixed eosinophils are typically seen (Figure 9.12).[27]

LCS typically consists of pleomorphic or epithelioid-type cells with substantial nuclear atypia (Figure 9.13). The tumors share considerable morphologic overlap with other pleomorphic sarcomas, and diagnosis is primarily based on its immunophenotype.[2]

Phenotype

Immunohistochemically, the cells in LCH show a staining pattern similar to that of benign Langerhans cells and are positive for CD68 (Golgi staining), S100, CD1a, and langerin (Figure 9.14). They show diffuse expression of cyclin D1.[30] OCT2 is negative, in contrast to RDD. They are commonly negative for CD163. The BRAFV600E stain is useful for identifying cases

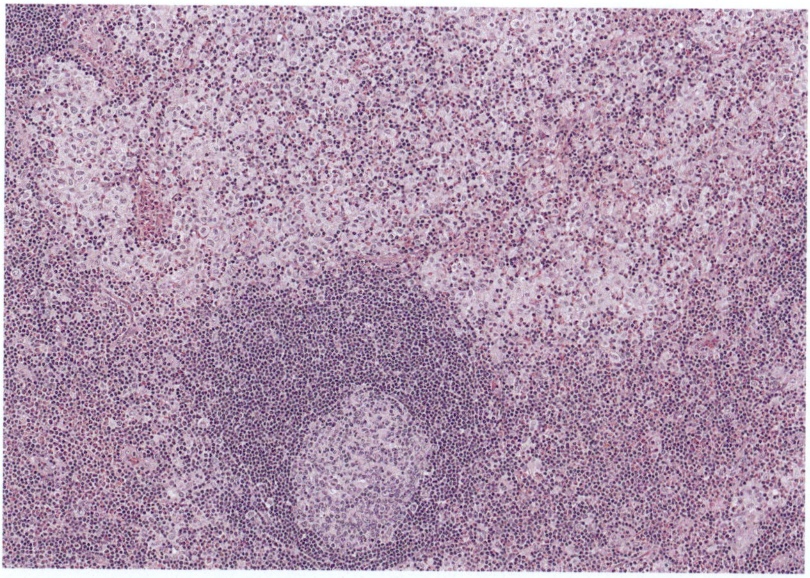

FIGURE 9.11 **Langerhans cell histiocytosis in a lymph node.** Sinuses are distended by a proliferation of pale Langerhans cells.

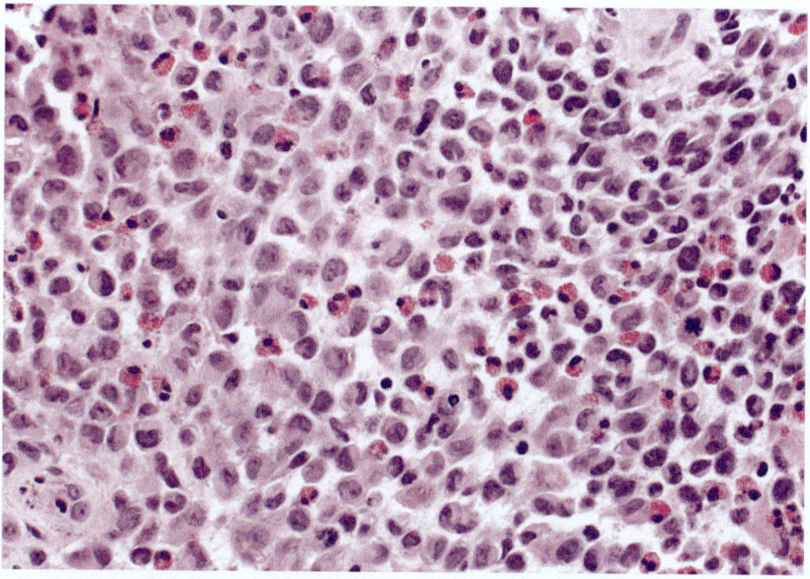

FIGURE 9.12 **Neoplastic Langerhans cells have folded, vesicular nuclei and pale cytoplasm.** Scattered eosinophils are seen in the background.

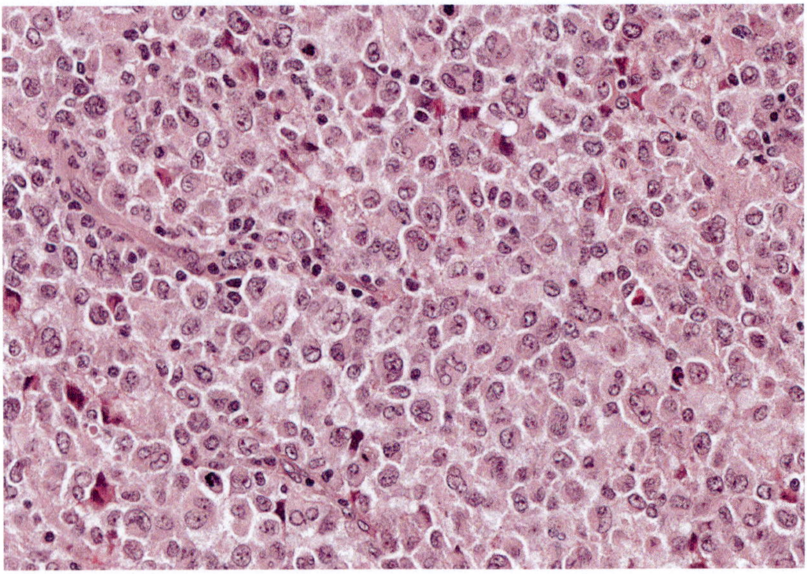

FIGURE 9.13 Langerhans cell sarcoma shows diffuse infiltration of large atypical cells with irregular vesicular nuclei, focally prominent nucleoli, and abundant eosinophilic cytoplasm.

with the mutation, although reports of sensitivity vary. The phenotype of LCS is less well established; however, to distinguish LCS from HS the majority of the tumor cells should express Langerhans cell markers such as CD1a and langerin (Figure 9.15). Given the positivity for S100 in LCH and LCS, the differential diagnosis includes metastatic melanoma to the lymph node. However, LCH and LCS lack expression of other melanocytic markers such as SOX10, melan A, and HMB45.

Genetics

The *BRAF* V600E mutation has been identified in approximately half of LCH cases. Furthermore, up to 25% of cases have *MAP2K1* mutation, which is mutually exclusive to *BRAF* mutation.[31] LCS has also been reported to have *BRAF* V600E mutation, although fewer data are available.[29]

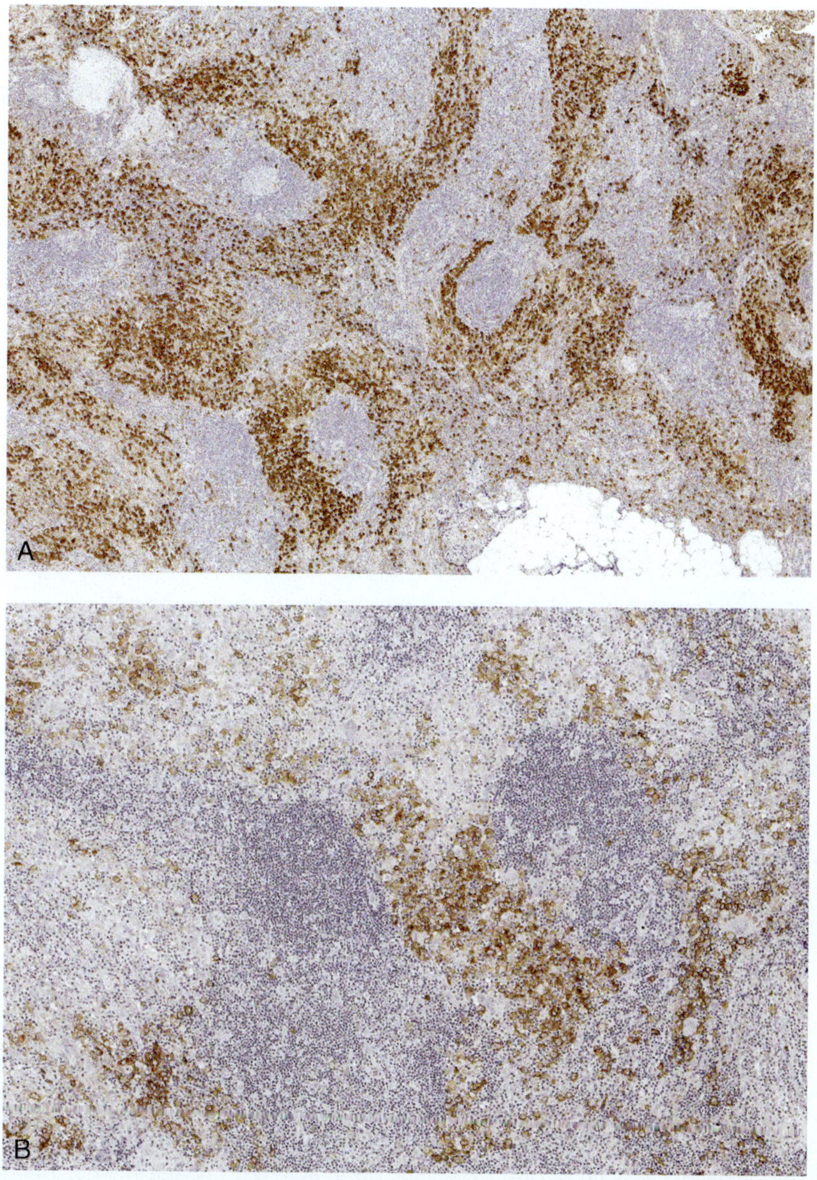

FIGURE 9.14 **Langerhans cell histiocytosis.** By immunohistochemistry, the cells are positive for S100, highlighting sinusoidal involvement (A), as well partially positive for CD1a (B).

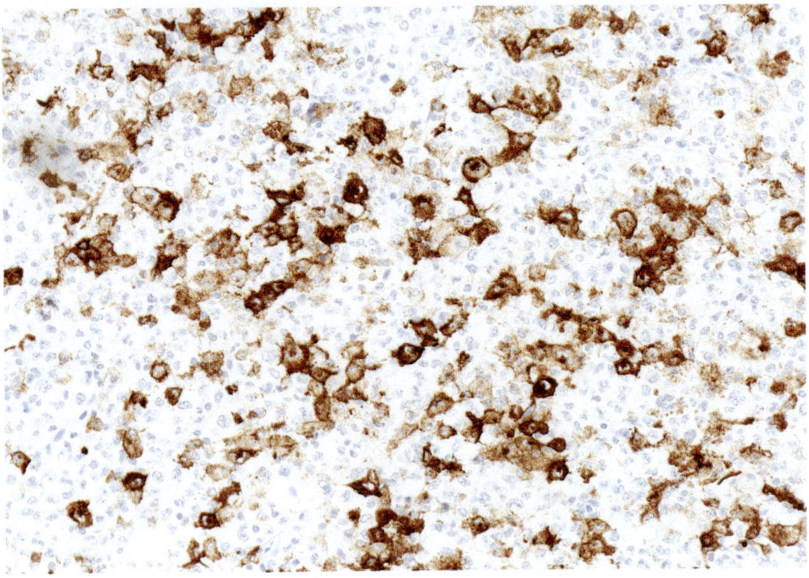

FIGURE 9.15 Langerhans cell sarcoma shows positivity for langerin.

REFERENCES

1. Campo E, Jaffe ES, Cook JR, et al. The International Consensus Classification of Mature Lymphoid Neoplasms: a report from the Clinical Advisory Committee. *Blood*. 2022;140(11):1229-1253. doi:10.1182/blood.2022015851
2. Medeiros LJ. *Ioachim's Lymph Node Pathology*. 5th ed. Wolters Kluwer; 2021.
3. Abla O, Jacobsen E, Picarsic J, et al. Consensus recommendations for the diagnosis and clinical management of Rosai-Dorfman-Destombes disease. *Blood*. 2018;131(26):2877-2890.
4. Ravindran A, Goyal G, Go RS, Rech KL; Mayo Clinic Histiocytosis Working Group. Rosai-Dorfman disease displays a unique monocyte-macrophage phenotype characterized by expression of OCT2. *Am J Surg Pathol*. 2021;45(1):35-44.
5. Baraban E, Sadigh S, Rosenbaum J, et al. Cyclin D1 expression and novel mutational findings in Rosai-Dorfman disease. *Br J Haematol*. 2019;186(6):837-844.
6. Garces S, Medeiros LJ, Patel KP, et al. Mutually exclusive recurrent KRAS and MAP2K1 mutations in Rosai-Dorfman disease. *Mod Pathol*. 2017;30(10):1367-1377.
7. Swerdlow SH, Campo E, Harris NL, Jaffe ES, et al. *WHO Classification of Tumours of Haematopoietic and Lymphoid Tissues*. IARC; 2017.
8. Hung YP, Qian X. Histiocytic sarcoma. *Arch Pathol Lab Med*. 2020;144(5):650-654.
9. Feldman AL, Minniti C, Santi M, Downing JR, Raffeld M, Jaffe ES. Histiocytic sarcoma after acute lymphoblastic leukaemia: a common clonal origin. *Lancet Oncol*. 2004;5(4):248-250.
10. Hornick JL. *Practical Soft Tissue Pathology: A Diagnostic Approach*. 2nd ed. Elsevier; 2018.
11. Shanmugam V, Griffin GK, Jacobsen ED, Fletcher CDM, Sholl LM, Hornick JL. Identification of diverse activating mutations of the RAS-MAPK pathway in histiocytic sarcoma. *Mod Pathol*. 2019;32(6):830-843.

12. Egan C, Nicolae A, Lack J, et al. Genomic profiling of primary histiocytic sarcoma reveals two molecular subgroups. *Haematologica*. 2020;105(4):951-960.
13. Facchetti F, Lorenzi L. Follicular dendritic cells and related sarcoma. *Semin Diagn Pathol*. 2016;33(5):262-276.
14. Jain P, Milgrom SA, Patel KP, et al. Characteristics, management, and outcomes of patients with follicular dendritic cell sarcoma. *Br J Haematol*. 2017;178(3):403-412.
15. Chan JK, Fletcher CD, Nayler SJ, Cooper K. Follicular dendritic cell sarcoma. Clinicopathologic analysis of 17 cases suggesting a malignant potential higher than currently recognized. *Cancer*. 1997;79(2):294-313.
16. Perry AM, Nelson M, Sanger WG, Bridge JA, Greiner TC. Cytogenetic abnormalities in follicular dendritic cell sarcoma: report of two cases and literature review. *In Vivo*. 2013;27(2):211-214.
17. Go H, Jeon YK, Huh J, et al. Frequent detection of BRAF(V600E) mutations in histiocytic and dendritic cell neoplasms. *Histopathology*. 2014;65(2):261-272.
18. Wright-Browne V, McClain KL, Talpaz M, Ordonez N, Estrov Z. Physiology and pathophysiology of dendritic cells. *Hum Pathol*. 1997;28(5):563-579.
19. Xue T, Jiang XN, Wang WG, Zhou XY, Li XQ. Interdigitating dendritic cell sarcoma: clinicopathologic study of 8 cases with review of the literature. *Ann Diagn Pathol*. 2018;34:155-160.
20. Fraser CR, Wang W, Gomez M, et al. Transformation of chronic lymphocytic leukemia/small lymphocytic lymphoma to interdigitating dendritic cell sarcoma: evidence for transdifferentiation of the lymphoma clone. *Am J Clin Pathol*. 2009;132(6):928-939.
21. Muhammed A, Ahmed ARH, Maysa H, Mohamed AES, Abd-ElLateef AA, Elnakib E. New insights inside the interdigitating dendritic cell sarcoma-pooled analysis and review of literature. *Ann Hematol*. 2019;98(12):2641-2651.
22. Berres ML, Merad M, Allen CE. Progress in understanding the pathogenesis of Langerhans cell histiocytosis: back to Histiocytosis X? *Br J Haematol*. 2015;169(1):3-13.
23. Edelweiss M, Medeiros LJ, Suster S, Moran CA. Lymph node involvement by Langerhans cell histiocytosis: a clinicopathologic and immunohistochemical study of 20 cases. *Hum Pathol*. 2007;38(10):1463-1469.
24. Egeler RM, Neglia JP, Puccetti DM, Brennan CA, Nesbit ME. Association of Langerhans cell histiocytosis with malignant neoplasms. *Cancer*. 1993;71(3):865-873.
25. Christie LJ, Evans AT, Bray SE, et al. Lesions resembling Langerhans cell histiocytosis in association with other lymphoproliferative disorders: a reactive or neoplastic phenomenon? *Hum Pathol*. 2006;37(1):32-39.
26. Pina-Oviedo S, Medeiros LJ, Li S, et al. Langerhans cell histiocytosis associated with lymphoma: an incidental finding that is not associated with BRAF or MAP2K1 mutations. *Mod Pathol*. 2017;30(5):734-744.
27. Rodriguez-Galindo C, Allen CE. Langerhans cell histiocytosis. *Blood*. 2020;135(16):1319-1331.
28. Moustafa MA, Jiang L, Tun HW. Langerhans cell sarcoma: the Mayo Clinic experience with an extremely rare disease. *J Clin Oncol*. 2020;38(15 suppl):e19543.
29. Howard JE, Dwivedi RC, Masterson L, Jani P. Langerhans cell sarcoma: a systematic review. *Cancer Treat Rev*. 2015;41(4):320-331.
30. Shanmugam V, Craig JW, Hornick JL, Morgan EA, Pinkus GS, Pozdnyakova O. Cyclin D1 is expressed in neoplastic cells of Langerhans cell histiocytosis but not reactive Langerhans cell proliferations. *Am J Surg Pathol*. 2017;41(10):1390-1396.
31. Brown NA, Furtado LV, Betz BL, et al. High prevalence of somatic MAP2K1 mutations in BRAF V600E-negative Langerhans cell histiocytosis. *Blood*. 2014;124(10):1655-1658.

APPENDIX 1

TABLE 1 2022 International Consensus Classification of Mature Lymphoid and Histiocytic/Dendritic Cell Neoplasms

Mature B-cell Neoplasms

Chronic lymphocytic leukemia/small lymphocytic lymphoma

Monoclonal B-cell lymphocytosis (CLL type and non-CLL type)

B-cell prolymphocytic leukemia

Splenic marginal zone lymphoma

Hairy cell leukemia

Splenic B-cell lymphoma/leukemia, unclassifiable

  Splenic diffuse red pulp small B-cell lymphoma

  Hairy cell leukemia-variant

Lymphoplasmacytic lymphoma

  Waldenström macroglobulinemia

IgM monoclonal gammopathy of undetermined significance (MGUS)

  IgM MGUS, plasma cell type

    IgM MGUS, NOS

Primary cold agglutinin disease

Heavy chain diseases

  Mu heavy chain disease

  Gamma heavy chain disease

  Alpha heavy chain disease

Plasma cell neoplasms

  Non-IgM monoclonal gammopathy of undetermined significance

  Multiple myeloma (plasma cell myeloma)

    Multiple myeloma, NOS

    Multiple myeloma with recurrent genetic abnormality

      Multiple myeloma with *CCND* family translocation

      Multiple myeloma with *MAF* family translocation

      Multiple myeloma with *NSD2* translocation

      Multiple myeloma with hyperdiploidy

  Solitary plasmacytoma of bone

  Extraosseous plasmacytoma

(*Continued*)

TABLE 1 2022 International Consensus Classification of Mature Lymphoid and Histiocytic/Dendritic Cell Neoplasms (*Continued*)

Monoclonal immunoglobulin deposition diseases
Immunoglobulin light chain amyloidosis (AL)
Localized AL amyloidosis
Light chain and heavy chain deposition disease
Extranodal marginal zone lymphoma of mucosa-associated lymphoid tissue (MALT lymphoma)
Primary cutaneous marginal zone lymphoproliferative disorder
Nodal marginal zone lymphoma
Pediatric nodal marginal zone lymphoma
Follicular lymphoma
In situ follicular neoplasia
Duodenal-type follicular lymphoma
BCL2-R negative, CD23-positive follicle center lymphoma
Primary cutaneous follicle center lymphoma
Pediatric-type follicular lymphoma
Testicular follicular lymphoma
Large B-cell lymphoma with *IRF4* rearrangement
Mantle cell lymphoma
In situ mantle cell neoplasia
Leukemic nonnodal mantle cell lymphoma
Diffuse large B-cell lymphoma (DLBCL), not otherwise specified (NOS)
Germinal center B-cell subtype
Activated B-cell subtype
Large B-cell lymphoma with 11q aberration
Nodular lymphocyte predominant B-cell lymphoma
T cell/histiocyte-rich large B-cell lymphoma
Primary DLBCL of the central nervous system
Primary DLBCL of the testis
Primary cutaneous DLBCL, leg type
Intravascular large B-cell lymphoma
HHV-8 and EBV-negative primary effusion-based lymphoma
EBV-positive mucocutaneous ulcer
EBV-positive DLBCL, NOS
DLBCL associated with chronic inflammation
Fibrin-associated DLBCL

TABLE 1 2022 International Consensus Classification of Mature Lymphoid and Histiocytic/Dendritic Cell Neoplasms (*Continued*)

Lymphomatoid granulomatosis
EBV-positive polymorphic B-cell lymphoproliferative disorder, NOS
ALK-positive large B-cell lymphoma
Plasmablastic lymphoma
HHV8-associated lymphoproliferative disorders
  Multicentric Castleman disease
  HHV8-positive germinotropic lymphoproliferative disorder
  HHV8-positive DLBCL, NOS
  Primary effusion lymphoma
Burkitt lymphoma
High-grade B-cell lymphoma, with MYC and BCL2 rearrangements
High-grade B-cell lymphoma with MYC and BCL6 rearrangements
High-grade B-cell lymphoma, NOS
Primary mediastinal large B-cell lymphoma
Mediastinal gray-zone lymphoma

Classic Hodgkin Lymphoma
Nodular sclerosis classic Hodgkin lymphoma
Lymphocyte-rich classic Hodgkin lymphoma
Mixed cellularity classic Hodgkin lymphoma
Lymphocyte-depleted classic Hodgkin lymphoma

Mature T- and NK-cell Neoplasms
T-cell prolymphocytic leukemia
T-cell large granular lymphocytic leukemia
Chronic lymphoproliferative disorder of NK cells
Adult T-cell leukemia/lymphoma
EBV-positive T/NK LPD of childhood
  Hydroa vacciniforme LPD
    Classic
    Systemic
  Severe mosquito bite allergy
  Chronic active EBV disease (T- and NK-cell phenotype)
  Systemic EBV-positive T-cell lymphoma of childhood
Extranodal NK-/T-cell lymphoma, nasal type
Aggressive NK-cell leukemia
Primary nodal EBV-positive T-/NK-cell lymphoma

(*Continued*)

TABLE 1 2022 International Consensus Classification of Mature Lymphoid and Histiocytic/Dendritic Cell Neoplasms (*Continued*)

Enteropathy-associated T-cell lymphoma
Type II refractory celiac disease
Monomorphic epitheliotropic intestinal T-cell lymphoma
Intestinal T-cell lymphoma, NOS
Indolent clonal T-cell lymphoproliferative disorder of the gastrointestinal tract
Indolent NK-cell lymphoproliferative disorder of the gastrointestinal tract
Hepatosplenic T-cell lymphoma
Mycosis fungoides
Sézary syndrome
Primary cutaneous CD30-positive T-cell lymphoproliferative disorders
Lymphomatoid papulosis
Primary cutaneous anaplastic large cell lymphoma
Primary cutaneous small/medium CD4-positive T-cell lymphoproliferative disorder
Subcutaneous panniculitis-like T-cell lymphoma
Primary cutaneous gamma-delta T-cell lymphoma
Primary cutaneous acral CD8-positive T-cell lymphoproliferative disorder
Primary cutaneous CD8-positive aggressive epidermotropic cytotoxic T-cell lymphoma
Peripheral T-cell lymphoma, NOS
Follicular helper T-cell lymphoma
Follicular helper T-cell lymphoma, angioimmunoblastic type (angioimmunoblastic T-cell lymphoma)
Follicular helper T-cell lymphoma, follicular type
Follicular helper T-cell lymphoma, NOS
Anaplastic large cell lymphoma, ALK positive
Anaplastic large cell lymphoma, ALK negative
Breast implant–associated anaplastic large cell lymphoma
Immunodeficiency-Associated Lymphoproliferative Disorders
Posttransplant lymphoproliferative disorders (PTLDs)
Nondestructive PTLD
Plasmacytic hyperplasia PTLD
Infectious mononucleosis PTLD
Florid follicular hyperplasia PTLD
Polymorphic PTLD
Monomorphic PTLD (B-and T-/NK-cell types)
Classic Hodgkin lymphoma PTLD
Other iatrogenic immunodeficiency-associated lymphoproliferative disorders

TABLE 1 2022 International Consensus Classification of Mature Lymphoid and Histiocytic/Dendritic Cell Neoplasms (*Continued*)

Histiocytic and Dendritic Cell Neoplasms
Histiocytic sarcoma
Langerhans cell histiocytosis
Langerhans cell sarcoma
Indeterminate dendritic cell histiocytosis
Interdigitating dendritic cell sarcoma
ALK-positive histiocytosis
Disseminated juvenile xanthogranuloma
Erdheim-Chester disease
Rosai-Dorfman-Destombes disease
Follicular dendritic cell sarcoma
Fibroblastic reticular cell sarcoma
EBV-positive inflammatory follicular dendritic cell/fibroblastic reticular cell tumor

In italics are provisional entities.

Source: Reproduced with permission from Campo E, Jaffe ES, Cook JR, et al. The International Consensus Classification of Mature Lymphoid Neoplasms: a report from the Clinical Advisory Committee. *Blood*. 2022;140(11):1229-1253. doi:10.1182/blood.2022015851.

TABLE 2 The 5th edition on the World Health Organization Classification of Hematolymphoid Tumors: Lymphoid Neoplasms

B-cell lymphoid proliferations and lymphomas
Tumor-like lesions with B-cell predominance
Reactive B-cell-rich lymphoid proliferations that can mimic lymphoma
IgG4-related disease
Unicentric Castleman disease
Idiopathic multicentric Castleman disease
KSHV/HHV8-associated multicentric Castleman disease
Precursor B-cell neoplasms
B-cell lymphoblastic leukemias/lymphomas
B-lymphoblastic leukemia/lymphoma, NOS
B-lymphoblastic leukemia/lymphoma with high hyperdiploidy
B-lymphoblastic leukemia/lymphoma with hypodiploidy
B-lymphoblastic leukemia/lymphoma with iAMP21
B-lymphoblastic leukemia/lymphoma with *BCR-ABL1* fusion

(*Continued*)

TABLE 2 The 5th edition on the World Health Organization Classification of Hematolymphoid Tumors: Lymphoid Neoplasms (*Continued*)

B-lymphoblastic leukemia/lymphoma with *BCR-ABL1*-like features
B-lymphoblastic leukemia/lymphoma with *KMT2A* rearrangement
B-lymphoblastic leukemia/lymphoma with *ETV6-RUNX1* fusion
B-lymphoblastic leukemia/lymphoma with *ETV6-RUNX1*-like features
B-lymphoblastic leukemia/lymphoma with *TCF3-PBX1* fusion
B-lymphoblastic leukemia/lymphoma with *IGH-IL3* fusion
B-lymphoblastic leukemia/lymphoma with *TCF3-HLF* fusion
B-lymphoblastic leukemia/lymphoma with other defined genetic abnormalities
Mature B-cell neoplasms
Preneoplastic and neoplastic small lymphocytic proliferations
Monoclonal B-cell lymphocytosis
Chronic lymphocytic leukemia/small lymphocytic lymphoma
Splenic B-cell lymphomas and leukemias
Hairy cell leukemia
Splenic marginal zone lymphoma
Splenic diffuse red pulp small B-cell lymphoma
Splenic B-cell lymphoma/leukemia with prominent nucleoli
Lymphoplasmacytic lymphoma
Marginal zone lymphoma
Extranodal marginal zone lymphoma of mucosa-associated lymphoid tissue
Primary cutaneous marginal zone lymphoma
Nodal marginal zone lymphoma
Pediatric marginal zone lymphoma
Follicular lymphoma
In situ follicular B-cell neoplasm
Follicular lymphoma
Pediatric-type follicular lymphoma
Duodenal-type follicular lymphoma
Primary cutaneous follicle center lymphoma
Mantle cell lymphoma
In situ mantle cell neoplasm
Mantle cell lymphoma
Leukemic nonnodal mantle cell lymphoma
Transformations of indolent B-cell lymphomas
Large B-cell lymphomas
Diffuse large B-cell lymphoma, NOS

TABLE 2 The 5th edition on the World Health Organization Classification of Hematolymphoid Tumors: Lymphoid Neoplasms (*Continued*)

T-cell/histiocyte-rich large B-cell lymphoma
Diffuse large B-cell lymphoma/high-grade B-cell lymphoma with *MYC* and *BCL2* rearrangements
ALK-positive large B-cell lymphoma
Large B-cell lymphoma with *IRF4* rearrangement
High-grade B-cell lymphoma with 11q aberrations
Lymphomatoid granulomatosis
EBV-positive diffuse large B-cell lymphoma
Diffuse large B-cell lymphoma associated with chronic inflammation
Fibrin-associated large B-cell lymphoma
Fluid overload-associated large B-cell lymphoma
Plasmablastic lymphoma
Primary large B-cell lymphoma of immune-privileged sites
Primary cutaneous diffuse large B-cell lymphoma, leg type
Intravascular large B-cell lymphoma
Primary mediastinal large B-cell lymphoma
Mediastinal gray zone lymphoma
High-grade B-cell lymphoma, NOS
Burkitt lymphoma
KSHV/HHV8-associated B-cell lymphoid proliferations and lymphomas
Primary effusion lymphoma
KSHV/HHV8-positive diffuse large B-cell lymphoma
KSHV/HHV8-positive germinotropic lymphoproliferative disorder
Lymphoid proliferations and lymphomas associated with immune deficiency and dysregulation
Hyperplasias arising in immune deficiency/dysregulation
Polymorphic lymphoproliferative disorders arising in immune deficiency/dysregulation
EBV-positive mucocutaneous ulcer
Lymphomas arising in immune deficiency/dysregulation
Inborn error of immunity-associated lymphoid proliferations and lymphomas
Hodgkin lymphoma
Classic Hodgkin lymphoma
Nodular lymphocyte predominant Hodgkin lymphoma
Plasma cell neoplasms and other diseases with paraproteins
Monoclonal gammopathies
Cold agglutinin disease

(*Continued*)

TABLE 2 The 5th edition on the World Health Organization Classification of Hematolymphoid Tumors: Lymphoid Neoplasms (*Continued*)

IgM monoclonal gammopathy of undetermined significance
Non-IgM monoclonal gammopathy of undetermined significance
Monoclonal gammopathy of renal significance
<u>Diseases with monoclonal immunoglobulin deposition</u>
Immunoglobulin-related (AL) amyloidosis
Monoclonal immunoglobulin deposition disease
<u>Heavy chain diseases</u>
Mu heavy chain disease
Gamma heavy chain disease
Alpha heavy chain disease
<u>Plasma cell neoplasms</u>
Plasmacytoma
Plasma cell myeloma
Plasma cell neoplasms with associated paraneoplastic syndrome
POEMS syndrome
TEMPI syndrome
AESOP syndrome
<u>T-cell and NK-cell lymphoid proliferations and lymphomas</u>
Tumor-like lesions with T-cell predominance
Kikuchi-Fujimoto disease
Indolent T-lymphoblastic proliferation
Autoimmune lymphoproliferative syndrome
Precursor T-neoplasms
<u>T-lymphoblastic leukemia/lymphoma</u>
T-lymphoblastic leukemia/lymphoma, NOS
Early T-precursor lymphoblastic leukemia/lymphoma
Mature T-cell and NK-cell neoplasms
<u>Mature T-cell and NK-cell leukemias</u>
T-prolymphocytic leukemia
T-large granular lymphocytic leukemia
NK-large granular lymphocytic leukemia
Adult T-cell leukemia/lymphoma
Sézary syndrome
Aggressive NK-cell leukemia
<u>Primary cutaneous T-cell lymphomas</u>

TABLE 2 The 5th edition on the World Health Organization Classification of Hematolymphoid Tumors: Lymphoid Neoplasms (*Continued*)

Primary cutaneous CD4-positive small or medium T-cell lymphoproliferative disorder
Primary cutaneous acral CD8-positive lymphoproliferative disorder
Mycosis fungoides
Primary cutaneous CD30-positive T-cell lymphoproliferative disorder: lymphomatoid papulosis
Primary cutaneous CD30-positive T-cell lymphoproliferative disorder: primary cutaneous anaplastic large cell lymphoma
Subcutaneous panniculitis-like T-cell lymphoma
Primary cutaneous gamma-delta T-cell lymphoma
Primary cutaneous CD8-positive aggressive epidermotropic cytotoxic T-cell lymphoma
Primary cutaneous peripheral T-cell lymphoma, NOS
Intestinal T-cell and NK-cell lymphoid proliferations and lymphomas
Indolent T-cell lymphoma of the gastrointestinal tract
Indolent NK-cell lymphoproliferative disorder of the gastrointestinal tract
Enteropathy-associated T-cell lymphoma
Monomorphic epitheliotropic intestinal T-cell lymphoma
Intestinal T-cell lymphoma, NOS
Hepatosplenic T-cell lymphoma
Anaplastic large cell lymphoma
ALK-positive anaplastic large cell lymphoma
ALK-negative anaplastic large cell lymphoma
Breast implant–associated anaplastic large cell lymphoma
Nodal T-follicular helper (TFH) cell lymphoma
Nodal TFH cell lymphoma, angioimmunoblastic type
Nodal TFH cell lymphoma, follicular-type
Nodal TFH cell lymphoma, NOS
Peripheral T-cell lymphoma, NOS
EBV-positive NK/T-cell lymphomas
EBV-positive nodal T-and NK-cell lymphoma
Extranodal NK/T-cell lymphoma
EBV-positive T- and NK-cell lymphoid proliferations and lymphomas of childhood
Severe mosquito bite allergy
Hydroa vacciniforme lymphoproliferative disorder
Systemic chronic active EBV disease
Systemic EBV-positive T-cell lymphoma of childhood

(*Continued*)

TABLE 2 The 5th edition on the World Health Organization Classification of Hematolymphoid Tumors: Lymphoid Neoplasms (*Continued*)

Stroma-derived neoplasms of lymphoid tissues
Mesenchymal dendritic cell neoplasms
Follicular dendritic cell sarcoma
EBV-positive inflammatory follicular dendritic cell sarcoma
Fibroblastic reticular cell tumor
Myofibroblastic tumor
Intranodal palisaded myofibroblastoma
Spleen-specific vascular-stromal tumors
Littoral cell angioma
Splenic hamartoma
Sclerosing angiomatoid nodular transformation of spleen

Source: Modified with permission from Alaggio R, Amador C, Anagnostopoulos I, et al. The 5th edition of the World Health Organization Classification of haematolymphoid tumours: lymphoid neoplasms. *Leukemia*. 2022;36(7):1720-1748.

INDEX

Note: Page numbers followed by "*f*" indicate figures and "*t*" indicate tables.